NEONATAL DERMATOLOGY

LAWRENCE M. SOLOMON, M.D.

Professor and Head of Dermatology,
The Abraham Lincoln School of the
University of Illinois College of Medicine,
Chicago, Illinois
Consultant in Dermatology to the Center for
Craniofacial Anomalies of the University of
Illinois, the Illinois State Pediatric Institute, and
Dixon State Hospital of the Department of Mental
Health, State of Illinois
Attending Physician, University of Illinois Hospital,
Hines Veterans Administration Hospital and West
Side Veterans Administration Hospital

NANCY B. ESTERLY, M.D.

Associate Professor of Pediatrics,
Pritzker School of Medicine,
University of Chicago
Director, Division of Dermatology,
Department of Pediatrics, Michael
Reese Hospital and Medical Center,
Chicago, Illinois

Volume IX in the Series

MAJOR PROBLEMS IN CLINICAL PEDIATRICS

ALEXANDER J. SCHAFFER
Consulting Editor

W. B. Saunders Company • Philadelphia • London • Toronto

W. B. Saunders Company: West Washington Square
Philadelphia, PA 19105

1 St. Anne's Road
Eastbourne, East Sussex BN21 3UN, England

1 Goldthorne Avenue
Toronto, Ontario M8Z 5T9, Canada

Listed here is the latest translated edition of this book together
with the language of the translation and the publisher.

Spanish (1st Edition) — Editorial Medica Panamericana,
Buenos Aires, Argentina

Neonatal Dermatology   ISBN 0-7216-8490-4

Print No.:   9   8   7   6   5

To our parents, spouses, and children,
Sarah, Anne, Debbie, John, Henry, and Marc.

Foreword

I have long wanted to own, and keep handy for quick reference, a monograph on neonatal dermatology. The descriptions of these disorders in textbooks devoted to general pediatrics or general neonatology are of necessity limited by two factors. One is simply that they must be brief; not too many pages can be allowed dermatology when there are so many other systems to be covered. More important is the fact that few generalists are finished dermatologists. These considerations too often result in a product which is limited to the commoner disorders, the discussions of which are superficial to the extent that vital matters concerning pathogenesis, pathology, physiology and pathophysiology receive scant attention.

Dr. Lawrence Solomon is a fine physician and one of the leading dermatologists in the country. Trained in Geneva, Montreal and Philadelphia, he has taught in Chicago since 1966, where he is now Associate Professor of Dermatology at the University of Illinois. He has written extensively on many aspects of dermatology, with emphasis on atopic dermatitis and, more recently, on skin diseases in the newborn. Dr. Nancy Esterly studied at The Johns Hopkins School of Medicine and served her residency in pediatrics at the Harriet Lane Home. She then chose pediatric dermatology as her subspecialty, receiving her indoctrination at Johns Hopkins, but also eventually coming to the University of Illinois. She is now Associate Professor of Pediatrics and Dermatology at that institution. From personal experience I can attest to her excellence as a pediatrician. Her bibliography is as long and as widely ranging as is that of Dr. Solomon, and within the past few years her interest too has been directed increasingly toward the newborn.

The book is instructive, thorough, liberally illustrated and interestingly written. We welcome this addition to our series.

ALEXANDER J. SCHAFFER, M.D.

Preface

A careful evaluation of the skin often affords a superb opportunity for early diagnosis of both acute and chronic disease. Widespread recognition of this fact has led to increasing interest in cutaneous medicine by physicians of diverse specialties. In 1970 we wrote two reviews on some aspects of neonatal dermatology, and the enthusiastic response to these reviews encouraged us to expand the subject and compile it in book form. The Saunders series, *Major Problems in Clinical Pediatrics*, seemed to us an ideal vehicle for this presentation because of its emphasis on the newborn. Cutaneous disease in the infant may have serious long-term consequences and frequently presents diagnostic difficulties unique to that age group. Obviously, because of limitations of space, we were not able to include every rare disorder or syndrome with cutaneous findings, but we did attempt to be comprehensive enough to interest pediatricians, dermatologists, family practitioners, and residents training in these disciplines.

We deliberately avoided the temptation to deal with the subject of neonatal skin disease in the form of an atlas, although we have included a liberal sampling of illustrative material. There are several reasons for this approach. Dermatology is a specialty in which visual clues are only one of several types of data required for diagnosis; the manner of gathering data (history and diagnostic techniques) is as important as recognizing the lesion. Pictures are often misleading and, in fact, cannot supplant clinical experience in mastering the skill of visual recall. Treatment, often a confusing aspect in this age group, requires some discussion, but we have purposely refrained from advocating specific dosages, particularly of systemic medications, since we feel these decisions must be individualized for each infant.

Diseases were assigned to each chapter on the basis of the most frequent and obvious presenting sign during the neonatal period. For example, disorders such as neurofibromatosis and tuberous sclerosis are dealt with in the chapter on pigmentary disorders although they are clearly hereditary and known to affect primarily neural and vascular structures. Because of numerous preferences of this nature on our part, the chapter on hereditary diseases is perforce quite brief. In addition, a number of hereditary entities have been omitted because they are not apparent during the neonatal period. By using cross-references we have attempted to keep duplication to a minimum.

We enjoyed writing this monograph and hope it will focus further deserved attention on the skin of newborn infants and dispel some of the mystery which frequently surrounds their cutaneous disorders. We also hoped to place the skin in its proper perspective as an integral part of the human organism.

Thanks are due Mrs. Mary Mungovan and Mrs. Marie Ehrlicher for their patient and efficient transcription of our illegible notes, and to Dr. Samuel Pruzansky and the Center for Craniofacial Anomalies for supporting this book. We are grateful to Drs. Ruth Seeler, David Fisher, John Paton, Alan Lasser, David Fretzin, Lewis Shapiro, Henry Mangurten, Samuel Pruzansky, Thomas Rea, Robert Morgan, James Ertle, Mark Everett, Marvin Chernosky, Eugene Bodian, Hermine Pashayan, McLemore Birdsong, J. Martin Beare, Tulio Briceño-Maaz, and Frank Netter for their generous contributions to our illustrative material, and to Mr. A. C. Lonert of Turtox for the photomicrographs of normal skin. Drs. Maria Medenica, Louise Tavs, Hermine Pashayan and Nancy Furey also provided expert advice in certain specialized areas. Some of the studies reported in this text were supported in part by a grant from the National Institutes of Health (DE–02872).

LAWRENCE M. SOLOMON

NANCY B. ESTERLY

Contents

Introduction

Specialization in medicine, although having obvious advantages, at times makes orphans of certain disease conditions. These are usually diseases that occur at the boundary of two specialties. Customarily, members of both specialties treat such conditions, but usually treat them inadequately because knowledge of both fields is required. Such is the case with skin diseases in the young child and, more specifically, in the neonate. The pediatrician, who as a rule sees these cases, understands the neonate but not skin diseases, and the dermatologist, if he sees the patient, does not understand that skin diseases may be expressed differently in neonatal skin. Over the years there have been several books on pediatric dermatology; however, few have been very successful. To my knowledge, there never has been a book focusing on skin diseases in the newborn. The present text very adequately satisfies the need for such a work. The authors are both Board-certified dermatologists; one of them is also a Board-certified pediatrician, and the other has a special interest in cutaneous diseases and maldevelopment in the newborn. Consequently, they have an especial expertise in this area. I believe this book will prove very useful in the practice of medicine.

ADOLPH ROSTENBERG, JR., M.D.

*Professor and Head of the Department
of Dermatology, University of Illinois*

Chapter One

STRUCTURE OF FETAL AND NEONATAL SKIN

The dividing line between a pathological and physiological reaction in the skin of the newborn is indistinct. As a result, neonatal skin may present a bewildering variety of lesions; some innocent, temporary, and the result of a physiological response; others the result of an episodic disease; and still others indicative of a serious, often fatal, underlying disorder. The presence of a cutaneous abnormality is usually evident on inspection, but a definitive diagnosis of specific skin lesions requires some understanding of the structure of infant skin and its physiological characteristics, and recognition of primary skin lesions as well as knowledge of their significance.

This chapter will review the structural characteristics of the skin at birth and relate them to what has preceded during intrauterine life and what is to follow.

STRUCTURE OF THE EPIDERMIS

Human skin is a complex organ which has two distinct structural compartments, the epidermis and dermis, and each contains several substructures, some permanent, others temporary (Plate I, page 81). The epidermis and dermis are interdependent and together provide a highly evolved, regenerative and protective coat which plays an important role in defense, temperature regulation and sexuality.

The epidermis evolves from a villous ectodermal envelope which at the fourth week of embryonic life is two cells thick (Serri, 1962). The outer periderm serves as a tempo-rary barrier and as an active transport membrane between the embryo and its amniotic environment (Pinkus, 1910; Breathnach, 1971); the inner layer, the stratum germinativum, gives rise to the epidermis and its appendages (Fig. 1–1). At about 11 weeks another layer is generated by the germinative layer and is interposed between it and the periderm (Fig. 1–2). At this time the three- to four-month epidermis shows marked accumulation of glycogen stores (Ebling, 1970). Glycogen is normally present in embryonic or fetal skin (Braun-Falco, 1961), but appears postnatally only if the epidermis is injured (Pass et al., 1965). The anaerobic glycolytic pathway is apparently preferentially used as an energy source for rapid epidermal growth, development and repair. Except for the presence of some glycogen, the epidermis has attained its adult keratogenous structure by the 17th week. There is marked regional variation in epidermal thickness, color, permeability and surface chemistry.

The postnatal epidermis results from a compact layering of two cell types, the keratinocyte and melanocyte. Recently a third distinct cell type, the Langerhans cell, has been recognized. We will consider the epidermal components separately.

The Keratinocyte

Young keratinocytes in the basal (innermost) layer contain a filamentous protein and lie adjacent to, but separated from, the dermis by a narrow basement membrane. The basal keratinocytes usually divide only

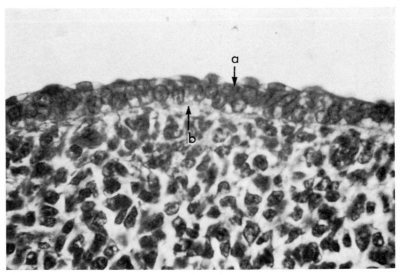

Figure 1–1. Cross section of skin from a 13 mm embryo. The periderm (a) and stratum germinativum (b) are visible at this stage of development.

once and as the keratinocytes migrate toward the surface, their cellular structure is replaced by their proteinaceous product, keratin. The cells become dehydrated, flattened and adhere to each other with such tenacity that within the 10-micron thick exterior layer, the stratum corneum, they form a tough, resilient and relatively impermeable membrane without which "dry land life would be impossible" (Kligman, 1964). The cells which comprise the stratum corneum become flattened, dehydrated and anuclear. They increase in size with age and are larger in females than in males. In infants the cells of this horny layer are more uniform in size than in children or adults (Plewig, 1970).

The keratinocyte in the basal layer of the epidermis is a columnar cell which contains the usual complement of organelles common to most cells, as well as five to eight Å wide

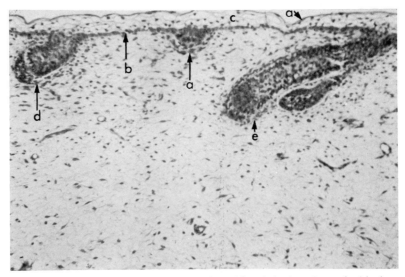

Figure 1–2. Cross section of skin from 9.5 cm fetus. The epidermis is three-layered with the periderm (a) still present; there is a stratum germinativum (b) and stratum intermedium (c) present. Several germinative buds (d) have begun to form appendageal structures, including a hair follicle (e).

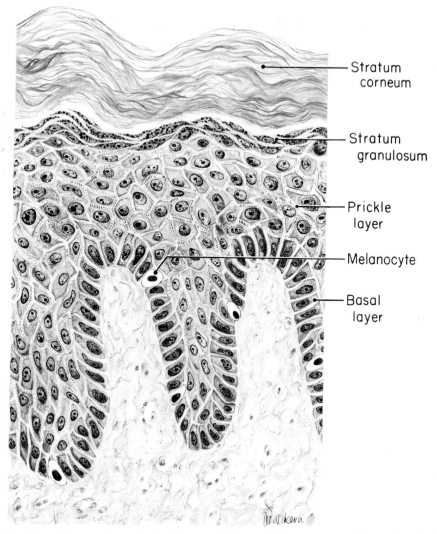

Figure 1–3. The epidermis. (From D. M. Pillsbury: A Manual of Dermatology. Philadelphia. W. B. Saunders Co., 1971.

strands of a fibrillar substance, the tonofibrils of early keratin, and melanin transferred from the melanocyte. In the prickle layer (stratum spinosum) the cells become polyhedric; the tonofibrils of keratin form a lacey network which extends from the cellular nucleus to its peripheral membrane and attach by way of desmosomes to the tonofibrils of adjacent cells. There is no direct continuity of keratin fibrils from one cell to the next, but the desmosome makes a strong bridge. As the keratinocyte matures it traverses the granular layer (stratum granulosum), where it acquires an amorphous matrix in the form of a hematoxylinophilic material, keratohyalin. The role of keratohyalin is not clear, but at this point in its maturation the cell loses its organ-

elles and enters the stratum corneum replete with keratin and dehydrated by loss of 85 per cent of its water content (Baden et al., 1971). The time of transit for a cell from the basal layer through the corneal layer normally takes about 28 days (Weinstein et al., 1971). Gerstein (1971) has recently shown that the rate of DNA synthesis in fetal skin is not very different from adult skin (Fig. 1–3).

The Melanocyte

The second important component of the epidermis is the melanocyte, a cell with a dendritic structure capable of producing melanin (Fitzpatrick et al., 1967). The melanocyte has its origin in the neural crest of the

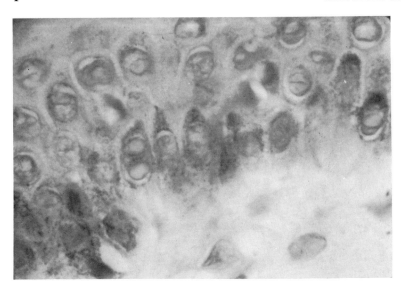

Figure 1-4. High power view of the epidermis. The basal cells are pigmented. Several "clear cells" or melanocytes may be seen. They contain a dark nucleus and clear cytoplasm. The prickle cells lie above.

human embryo in common with the dorsal root, the cranial ganglia and the sympathetic nervous system (Boyd, 1960). As the embryo matures the melanoblasts are lost in the mesenchyme of the somites and at about the fourth month of gestation melanin begins to appear in some melanoblasts, converting them to melanocytes (Figs. 1–4 and 2–2, page 21) (Sims, 1970). By this time melanocytes have migrated to many parts of the body, but particularly to the dermal-epidermal junction where they begin functioning inside the basal layer at six months of fetal age. Szabo (1967) has calculated the number of melanocytes in adult human skin to be about 2×10^9. The density of melanocytes is highest in the first 15 years, particularly in areas of light exposure and on the penile skin, scalp and cheek. Melanin provides an effective, protective umbrella against ultraviolet radiation damage to vital nuclear DNA. Melanin granules are formed in the melanocytic cytoplasm as watermelon-shaped melanosomes and move via the dendritic processes into the basal cells. The melanosome of a dark haired person measures about $8 \times 3\text{Å}$, and is replete with melanin. Its internal structure is not visible. The blonde individual has less melanin deposited in his melanosome, but the structure of the organelle is similar. The red-haired individual has a round melanosome five Å in diameter (Birbeck, 1963). The mechanism of melanin transfer from melanocytic dendrite to basal cell most probably takes place by a process in which the periphery of the dendrites are phagocytosed by the recipient basal cell (Prunieras, 1969; Klaus,

1969). As the basal keratinocyte matures its melanin content is dispersed as a fine intracellular granular dust which may be visualized on examination of Scotch tape strippings of the horny layer.

The Langerhans cell is a recently discovered epidermal cell with peculiar racquet-shaped intracellular organelles. The function of this cell remains unknown. Previously thought to be an "effete melanocyte," recent studies suggest it may in fact be related to the histiocyte (Tarnowski et al., 1967).

THE APPENDAGES

These structures result from an invagination or downgrowth of epidermis or epidermal germinative buds into the dermis (Fig. 1–5). The sebaceous and apocrine glands usually differentiate from the germinative bud that gives rise to the hair follicle. The arrector pili muscle is attached to the hair follicle. The eccrine gland differentiates from the epidermis itself.

Hair

Hair develops during the third foetal month. After birth few new follicles are formed so that any loss of follicles becomes permanent except for facial hair (Muller, 1971). Each hair follicle, by virtue of its genetic type hormonal influences, nutritional and environmental factors, produces a hair of a given caliber and length (Fig. 1–6). The earliest down (lanugo hair) is fine, soft,

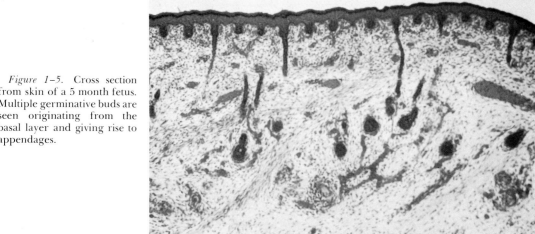

Figure 1–5. Cross section from skin of a 5 month fetus. Multiple germinative buds are seen originating from the basal layer and giving rise to appendages.

poorly pigmented and unmedullated, and grows to only several centimeters in length. At birth, in the premature neonate, it frequently covers the scalp and brow and the scalp line may be poorly demarcated. Scalp hair varies considerably but is usually somewhat coarser and more mature in dark-haired infants. Lanugo hair may also cover the face. The term "lanugo" hair is often used interchangeably with "vellus" hair. Strictly speaking, the latter term refers to the facial hair of children and women. It is similar in appearance to lanugo hair. The mature adult hair is called terminal hair. It is pigmented, medullated, and of varying length, depending on the site.

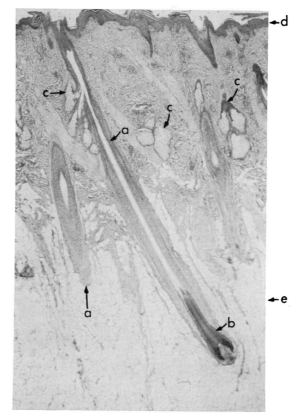

Figure 1–6. Cross section from the scalp: (a) a pilosebaceous follicle in longitudinal section; (b) hair bulb; (c) sebaceous glands; (d) epidermis; (e) hypodermic fat.

On the scalp the hair undergoes several phases. The generative or active growth phase (anagen) lasts two to five years; the follicle then undergoes a period of partial degeneration (catagen) which may take 10 to 14 days, and this is immediately followed by a three to four month resting phase (telogen). Normally, 80 per cent of the scalp hair is actively growing. Fifty to 100 hairs are shed each day and are simultaneously replaced (Kligman, 1961).

In the newborn the phases of the hair follicles are usually synchronized, and 80 per cent of the follicles are in the resting state. During the first few months of life hair loss and regrowth loses its lockstep phase synchrony and the hair becomes coarser and thicker, and has an adult distribution. During the course of dysynchronization of hair growth a temporary alopecia may occur. (Barman et al., 1967). There is also a sex difference in that boys' hair grows faster than girls' hair. In both sexes the scalp hair grows slower at the crown (Pecoraro, 1964).

The normal hair is a piston-like structure in a cylindrical follicle (Plate II–A). The adult hair has a small medulla, large perforated cortex, and is enveloped by a cuticle which usually has a simple, pigment free layer (Fig. 1–7). Near the bulb the cuticular cells of the hair itself interlock with the innermost layer of cells of the follicle, forming the internal root sheath (Fig. 1–8). The hair follicle has several layers which resemble the epidermal layers. The hair cells are produced in the matrix of the bulb, the region which also gives rise to the cuticular cells.

The Nail

The nail develops in the nine week embryo from a groove formed by an epidermal invagination on the distal phalanx. Its formation is complete by the fifth fetal month (Zaias, 1963, 1965). The nail is made of hard keratin which is contained in tightly packed cells originating in a groove transversely located behind the visible portion of the nail (the nail plate). The posterior nail groove or fold has a floor and roof. It extends laterally so that the nail plate is set within a hollow crescent, the posterior part of which produces the nail (Fig. 1–9).

The lateral parts of the nail groove (lateral

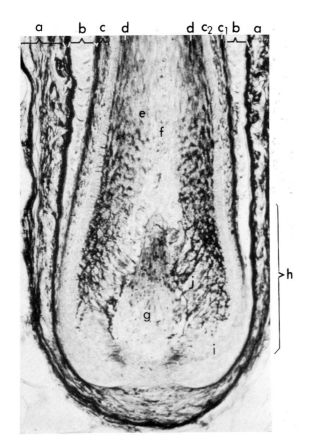

Figure 1–7. Diagram showing construction of hair root. (a) Connective tissue sheath of the follicle, (b) external root sheath, (c) internal root sheath, (c_1) Huxley's layer, (c_2) cuticular cells of the internal root sheath, (d) cuticle cells of the hair, (e) cortex of the hair, (f) medulla of the hair, (g) papilla, containing a blood vessel, (h) hair bulb, (i) lower bulb, where the cells produce both the internal root sheath and the cuticle of the hair. There are no melanocytes in this area. (j) upper bulb area. Here, the cells make the hair cortex containing keratinocytes and melanocytes.

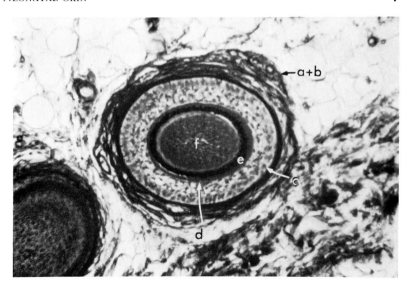

Figure 1–8. Hair in cross section (Refer to letters of Figure 1–7.) The medulla is much larger than that seen in human terminal hair.

nail fold) envelop the nail, add to its stability and protect its border (Fig. 1–10). The cells producing the nail plate form the nail matrix. Viewed from the top, and particularly on the thumb, an opaque white semilunar area may be seen through the plate. This represents the visible portion of matrix (the lunula). The nail plate adheres closely to, and rides over, the nail bed which in turn closely adheres to the periosteal tissue. As the nail plate rides over its bed it pulls with it the desquamating cells of the bed's epithelium (Zaias, 1967). This debris is usually found under the distal free edge of the nail. Proximal to the nail plate is the cuticle which is made up of the su-perficial layers of epidermis forming the pos-terior nail fold.

The nail plate is translucent, and its cells are anuclear. Small imperfections in nail cell formation may result in retention of nuclei and these are seen as white spots. Serious in-flammatory, genetic or traumatic damage to the matrix may result in pits, ridging, gross hypertrophic deformity or agenesis of the nail. The toenails grow more slowly than fingernails, which elongate at about 3.5 mm per month. Nail growth is slower in winter and in malnourished children. As Pillsbury (1971) has pointed out, dietary and vitamin deficiency are rarely a cause of nail splitting,

Figure 1–9. Longitudinal section of a finger tip: (a) Nail bed; (b) nail matrix; (c) nail plate; (d) posterior nail fold; (e) cuticle of the nail.

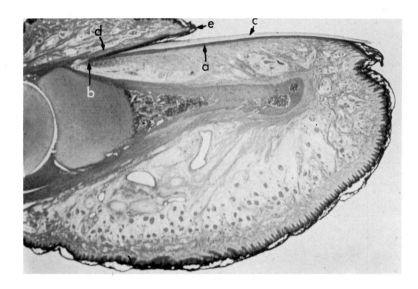

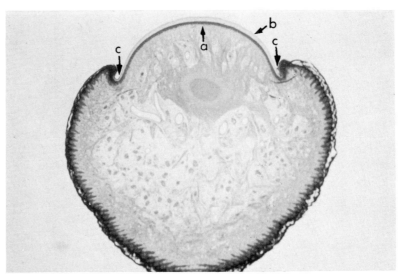

Figure 1–10. Cross section of finger tip: (a) nail bed; (b) nail plate; (c) lateral nail fold. (Courtesy of A. C. Lonert, Director of Research, General Biological, Inc.)

fragility or brittleness, contrary to popularly held conceptions.

GLANDS OF THE SKIN

The Eccrine Gland

The eccrine sweat glands are distributed throughout the entire skin (Fig. 1–11). Embryologically, they are derived from an epidermal downgrowth beginning at about the sixth week. The eccrine glands are more or less completely formed by the fifth fetal month. The adult complement of glands is densely and evenly distributed over the body surface. About three million glands are present in the normal individual. As the individual grows, the face, palms and soles acquire a proportionately greater number of glands (Szabo, 1967).

The eccrine gland is independent of the hair follicle. It has three structural portions: a deep dermal coiled portion; a straight duct heading toward the epidermis; and a tortuous intraepidermal sweat duct ending in a funnel-shaped opening on the surface, seen as a pore (Figs. 1–12 and 1–13). The coiled portion contains the secretory gland which is lined by a single layer of cells of two types: numerous large clear cells containing glycogen and responsible for sweat production; and smaller, less numerous granular dark

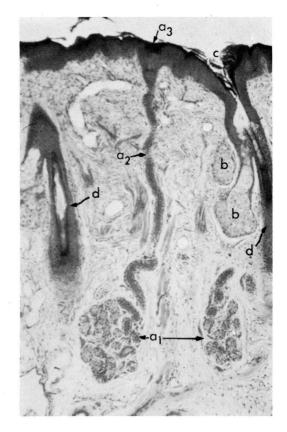

Figure 1–11. Cross section of skin showing a complete eccrine sweat gland (a). (a_1) Coiled intradermal portion; (a_2) straight ductal portion; (a_3) intraepidermal sweat duct; (b) sebaceous gland; (c) pilosebaceous orifice; (d) cross section of hair.

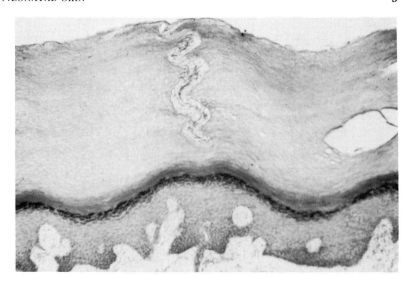

Figure 1-12. Cross section of epidermis from the palm. The spiral nature of the intraepidermal sweat duct is illustrated.

cells whose function is probably mucin secretion. Small canaliculi leading into the lumen of the gland are found between the lining cells. All of the cells are attached to a basement membrane which also engulfs some myoepithelial cells and filaments (Montagna, 1962). The function of these contractile elements is not clear in spite of the compelling logic to regard them as a physical "pump." Part of the coiled portion contains a ductile element leading into a straight duct. The duct has two or three layers of metabolically active cuboidal cells which may reabsorb water from sweat and provide transport for some vasoactive substances and electrolytes into the dermis. The epidermal portion is lined by two layers of cells similar to those of the straight duct. These cells produce keratin, which rings the opening onto the surface. The ductal and coiled portion are both richly vascularized. The gland is innervated by the sympathetic nervous system but the neurotransmitter is acetylcholine.

Sebaceous and Apocrine Glands

Most sebaceous glands (Ebling, 1970; Hurley et al., 1960) differentiate from the epithelial portion of the hair follicle at about thirteen to fifteen weeks and almost immediately begin to function by producing sebum in all hairy areas and occasionally, ectopically on the buccal mucosa, esophagus, vagina and lips (Montagna, 1962). The size of the indi-

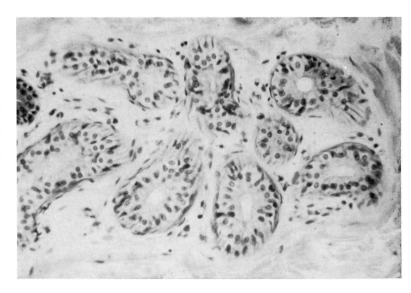

Figure 1-13. The coiled glandular portion of the eccrine sweat gland. Each acinus contains large clear cells and smaller dark cells. The acini are surrounded by elongated myoepithelial cells.

vidual glands tends to be greatest in the areas where the glands are most densely concentrated (Strauss et al., 1968). Their rapid growth and activity up to and immediately after birth is governed, in part, by maternal androgens, and possibly also by endogenous steroid production by the fetus. Androgens are the only hormones unequivocably shown to have a stimulating effect on the glands, whereas estrogens depress their growth (Strauss et al., 1968). The gland develops as a solid outpouching from the upper third of the hair follicle. These solid buds become filled with liquid centrally as the cells disintegrate; as the acini and ducts develop, they open most frequently into the canal located between the hair follicle and hair shaft.

The sebaceous gland is holocrine. It usually has several lobules which, in the infant, are small and few in number. The lobules have no lumen but are filled with disintegrated sebaceous cells and empty into the excretory duct, which has a stratified squamous epithelium. Each lobule is surrounded by a layer of young cuboidal (basophilic) cells which do not have a granular structure. The cells located toward the center of the acini contain lipid globules (Lever, 1967). There are two views concerning the function of the peripheral cells; one postulates that they replace the acini, (Montagna, 1963); another (Epstein et al., 1966), suggests that the peripheral cells directly replenish those lost in the centro-acinar holocrine function. The average renewal time for the sebaceous gland is about one week.

The shedding of sebaceous gland cells into the amniotic fluid late in gestation forms the basis for one of the tests of fetal maturity. These lipid-laden cells stain orange or brown with Nile blue sulfate in contrast to the fetal squames, which stain blue. A cytological count of 10 per cent fat-laden cells indicates a gestational age of 36 weeks, whereas a 20 per cent count indicates a 40 week pregnancy (Andrews, 1970).

The apocrine glands, relatively voluminous organs larger than eccrine glands, originate from, and empty into, the hair follicle. They develop somewhat later embryologically than the eccrine glands. Apocrine development is well advanced at the seventh or eighth foetal month, when they begin to produce a milky white fluid containing water, lipids, protein, reducing sugars, ferric iron and ammonia. The biological function of the gland is unknown but may be related to sexuality. The glands are distributed in the axillae, groin, pudenda, midline abdomen, external ear, nasal vestibule and eyelids. The apocrine gland, like the eccrine gland, is a tubular organ whose cells, as the name suggests, secrete in an apocrine (by decapitation) manner.

The acini have a single layer of secretory cells. In the infant these may be cuboidal, but become cylindrical as age and function increase. The mature cells have an eosinophilic cytoplasm containing mucopolysaccharides and iron granules. They contain little glycogen. The acini have a large lumen and are surrounded by myoepithelial contractile elements which respond to adrenergic agents, although sympathetic innervation has not been demonstrated (Hurley et al., 1954). In the newborn the acini are well formed; the coiled secretory portion has a periglandular connective tissue capsule, but myoepithelial elements have not been seen postnatally (Montagna, 1962). The histological features of the ductal portion are identical to those seen in the eccrine duct. When the duct empties onto the surface by way of a direct epidermal route, the intraepidermal portion is straight rather than tortuous as in the structure of the intraepidermal eccrine sweat duct unit. Breast glandular tissue results from modification of the apocrine glands.

The Dermo-Epidermal Junction

The epidermis firmly adheres to the underlying dermis. Anyone working with skin in a laboratory knows of the great difficulty incurred in separating epidermis from dermis. This attachment is most secure in the adult and least secure in the newborn and the very aged (although for different reasons). The basal layer is anchored to a basement membrane or lamina by hemidesmosomes which protrude podal–like from the undersurface of the basal cells. The basal membrane probably contains a number of polysaccharides of the branched type. The resistance of the dermo-epidermal junction to shearing stress is enhanced by the undulation characteristic of its structure (Odland et al., 1971).

THE DERMIS

In the past, the dermis and its constituents had been considered relatively inactive structures; however, recent evidence has shown that both the appendages and the cellular, collagenous and ground substance components of the dermis have a high degree of metabolic activity. The whole dermis remains in symbiotic relation to, and perhaps exerts a controlling influence on, the epidermis (Briggaman et al., 1968). It has been shown experimentally that the dermal mesenchyme induces differentiation of the keratinocytic cells from the undifferentiated ectoderm in the chick embryo and that epidermis from one area (limb) transplanted to a different site (gizzard) acts under the influence of the receptor mesenchyme to produce a receptor site type of epithelium (Flaxman, 1971). Although it is suspected that a dermal chemical component functions as the controlling substance, its nature has not yet been elucidated. Once the epidermis has been differentiated, the isolated basal cell layer can produce a basement membrane and continue to function (Flaxman, 1971).

The Structure of the Dermis

A rapid review of the embryology and structure of the dermis and its constituents is essential prior to a discussion of the peculiarities of neonatal dermis. The dermis of the two-month embryo is an undifferentiated cellular myxomatous tissue without a fibrillar structure. Fibrils become apparent between two and four months of age, when they replace some of the cells. A moderate number of elastic and collagen fibers is found from the 20th to 40th weeks. During this period the fetal dermis makes a transition from an organ rich in water, sugars and hyaluronic acid to one composed mainly of collagen and sulfated mucopolysaccharide (Odland et al., 1971).

At birth the dermis is one to four mm thick and contains fibrous elements, amorphous ground substance, free cells, nerves, blood vessels and lymphatic vessels. The fibrinous elements are collagen and elastic tissue. The fatty panniculus is hypodermic.

Collagen

Collagen comprises more than 90 per cent of the dermal connective tissue. It has a characteristic structure, the smallest element of which is filamentous tropocollagen (Jackson, 1970). Tropocollagen molecules produced by the fibroblast measure 2800 Å $\times$ 15 Å and have a molecular weight of 300,000 (Gross, 1961). These molecules condense into fibrils which aggregate to form fibers; the fibers in turn aggregate into parallel inextensible bundles. The fibrils, about 1000 Å in width, show cross striations under high-power light microscopy that have a distinct periodicity of 640 Å (Zelickson, 1965). The fibrils have a triple helical structure and, uniquely, contain hydroxyproline and hydroxylysine.

Young collagen is extractable with neutral buffers. With increasing age collagen becomes progressively less soluble, and its constituent amino acids have a slower turnover time. In other words, collagen becomes more stable with age. It has been proposed that this phenomenon can be attributed to an increase in more stable interfibrillar and interfiber ester bonds which may occur with maturation (Gallap, 1964).

Reticulin fibers are fine branching, argyrophilic fibers which are probably identical to young collagen and should not be considered a separate type of fiber.

Elastic Fibers

The structural morphology and chemical and physical properties of cutaneous elastic fibers are different from collagen (Smith, 1963; Partridge, 1970). Elastic fibers branch, wave and curl, are extensible, amorphous and do not form bundles, whereas collagen fibers are inelastic, nonbranching and straight, show periodicity and form bundles. Histochemically, the two types of fibers are also distinct. Collagen is soluble in many solvents and is digested by collagenase. Elastic tissue (even "young" fibers) is relatively insoluble, contains desmosine and isodesmosine and is digested by elastase. Little factual information is available on the elastic content of newborn skin except that elastic tissue is known to increase postnatally and to contain less lysine than fetal tissue. There has been interesting speculation about elastic fiber abnormalities in those entities showing clinical alteration in cutaneous elasticity. The clinical changes may be related to the arrangement of elastic tissue in the skin (Shellow et al., 1967), as well as to a qualitative, rather than quantitative, change in the elastic fibers or collagen.

Ground Substance

The properties of the amorphous substance in which cellular and fibrous elements of the dermis are suspended are slowly acquiring greater definition (Bentley, 1970;

Elden, 1970). Mucopolysaccharides and water are two of the major constituents of this ground substance. In skin the major mucopolysaccharides are hyaluronic acid and chondroitin sulfate B (dermatan sulfate). The ground substance forms a gelatinous mass which profoundly influences the organs and cells suspended therein, as well as the movement of varying-sized molecules, proteins and electrolytes through it.

The water-binding properties and the nature of the ground substance change dramatically after birth. Neonatal skin is often edematous — clinical evidence of a cutaneous excess of water and sodium. Within a few days the skin loses most of the excess water and sodium. Although there are conflicting data, during infancy the skin probably decreases its hexosamine content while markedly increasing its collagen, which becomes relatively more insoluble.

The ground substance is affected by a variety of substances including corticoids, estrogens, androgens, thyroid hormones, antidiuretic hormone and vitamins A and C. Ultraviolet and x-irradiation alter the cross-linking of collagen and its perifibrillar mucoproteins. Infections, immune mechanisms and the pharmacologic mediators of inflammation probably also play a role in altering ground substance structure. Finally, enzymes such as hyaluronidase, which lyse mucin, play a role in ground substance permeability. Abnormalities in mucopolysaccharide metabolism have now been identified in a series of well-recognized, genetically determined disorders (see Chapter 15).

Cellular Components of the Dermis

The fibroblasts are the most numerous cells in the dermis. They are mesenchymal in origin, and are responsible for the formation of collagen and probably the mucopolysaccharides of ground substance. Their role in elastin formation remains controversial. Also normally present in the dermis are mast cells (which produce heparin and histamine), histiocytes, macrophages, a few lymphocytes, neutrophils and an occasional plasma cell and eosinophil.

THE BLOOD AND LYMPHATIC VESSELS

The vascular needs of the skin are dictated in part by its size (in the adult, skin accounts for about 10 per cent of body weight and equals about two square meters), and in part by its thermoregulatory function. It is equally apparent that these needs will vary considerably with the internal and external environmental conditions the subject encounters. As a result, the cutaneous vasculature demonstrates remarkable physiologic capabilities, with blood flow ranging from 0.3 to 150 ml per 100 mg tissue per minute (Champion et al., 1968).

The vascular network develops in early embryonic life from the mesoderm and forms a complex series of tubular structures in the skin. The dermis and epidermis are served by networks of anastomosing arteries at three levels: a subepidermal or papillary plexus; a dermal (or subpapillary) plexus; and a third plexus at the junction of the dermis and subcutaneous panniculus (fascial network) (Moretti, 1968). The subpapillary network is disorderly at birth and gradually develops an orderly adult structure during the first 17 weeks of life (Perera et al., 1970).

The veins form five plexuses. Direct arteriovenous anastomoses are present in abundance, and the glomerular organs apparently are responsible for thermoregulatory shunting. The appendages also have special vascular networks: perifollicular and follicular papillary networks; eccrine gland; apocrine, and sebaceous gland networks are all present.

The Lymphatic Vessels

Because of the difficulty in visualizing and identifying these vessels, the structure of the cutaneous lymphatic system has only recently been studied in detail by means of microlymphangiography and electron microscopy (Champion, 1970).

The embryonic veins give rise to the lymphatic vessels. In the adult new vessels can form from the ruptured ends of existing lymphatics but not from veins or other blood vessels.

A single lymphatic vessel ends blindly in each dermal papilla. From here the lymphatic drainage proceeds toward a superficial lymphatic plexus and then spills into a deeper plexus of larger bore vessels containing valves. The deeper vessels follow the major arteries and veins to the regional nodes and proceed to the lymphatic trunks. The vessel walls appear to be simpler than those of the veins containing no internal projections; the endothelial intercellular junctions capable of opening are readily bridged by relatively large molecules in contrast to the tightly joined endothelial cells of the venous walls.

CUTANEOUS INNERVATION

Since 1956 (Lele et al.) it has become increasingly evident that the older concept of a specific nerve ending structure correlating with a specific function probably is not realistic. According to current thinking the networks of cutaneous nerves serve overlapping cutaneous areas so that activation of one nerve in the skin does not necessarily cause stimulation of one spot on the cerebral cortex. Sensation is probably a composite of several types of input, including spatial and temporal patterns of nerve stimulation in skin and spinal cord (Winkelmann, 1960), local chemical factors in the skin, previous experience, the state of cortical arousal and genetic factors relating to nerve stimulation thresholds.

Nerve networks develop in the dermis at a very early embryological age and are distributed in an entirely random fashion (Winkelmann, 1960). The most superficial nerves have the smallest diameter; the thicker nerve fibers and more completely myelinized fibers are found deeper in the dermis. At the papillary level sensory nerves cannot be distinguished from autonomic nerve fibers with the light or electron microscope.

Apart from the dermal nerve network, which may show considerable regional variation, nerve fibers may go directly to particular regions or structures such as hair follicles, eccrine glands, arrector pili muscles and the subepidermal zone. The sebaceous glands are not innervated. Winkelmann (1956) found that, in the prepuce, the nerve networks are more delicate, less myelinated and more densely grouped in the neonate than in the adult.

Special neurologic structures include a dense perifollicular nerve network with exquisite tactile sensory properties and mucocutaneous end organs which are highly concentrated in erogenous zones. Meissner's corpuscle, found most frequently on palms and fingertips, has an exclusive, undisputed function in two-point tactile discrimination (Fig. 1–14). Meissner's tactile organs are found in newborn skin as undeveloped structures which become organized after birth (Cauna, 1965).

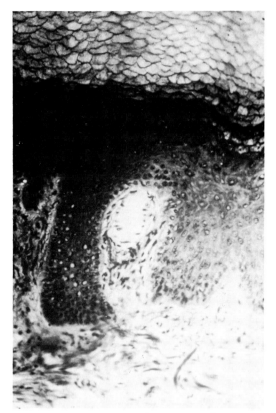

Figure 1–14. A Meissner corpuscle.

The Merkel-Ranvier corpuscles are found in the distal skin of the limbs. They are disc-shaped terminals which are seen lying in great numbers under the epidermis in the 28-week foetus. After birth the receptors undergo little alteration and are found around the sweat pores of hairless skin.

Vater-Pacini bodies are found around the digits, palms, periosteum and genitalia. They are present in great numbers at birth, fully formed (Cauna, 1965). Their function may be that of a vascular shunt control organ. The evidence for the presence of intraepidermal nerve endings is reasonably strong; however, some authors feel the data is not yet conclusive

The Autonomic Nervous System

Sympathetic nerves are abundant in the skin. The arrector pili muscle is richly innervated by sympathetic nerves with norepinephrine acting as the neurotransmitter. The arterioles are similarly innervated. The eccrine glands have some sympathetic nerve fibers around them, but acetylcholine transmits the impulse. Parasympathetic fibers may accompany the sensory nerves in the vessel walls and may cause active vasodilation.

The Subcutaneous Tissue

The hypodermis is a highly active tissue metabolically, consisting of fat cells, fibrous tissue, nerves, vessels, reticuloendothelial cells and transient white blood cells (Cairns, 1968).

The subcutaneous fat first appears at about the 14th week of foetal life as a differentiation of the primitive mesenchymal cell located adjacent to the blood vessels (Wasserman, 1964). The cytoblast contains lipid droplets and slowly matures to become replete with fat, pushing the nuclear material to its periphery. Foetal fat has certain metabolic peculiarities which have caused some authors to liken it to the heat producing brown fat (hibernoma) of some hibernating animals.

The preterm infant has a poorly developed fat supply. Within several weeks, however, the fat pad develops in the subcutis. The structure of this fat panniculus is lobular with a surrounding net of fibrous tissue containing collagen. The interlobular septa are traversed by an abundant vasculature with an artery and two veins present for each lobule. The larger vessels divide into smaller vessels so that ultimately, each fat cell contains an encircling capillary ring. The transfer of lipids across the basement membrane of the capillary to and from the lipocyte is regulated by a multitude of physical and hormonal factors including heat, norepinephrine, insulin, corticosteroids, thyroxin and lipolytic hormones.

DERMATOGLYPHICS

Dermatoglyphics is the descriptive term for the patterns formed by the epidermal ridges on the palms, soles, and digits. Although influenced in part by genetic factors (Cummins, 1964), these configurations are best understood by consideration of fetal anatomy and embryology. The ridge patterns are localized to the tips of the digits, the thenar and hypothenar areas of the palms and soles and the calcar area of the sole. Each area is the site of a fetal mound or pad which develops during the sixth week of gestation. These mounds appear when the hands and feet are still relatively undifferentiated and persist until the 30th week of gestation, when they

begin to regress. Formation of the epidermal ridges occurs simultaneously with involution of the fetal mounds. The ridge patterning is largely complete in the hand by the 19th fetal week; however, the embryogeneisis of the foot lags behind that of the hand by two to three weeks.

The pattern of epidermal ridges is characteristic for a given individual, cannot be altered after the formative period, and is probably determined by the growth and topography of the fetal hands and feet during that period. The ridges are thought to develop parallel and at right angles to the plane of growth forces; thus, the ultimate configuration reflects the surface distortion, height and curvature of the fetal mounds during their regression. Evidence in support of this postulate derives from embryological studies in primates and humans, theoretical mathematics and analysis of fingerprints of malformed hands (Mulvihill, 1969).

The study of dermatoglyphics is most often applied to the hands because patterning on the sole is more difficult to delineate and record. Dermatoglyphic analysis usually includes documentation of patterns on the digital tips (arches, loops and whorls), hypothenar and thenar eminences, interdigital patterns, localization of the digital and axial triradii (points at which these epidermal ridge fields meet), and total finger ridge counts. Abnormalities in the flexion crease lines of the palm, although anatomically of different derivation, often coexist with anomalies of epidermal ridge patterns, and observations on the flexion creases are usually included in a study of dermatoglyphics.

Aberrations in dermatoglyphics have been reported with increasing frequency in a number of chromosomal disorders and congenital malformations (Verbov, 1970). While certain unusual ridge patterns undoubtedly occur in a significantly increased incidence in these disorders, it is important to realize that the alterations are in themselves nonspecific and reflect a disturbance in development during a particular period of fetal life. It must be stressed that no one feature is pathognomonic for a particular entity, and abnormal patterns are occasionally present in otherwise normal individuals.

REGIONAL VARIATIONS

Some of the more difficult questions frequently posed by the dermatological neophyte concern the reasons for the peculiar distribution on the body surface of the lesions of certain diseases. Why, in the adult, is psoriasis a disease of extensor surfaces while atopic dermatitis is localized to the flexor areas, and why is this distribution frequently the inverse in the infant? The answers are unknown for the moment but the solution may, in part at least, rest with regional differences in cutaneous physiology and anatomy. Most of the localized physical and chemical attributes of skin (for example, scalp, lip and palm), are innate, apparent in foetal life, and remain so even under conditions of transplantation. A classic example of tenacity of dermal control over epidermal proliferation may be found in the epidermal nevus (see Chap. 8). Within a 2 mm area one may see normal epidermis becoming a warty, disfigured excrescence; the normal and abnormal coexist side by side with little tendency to affect each other over a life span.

Without going into great detail, the reader should note that there are marked regional differences in topography, epidermal thickness, stratum corneum thickness (Fig. 1–15), number and activity of melanocytes, dermal thickness, collagen and elastic tissue content, sweat glands, sebaceous glands, apocrine glands, vessel structure and nerve structure. Physiologically these variations may result in differences of permeability, microbial flora, thermoregulation, itch threshhold, pharmacological sensitivity of the skin and in the defenses of the skin against infection by microbial and other parasites.

REFERENCES

Andrews, B. F.: Amniotic fluid studies to determine maturity. Pediat. Clin. N. Amer., 17:49, 1970.

Baden, H. P., and Freedberg, I. M.: Epidermal proteins. In Fitzpatrick, T. B., Arndt, K. A., Clark, W. H., Eisen, A. Z., Van Scott, E. J., and Vaughan, J. H. (eds.): Dermatology in General Medicine. New York, McGraw-Hill-Blakiston, 1971, pp. 87–95.

Barman, J. M., Pecoraro, V., Astore, I., and Ferrer, J.: The first stage in the natural history of the human scalp hair cycle. J. Invest. Derm., 48:138–142, 1967.

Bentley, J. P.: The biological role of the ground substance mucopolysaccharides. In Montagna, W., Bentley, J. P., and Dobson, R. L. (eds.): The Dermis. New York, Appleton-Century-Crofts, Inc., 1970, pp. 103–121.

Birbeck, M. S. C.: Electron microscopy of melanocytes. Ann. N. Y. Acad. Sci., 100:540, 1963.

Boyd, J. D.: The embryology and comparative anatomy of the melanocyte. In Rook, A. (ed.): Progress in the Biological Sciences in Relation to Dermatology. London, Cambridge University Press, 1960, pp. 3–14.

Braun-Falco, O.: Histochemie der Haut. In Gottron, H. A., and Schönfeld, W. (eds.): Dermatologie und Venereologie. Vol. 1, Part 1. Stuttgart, Georg Thieme, 1961.

Breathnach, A. S.: Embryology of human skin. J. Invest. Derm., 57:133, 1971.

Briggaman, R., and Wheeler, C., Jr.: Epidermal-dermal interaction in adult human skin: Role of dermis in epidermal maintenance. J. Invest. Derm., 51:454–465, 1968.

Cairns, R. J.: The subcutaneous fat. In Rook, A., Wilkinson, D. S., and Ebling, F. J. G. (eds.): Textbook of Dermatology. Philadelphia, F. A. Davis Co., 1968.

Cauna, N.: The effects of aging on the receptor organs of the human. In Montagna, W. (ed.): Advances in Biology of the Skin. Vol. 6. New York, Pergamon Press, 1965, p. 63.

Champion, R. H.: Blood vessels and lymphatics of the skin. In Champion, R. H., Gillman, T., Rook, A. J., and Sims, R. T. (eds): An Introduction to the Biology of the Skin. Philadelphia, F. A. Davis Co., 1970, pp. 114–123.

Champion, R. H., and Wilkinson, D. S.: Disorders affecting blood vessels. In Rook, A., Wilkinson, D. S., and Ebling, F. J. G. (eds.): Textbook of Dermatology. Philadelphia, F. A. Davis Co., 1968, p. 397.

Ebling, F. J. G.: The embryology of skin. In Champion, R. H., Gillman, T., Rook, A. J., and Sims, R. T.

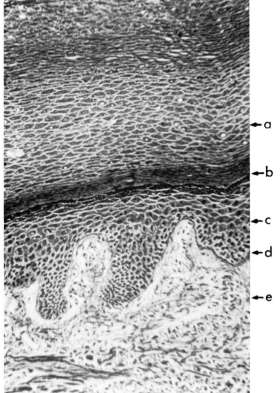

←a

←b

←c

←d

←e

Figure 1–15. Cross section of skin from the palm. Note the thickness of the stratum corneum. (a) Stratum corneum; (b) granular layer; (c) Malpighian (spiny or prickle) layer; (d) basal layer; (e) dermis.

(eds.): An Introduction to the Biology of the Skin. Philadelphia, F. A. Davis Co., 1970, p. 23.

Ebling, F. J. G.: Sebaceous glands. *In* Champion, R. H., Gillman, T., Rook, A. J., and Sims, R. T. (eds.): An Introduction to the Biology of the Skin. Philadelphia, F. A. Davis Co., 1970, p. 184.

Elden, H. R.: Biophysical properties of aging skin. *In* Montagna, W., Bentley, J. P., and Dobson, R. L. (eds.): The Dermis. New York, Appleton-Century-Crofts, Inc., 1970, pp. 231–252.

Epstein, E. H., Jr., and Epstein, W. L.: New cell formation in human sebaceous glands. J. Invest. Derm., *46*:453, 1966.

Fitzpatrick, T. B., Miyomoto, M., and Ishikawa, K.: The evolution of concepts of melanin biology. Arch. Derm., *96*:305–323, 1967.

Flaxman, A. B.: Principles of skin development. *In* Fitzpatrick, T. B., Arndt, K. A., Clark, W. H., Eisen, A. Z., Van Scott, E. J., and Vaughan, J. H. (eds.): Dermatology in General Medicine. New York, McGraw-Hill-Blakiston, 1971, p. 54.

Gallap, P. M.: Concerning some special structural features of the collagen molecule. Biophys. J., *4*:79, 1964.

Gerstein, W.: Cell proliferation in human fetal epidermis. J. Invest. Derm., *57*:262, 1971.

Gross, J.: Collagen. Sci. Amer., *204*:121, 1961.

Hurley, H. J., Jr., and Shelley, W. B.: The Human Apocrine Gland in Health and Disease. Springfield, Charles C Thomas, 1960.

Hurley, H. J., Jr., and Shelley, W. B.: The role of the myoepithelium of the human apocrine sweat gland. J. Invest. Derm., *22*:143, 1954.

Jackson, D. S.: Biological function of collagen in the dermis. *In* Montagna, W., Bentley, J. P., and Dobson, R. L. (eds.): The Dermis. New York, Appleton-Century-Crofts, Inc., 1970, pp. 39–48.

Klaus, S. N.: Pigment transfer in mammalian epidermis. Arch. Derm., *100*:757–762, 1969.

Kligman, A. M.: The biology of the stratum corneum. *In* Montagna, W., and Lobitz, W. C., Jr. (eds.): The Epidermis. New York, Academic Press, 1964, p. 387.

Kligman, A. M.: Pathologic dynamics of human hair loss. I. Telogen effluvium. Arch. Derm., *83*:175, 1961.

Lele, P. P., and Weddell, S.: The relationship between neurohistology and corneal sensitivity. Brain, *79*:119, 1956.

Lever, W. F.: Embryology of the skin. *In* Histopathology of the Skin. 4th ed. Philadelphia, J. B. Lippincott Co., 1967.

Montagna, W.: The sebaceous glands in man. *In* Montagna, W., Ellis, R. A., and Silver, A. (eds.): Advances in Biology of Skin, Vol. 4. New York, Pergamon Press, 1963, p. 19.

Montagna, W.: The Structure and Function of the Skin. 2nd ed. New York, Academic Press, 1962, p. 381.

Moretti, G.: The blood vessels of the skin. *In* Gans, O., and Steigleder, G. K. (eds.): Handbuch des Haut und Geschlecht-Krankheiten. New York, Springer-Verlag, 1968, p. 491.

Muller, S. A.: Hair neogenesis. J. Invest. Derm., *56*:1, 1971.

Odland, G. F., and Short, J. M.: Structure of the Skin. *In* Fitzpatrick, T. B., Arndt, K. A., Clark, W. H., Eisen, A. Z., Van Scott, E. J., and Vaughan, J. H. (eds.): Dermatology in General Medicine. New York, McGraw-Hill-Blakiston, 1971, pp. 39–48.

Partridge, S. M.: Biological role of elastin. *In* Montagna,

W., Bentley, J. P., and Dobson, R. L. (eds.): The Dermis. New York, Appleton-Century-Crofts, Inc., 1970, pp. 69–87.

Pass, F., Brophy, D., Pearson, M. L., and Lobitz, W. C.: Human epidermal glycogen after inflammatory stimuli. J. Invest. Derm., *45*:391–395, 1965.

Pecoraro, V., Astore, I., Barman, J., and Araujo, C. I.: The normal trichogram in the child before the age of puberty. J. Invest. Derm., *42*:427–430, 1964.

Perera, P., Kurban, A. K., and Ryan, T. J.: The development of the cutaneous microvascular system in the newborn. Brit. J. Derm., *82*(Suppl. 5):186, 1970.

Pillsbury, D. M.: Nails. *In* A Manual of Dermatology. Philadelphia, W. B. Saunders Co., 1971, p. 17.

Pinkus, F.: The development of the integument. *In* Keibel, F., and Mall, F. P. (eds.): Manual of Human Embryology. Philadelphia, J. B. Lippincott Co., 1910, pp. 243–291.

Plewig, G.: Regional differences in cell sizes in the human stratum corneum. Part II. Effects of sex and age. J. Invest. Derm., *54*:19–20, 1970.

Prunieras, M.: Interactions between keratinocytes and dendritic cells. J. Invest. Derm., *52*:1–14, 1969.

Serri, F., Montagna, W., and Mescon, H.: Studies of the skin of the fetus and the child. II. Glycogen and amylophosphorylase in the skin of the fetus. J. Invest. Derm., *39*:199–217, 1962.

Shellow, W. V. R., and Kligman, A. M.: Three dimensional visualization of elastic fibers in thick skin section. Arch. Derm., *95*:221–224, 1967.

Sims, R. T.: Melanocytes. *In* Champion, R. H., Gillman, T., Rook, A. J., and Sims, R. T. (eds.): An Introduction to the Biology of the Skin. Philadelphia, F. A. Davis Co., 1970, pp. 139–153.

Smith, J. G., Jr.: The dermal elastoses. Arch. Derm., *88*:382, 1963.

Strauss, J. S., and Pochi, P. E.: Histology, histochemistry and electron microscopy of sebaceous glands in man. *In* Gans, O., and Steigleder, G. K. (eds.): Handbuch des Haut und Geschlechts Krankheiten. New York, Springer-Verlag, 1968, p. 184.

Szabo, G.: The regional anatomy of the human integument. Phil. Trans. Roy. Soc., *252*:447, 1967.

Tarnowski, W. M., and Hashimoto, K.: Langerhans cell granules in histiocytosis X. Arch. Derm., *96*:298–304, 1967.

Wasserman, F.: *In* Rodahl, K. (ed.): Fat as a Tissue. London, McGraw-Hill, 1964.

Weinstein, G. D., and Frost, P.: Replacement kinetics. *In* Fitzpatrick, T. B., Arndt, K. A., Clark, W. H., Eisen, A. Z., Van Scott, E. J., and Vaughan, J. H. (eds.): Dermatology in General Medicine. New York, McGraw-Hill-Blakiston, 1971, pp. 78–87.

Winkelmann, R. K.: The cutaneous innervation of the human newborn prepuce. J. Invest. Derm., *26*:53–67, 1956.

Winkelmann, R. K.: Nerve Endings in Normal and Pathologic Skin. Contributions to the Anatomy of Sensations. Springfield, Charles C Thomas, 1960.

Zaias, N.: Embryology of the human nail. Arch. Derm., *87*:37, 1963.

Zaias, N.: The regeneration of the primate nail. Studies of the squirrel monkey, Saimiri. J. Invest. Derm., *44*:107, 1965.

Zaias, N.: The movement of the nail bed. J. Invest. Derm., *48*:402, 1967.

Zelickson, A. S.: Fibroblast development and fibrogenesis. Arch. Derm., *88*:497, 1963.

Chapter Two

FUNCTIONAL COMPONENTS OF THE SKIN

In the previous chapter we described the structural components of the newborn infant's skin and some of their functions. Here we will treat other important cutaneous functions requiring the concerted activity of several anatomical components of the skin.

THE SKIN SURFACE

The fetal epidermis is a glycogen rich organ which is covered with a mixture of desquamating cells, sebum, water and other substances derived from the amniotic fluid. This greasy film, the *vernix caseosa*, is lost during the early weeks of life due to the normal turnover of the epidermis and abetted by the washing with water and inunction with oil that is frequently the lot of the newborn infant. Glycogen present within the epidermal cells is lost from the skin surface after the sixth fetal month since the basal cells cease to produce it after this time. Basal layer glycogen may reappear during keratogenesis whenever the epidermis is injured and undergoing repair (Pass, 1965).

FUNCTIONS OF THE SKIN SURFACE

Skin pH

Determinations of skin pH are actually measurements of the hydrogen ion concentration in the aqueous phase of the surface emulsion. Although the surface pH over most of the body is acid in the child and adult, acidity of the skin surface is clearly an age-dependent phenomenon as shown by the detailed studies of Behrendt and Green (1971). In a large series of full-term infants a mean surface pH of 6.34 was obtained for the first two days of life, using combined data from three separate sites: shoulder, axilla and abdomen. During the subsequent four days, the mean pH dropped to 4.95, and between the seventh and 30th days further decreased to 4.70. It should be noted, however, that there was wide individual variation among infants with a range of from 3.4 to 8.5 on days one to two, 3.0 to 7.9 on days three to six, and 3.2 to 7.2 on days seven to 30. No sex or racial differences were noted. Data on low birth weight infants indicate a similar decline in surface pH with increasing postnatal age.

Presumably the neutrality of the surface coat at birth is influenced by the pH of the vernix caseosa and the amniotic fluid in which the infant has been immersed. Even after removal of the vernix, the skin pH remains high for the first day or two of life. The mechanism responsible for the pH shift during the subsequent several days is still unclear, but may be related to alteration in the composition of the surface lipids and in the functional capacity and activity of the eccrine glands.

Sebum

The occasional infant develops acne in the neonatal period. This possibly is the result of an idiosyncratic hyper-responsiveness of the infant's sebaceous glands to stimulation by maternal androgens. It is equally interesting to note that infants with the feminizing testis syndrome have sebaceous glands which are incapable of being stimulated by testosterone since they apparently lack the enzyme responsible for converting inactive testosterone to active 5-dihydrotestosterone. Children with feminizing testis syndrome never develop acne.

We previously discussed abnormal variants of sebaceous gland behavior (see Chap. 1). Ramasastry and his colleagues (1970) studied the effects of age on changes of normal skin surface lipids in 51 subjects five days to 15 years old. Using a microtechnique it was established that qualitatively and quantitatively, the skin surface lipids of the newborn are similar to those of adults. The values change slowly, so that at four years of age the lipids reflect relative inactivity by the sebaceous glands. In the first month, the surface film is rich in triglycerides, free fatty acids and wax esters (sebum) and low in cholesterol (epidermal lipids). By age four the predominant lipid is cholesterol, reflecting the quiescence of the sebaceous glands. At puberty the lipids change in character again as the result of activation of sebaceous gland function.

Skin Flora

The colonization of the newborn skin is a physiologic event occurring during the first hours and days of life and may be modified by environmental factors. In a study of the bacterial flora of infants at delivery, the skin was found to be colonized mainly by non-pathogenic coagulase-negative staphylococci and diphtheroid bacilli with coliforms occurring in about 10 per cent and streptococci in 4.5 per cent of infants (Sarkany, 1967). Neither *S. aureus* nor *C. albicans* were found in appreciable numbers. The skin of infants delivered by Caesarean section was routinely sterile. During the subsequent hours of life a sharp rise in the number of all types of flora was noted.

In an extensive study of colonization of the umbilical area, *Staphylococcus epidermidis* (coagulase-negative staphylococcus) was found to be the prevalent organism, while small numbers of *S. aureus*, gamma streptococci, *Pseudomonas, Klebsiella-Enterobacter* and a few other species were also cultured. An increasing number of infants were colonized by these organisms until day four, at which time approximately 80 per cent of the mature infant population was colonized at the umbilical site. Premature infants had a greater prevalence of *S. aureus* in the umbilical area than did full-term infants. No sex differences were noted (Evans, 1970).

The number and species of organisms found on infant skin can be profoundly altered by manipulation of the environmental conditions. Although routine washing with soap and water does not appear to influence either the rate or pattern of skin colonization, washing with hexachlorophene was found to cause marked suppression of the resident skin flora as well as a decrease in the numbers of *Staphylococcus aureus*. Little effect was noted on streptococci or *E. coli*. An average 20 per cent increase in the incidence of Proteus in all sites was also observed (Sarkany, 1970).

Infants who become heavily colonized with staphylococci and gram-negative bacilli are more prone to infection than those who are lightly colonized. Transfer of potentially pathogenic organisms may occur through handling by the mother and nursery personnel as well as by contact with organisms shed via skin scales and dispersed in the environment. *S. aureus* may be found with relative frequency in the groin, axillae and umbilicus. Acquisition of gram-negative organisms, particularly in the preterm infant, is encouraged when an atmosphere of high humidity is maintained in the isolette.

THE EPIDERMAL BARRIER

PERCUTANEOUS ABSORPTION

The physiologic barrier to skin penetration by exogenous substances is known to reside almost entirely in the stratum corneum, the compact outer layer of the epidermis. The phenomenon of percutaneous absorption is essentially one of diffusion of a substance through stratum corneum and epidermis into the dermis where passage into the microcirculation is accomplished (Fig. 2–1). Entry into the dermis may occur via the orifices of appendageal structures, which may act as shunts in this process, but their relative surface area is small (Scheuplein, 1971), and their contribution to overall epidermal permeability is limited except to permit entry of

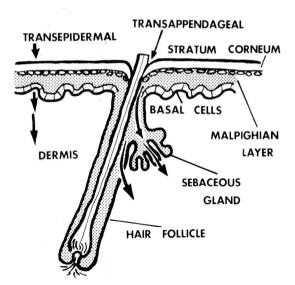

PERCUTANEOUS ABSORPTION

Figure 2–1. Routes of percutaneous absorption. The transepidermal route is the major pathway in humans.

certain large molecules. Variation in rates of permeability is probably also related to anatomic differences in the thickness of stratum corneum. However, absorption is also modified by genetic factors and other variables, such as lipid and water solubility of the penetrant, skin hyperemia and alterations in skin temperature and hydration.

Little is known about the permeability of fetal and neonatal skin. Recent studies of barrier function in fetal rat and guinea pig suggest that maturation of the epidermal barrier occurs during the last quarter of gestation, as evidenced by a decrease in water permeability, an increase in epidermal sulfhydryl content (as a measure of keratinization) and alterations in ultrastructure of the epidermal cells (Singer, 1971). Increased diffusion permeability of skin from fetuses under 24 weeks of age has also been demonstrated using *in vitro* preparations and isotopic water (Parmley, 1970).

In vivo studies support the contention that fetal skin may be more permeable than that of the adult. Nachman and Esterly (1971) assessed permeability by measuring the skin blanching response of infants of varying gestational ages to the topical application of a 10 per cent Neo-Synephrine solution. Infants 28 to 34 weeks gestational age had a rapid blanching response which could no longer be elicited after 21 days of postnatal life. Infants 35 to 37 weeks gestational age responded less dramatically and lost the blanching response by seven to 10 days of age. Term infants, in most instances, failed to exhibit blanching

even on the first day of life. Palms and soles of infants of any age did not appear to be permeable to Neo-Synephrine. More data on percutaneous absorption needs to be accumulated in the human fetus and newborn; unfortunately, animal studies yield results which are difficult to interpret since permeability is not directly comparable among the various mammalian species (Tregar, 1966).

Transepidermal Water Loss

Transepidermal water loss is dependent on a number of factors, including regional variability, hydration of stratum corneum, skin surface temperature, ambient humidity and neural control of eccrine sweating. Normally there is conservation of water loss in the newborn infant. Wildnauer and Kennedy (1970) have demonstrated a 30 per cent lower transepidermal water loss in this age group as compared to the infant a few weeks older. Although eccrine gland quiescence in this period may play some role in this phenomenon, the recent finding in preterm infants that phototherapy (for hyperbilirubinemia) causes an increase in transepidermal water loss (Wu, 1972) suggests that other factors such as vascular dilatation and photobiologic effects on the epidermis may be equally important.

Sweating

Eccrine sweat glands are distributed over the entire body. In the late stages of fetal development (about 28 weeks) these glands acquire secretory capabilities. At birth there is little or no functional sweating. During this time proper environmental control is essential for the maintenance of normal body temperature. In normal mature infants sweating begins on about the third postnatal day and rapidly approaches adult function, but complete activity is not achieved until two or three years later. Axillary apocrine sweating starts a few years before puberty.

Thermal Sweating (Kuno, 1956). Heat-stressed newborn term infants are not capable of lowering their skin temperature by sweating. An increase in rectal temperature is noted in such infants until the sweat response is initiated. In the majority this occurs between the second to fifth postnatal day. Preterm or low birth weight infants suffer a delay of from 21 to 33 days in onset of sweating.

Mental Sweating (Kuno, 1956). Emotionally induced sweating was studied in 18 newborn term infants and found to be initiated 38 to 97 days after birth. Kuno believed that induction of thermal sweating was dependent upon the maturation of a hypothalamic center and emotional sweating upon the maturation of the cerebral cortex.

CONSTITUENTS OF SWEAT. Sweat contains water, electrolytes and lactate. Glucose is found in minute concentrations (3 to 10 mg/100 ml). The pH of sweat is between 4.0 and 6.8. In cystic fibrosis, sweat sodium may rise well above the normal value of 60 mEq/L and often reaches 90 mEq/L or more.

Pharmacologic Responsiveness of the Newborn Eccrine Gland

Behrendt and Green (1969) studied the sudorific responses of neonatal eccrine glands to acetylcholine and adrenalin. After studying 125 neonates aged one to seven days, they concluded that sweat gland responsiveness to these agents was a function of gestational age. The less mature the infant, the higher the threshold to stimulation. Similarly, in a later study (1970) they found that the cholinesterase inhibitor, neostigmine, was less effective in stimulating sweating in term neonates than in mature newborn infants.

In summary, the eccrine sweat gland appears to be morphologically mature at 28 weeks of gestational age but functionally immature until about 38 to 40 weeks of life. It is not yet clear which component is responsible for lack of function.

VASOMOTOR TONE

Vasomotor tone is altered by a delicate and complex series of nervous and pharmacological control mechanisms. The sympathetic nervous system, norepinephrine, acetylcholine and histamine probably are operative at this level. Local mediators such as serotonin, vasoactive polypeptides, corticosteroids and prostaglandins also play a role in vasomotion and tone. The nervous control of thermoregulation includes participation by the hypothalamus, higher cerebral centers, autonomic and sensory nerves and the axon reflex. Venous circulation is similarly controlled by nervous, pharmacologic, local tissue changes and systemic hemodynamic conditions.

Most important, the peripheral circulatory tone may also reflect the profound hemodynamic changes occurring in the cardiopulmonary, umbilical and other major blood vessels during the first several hours to several days after birth (Schaffer, 1971). Furthermore, as the skin surface grows its capillaries proliferate in a disordered pattern and only slowly acquire the regular adult pattern (Perera, 1970). The blood pressure tends to be low and the blood is more viscous. The latter factors, combined with the immaturity of the vessel wall, lead to extravasation of fluid and result in dermal edema.

The premature infant shows exaggeration of all these responses, as well as deficits in sweating, shivering reflex and minimal fat pad insulation. The result is defective body temperature regulation and the need for careful environmental control in the low birth weight infant.

The Axon Reflex

The maturity of the peripheral nervous system is more nearly correlated with gestaional age and weight than with age as measured from the day of birth. Wilkes, Freedman and Hodgman (1966) studied the flare reaction to histamine (which together with the central erythema and subsequent wheal form the triple response of Lewis) in newborn infants as an indicator of axon reflex capability. They found the axon reflex reaction to be less consistently present in mature neonates than in adults and most difficult to elicit in premature infants.

NUTRITIONAL DEFICIENCIES AND THE SKIN

Gillman (1970) and Sims (1970) reviewed the cutaneous effects of malnutrition and most of the material contained in this brief comment may be found in amplified form in their own excellent reviews. We feel the problem of malnutrition is of overwhelming worldwide importance and that attention should be focused on this aspect of cutaneous biology.

Deficient feeding may start soon after birth and be aggravated by an imprudent diet following weaning. The systemic signs and symptoms of malnutrition are obviously more profound than those seen in the skin, and usually appear only during the following year. The rapidity with which the effects of malnutrition appear is related to the patient's genetic constitution, the climate, the nature of the deficient diet and the interactions of the infant's endocrine system as well as some of its mediators (e.g., the relation between arachidonic acid and prostaglandins). The effects of malnutrition on the skin are of several types: (1) pigmentary disturbances, both hyperpigmentation in light-exposed areas as well as hypopigmentation of hair; (2) scaling and exfoliation; (3) edema in the cutis; (4)

comedones and perifollicular hyperkeratosis; and (5) hair changes, including reductions in its diameter and linear growth, a function of decreased protein synthesis. The hair loses its curl, becomes softer and swells excessively when exposed to water. The stress-strain curve is also altered, indicating increased fragility of hair.

THE APPEARANCE OF NEWBORN SKIN

Within a few hours of birth the skin develops an intense red color which may remain for a period of several hours. With fading of this erythema, bluish mottling (livedo reticularis) becomes evident, particularly when the infant is exposed to a cool environment, with occasional associated acrocyanosis (Plate II-B, page 82). Localized mild edema may also be present over the pubis and the dorsa of the hands and feet, possibly as an additional manifestation of an unstable peripheral circulation.

Although the body surface tends to be less pigmented during the neonatal period than later in life, certain areas, such as the linea alba, the areolae and the scrotum, are often deeply pigmented as a result of high circulating levels of maternal and placental hor-

I. Biosynthesis of melanin
II. Premelanosome
III. Partially melanized melanosome
IV. Melanin granules inside dendrites phagocytosed by basal cell
V. Supranuclear melanin in basal cell

B.M. Basement membrane

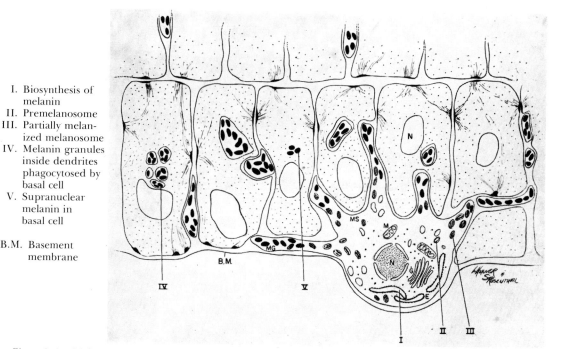

Figure 2–2. Melanin synthesis. (From: T. B. Fitzpatrick and A. S. Breathnach: Das epidermale Melanin-Einheit-System. *Derm. Wschr., 147*:481–489, May 1963.)

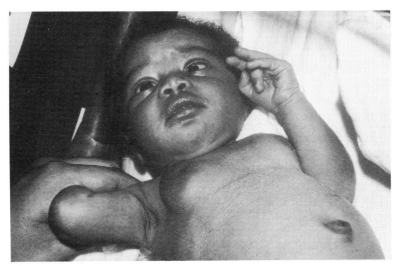

Figure 2–3. "Physiologic" breast engorgement. (Courtesy of Drs. David Fisher and John Paton.)

mones. Palpable nodules of breast tissue, active secretion by the mammary gland and a hyperplastic vaginal epithelium are additional normal end-organ responses to these hormones (Fig. 2–3).

The premature infant's skin may be readily distinguished from the full-term infant's skin. At birth the skin is more transparent and gelatinous and tends to be free of wrinkles. The premature infant may be covered with fine lanugo hair which in the full-term infant has been lost or, in some areas, replaced by vellus hair. Sexual hormonal effects are less conspicuous in the premature infant; the scrotum is less rugose and pigmented, the labia majora are less prominent, and nipples and areolae are less pigmented with less palpable breast tissue.

REFERENCES

Behrendt, H. and Green, M.: Drug-induced localized sweating in full-size and low birth weight neonates. Amer. J. Dis. Child. *117*:299, 1969.

Behrendt, H. and Green, M.: Patterns of Skin pH from Birth Through Adolescence. Springfield, Charles C Thomas, 1971.

Evans, H. E., Akpata, S. O. and Baki, A.: Factors influencing the establishment of the neonatal bacterial flora. I. The role of host factors. Arch. Environ. Health *21*:514, 1970.

Gillman, T.: Nutritional influences on the skin in man. *In* Champion, R. H., Gillman, T., Rook, A. S. and Sims, R. T. (eds.): An Introduction to the Biology of the Skin. Philadelphia, F. A. Davis Co., 1970, p. 355.

Green, M. and Behrendt, H.: Drug-induced localized sweating in neonates. Amer. J. Dis. Child. *120*:434, 1970.

Kuno, Y.: Human Perspiration. Springfield, Charles C Thomas, 1956, pp. 128–136.

Nachman, R. L. and Esterly, N. B.: Increased skin permeability in preterm infants. J. Pediat. *79*:628, 1971.

Parmley, T. H. and Seeds, A. E.: Fetal skin permeability to isotopic water (THO) in early pregnancy. Amer. J. Obstet. Gynec. *108*:128, 1970.

Pass, F., Brophy, D., Pearson, M. L. and Lobitz, W. C.: Human epidermal glycogen after inflammatory stimuli. J. Invest. Derm. *45*:391, 1965.

Perera, P., Kurban, A. K. and Ryan, T. J.: The development of the cutaneous microvascular system in the newborn. Brit. J. Derm. 82 (Suppl. 5):*86*, 1970.

Ramasastry, P., Downing, D. T., Pochi, P. E. and Strauss, J. S.: Chemical composition of human skin surface lipids from birth to puberty. J. Invest. Derm. *54*:139, 1970.

Sarkany, I. and Arnold, L.: The effect of single and repeated applications of hexachlorophene on the bacterial flora of the skin of the newborn. Brit. J. Derm. *82*:261, 1970.

Sarkany, I. and Gaylarde, C. C.: Skin flora of the newborn. Lancet *1*:589, 1967.

Schaffer, A. J. and Avery, M. E.: Diseases of the newborn. 3rd ed. Philadelphia, W. B. Saunders Co., 1971, p. 25.

Scheuplein, R. J. and Blank, I. H.: Permeability of the skin. Physiol. Rev. *51*:702, 1971.

Sims, R. T.: Hair as an indicator of incipient and developed malnutrition and response to therapy. *In* Champion, R. H., Gillman, T., Rook, A. J. and Sims, R. T. (eds.): An Introduction to the Biology of the Skin. Philadelphia, F. A. Davis Co., 1970, p. 408.

Singer, G. J., Wegman, P. C., Lehman, M. D., Christensen, M. J. and Vinson, L. J.: Barrier development, ultrastructure, and sulfhydryl content of the fetal epidermis. J. Soc. Cosmet. Chem. *22*:119, 1971.

Tregar, R. T.: Physical Functions of Skin. London, Academic Press, 1966.

Wildnauer, R. H. and Kennedy, R.: Transepidermal water loss of human newborns. J. Invest. Derm. *54*:483, 1970.

Wilkes, T., Freeman, R. I. and Hodgman, J.: The sensitivity of the axon-reflex in term and premature infants. J. Invest. Derm. *47*:491, 1966.

Wu, P. Y. K. and Hodgman, J. E.: Changes in insensible water loss in infants with and without phototherapy. Clin. Res. *20*:294, 1972.

Chapter Three

SKIN LESIONS

BASIC LESIONS

The ability to recognize the earliest form (basic lesions) of a particular disease is essential to the visual diagnosis of the patient's problem. The skin has a limited number of pathological notes to play, but manages to construct chords, and even symphonies, of disease. In this chapter we will deal with these pathological notes, or basic lesions, their configuration (to continue the analogy, the chords), and their distribution (theme). The basic lesions are: macules; papules; wheals; vesicles; pustules; bullae; comedones; nodules; plaques; patches; crusts; scales; erosions; ulcerations; and, atrophy.*

The macule is a colored spot without elevation, usually 1 cm in size or smaller, and its color may be brown as in a freckle, black as in junction nevi, red as in telangiectasia or purpura or white as in tuberous sclerosis (Plate II–C, page 82). Several macules may coalesce to form a patch which is similarly flat, but larger. Papules are solid, elevated, discrete lesions up to 1 cm in diameter (Fig. 3–1). They vaguely resemble large goose bumps, and milia are characteristic examples of these lesions (Fig. 17–16, page 198). The papules may have different shades and hues, depending on the nature of the lesion: red or flesh colored for hemangiomas or some dermal melanocytic nevi; tan for urticaria pigmentosa; or yellow in nevo-xanthoendothelioma. Plaques result from the coalescence of several papules. Nodules are larger papules, and may or may not be cystic, depending on their

contents and whether or not they have a wall (Fig. 3–2).

Vesicles are small blisters less than 1 cm in diameter. They contain a serous fluid. As the contents become cloudy the vesicle becomes a pustule. When the blister is larger than 1 cm the term "bulla" is used (Fig. 3–3). Vesicles and bullae are characteristic of chicken pox and insect bites, as well as of dermatitis herpetiformis and herpes simplex. The term vesicle implies the collection of fluid within or just beneath the epidermis, and lesions that appear vesicular in infancy may become urticarial or wheal-like in adulthood.

The wheal is due to fluid collection deep

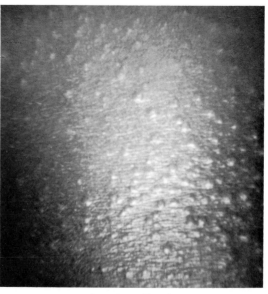

Figure 3–1. Papules.

---

*Adapted from Watt, T. L. and Jillion, D. T.: Arch. Derm. *90*:454, 1964.

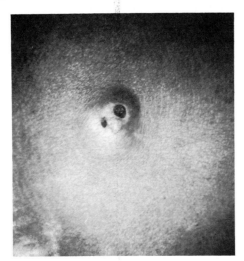

Figure 3–2. A cystic lesion (epidermoid inclusion cyst).

in the dermis. Since the infantile dermis is thinner than the adult dermis and the epidermal attachment to the dermis is less secure, a wheal in the newborn may give rise to a bulla. Blood collected in the dermis results in a hematoma or bruise (Fig. 3–4).

A comedo, or blackhead, results from plugging of a pilosebaceous orifice with keratin or sebum and is typical of acne.

Scales are the result of excess keratin, in contrast to crusts, which are composed of dried serum, blood or pus (Fig. 3–5). Scaling is typical of ichthyosis. Crusting, for example, follows the rupture of vesicles and pustules of impetigo.

Erosions result from a superficial loss of tis-

sue and usually heal without scarring. At the histological level this signifies a loss of epidermis, or part of the epidermis, leaving an epithelial remnant adequate to regenerate the entire epidermis. It can be likened to the loss of tissue in a superficial second degree burn or split thickness graft. An ulceration is a deeper lesion which usually leaves a scar. Ulceration may at times accompany infection, or a tumor such as cavernous hemangioma (Fig. 3–6).

Atrophy results from a uniform loss of tissue. In atrophy, the hair, sebaceous, apocrine and eccrine glands may disappear and the stability of the pigment can be disturbed. The skin turgor is decreased and the skin feels thinner. Atrophy is characteristic of ectodermal dysplasia and focal dermal hypoplasia. Epidermal hypertrophy, the opposite of atrophy, results in a warty appearance (a special type of papule or tumor) and may be seen in epidermal nevi (Fig. 3–7).

CONFIGURATION

The local pattern a group of lesions may take, or sometimes the evolution of a single lesion, can be extremely helpful in suggesting a diagnosis to the astute observer.

Iris Configuration. As a blister of erythema multiforme develops, it may lead to a lesion resembling a bull's eye: the older part of the lesion, the center, becomes cyanotic or hemorrhagic, and is surrounded by an area of erythema having a pale inner circle of vasoconstriction (Fig. 3–8).

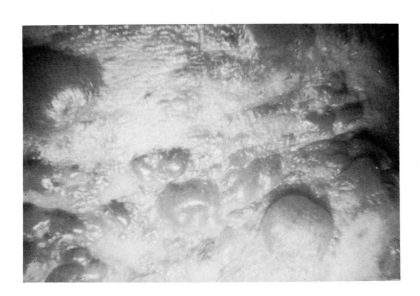

Figure 3–3. Bullous lesions (urticaria pigmentosa). (Courtesy of Dr. Alan Lasser.)

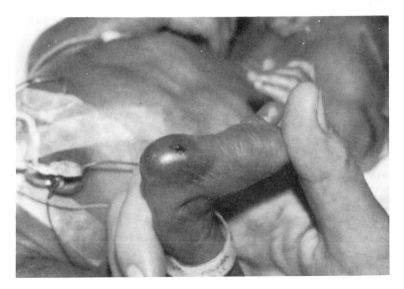

Figure 3-4. Ecchymosis (traumatic). (Courtesy of Drs. David Fisher and John Paton.)

Grouping. Herpes simplex, lymphangioma circumscriptum and dermatitis herpetiformis result in a grape-like cluster of vesicles on an erythematous or normal base, depending on the diagnosis. Verruca vulgaris may evolve as grouped papules.

Annularity. Certain diseases may be manifested by grouped primary lesions in an annular or arciform pattern which, when present, helps to narrow the diagnostic possibilities. Some of them are erythema annulare centrifugum, granuloma annulare, psoriasis, urticaria and erythema multiforme (Fig. 3-9).

Linearity. Linear streaks may occur as a result of contact with an irritant, or frequently, for completely mysterious reasons, from a disease involving cutaneous vessels or nerves. Such a linear configuration is typical of lichen striatus (Fig. 3-10).

Marbling. (See Plate IV-D). Some achromic nevi, ichthyosis hystrix or incontinentia pigmenti may result in a rather characteristic change resembling a marbled pattern, with swirls, streaks and sweeping, brush-like patterns which respect none of the cutaneous structural or developmental laws. In cutis marmorata the marbling effect may be due to a reticulated vascular distribution.

Distribution. In certain diseases groups of lesions tend to localize to given areas (Fig. 3-11). Examples of localized lesions are:

Diaper area: primary irritant dermatitis; candidal dermatitis.

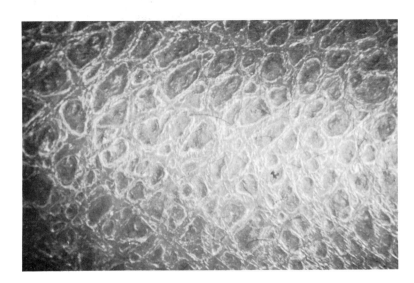

Figure 3-5. Scales (ichthyosis).

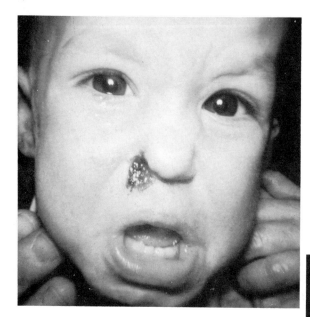

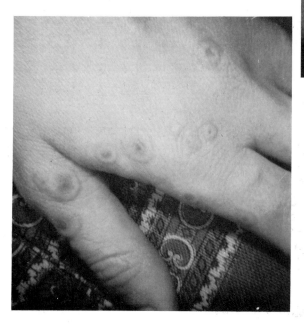

Figure 3-6. An ulcer (Pseudomonas infection).

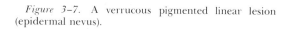

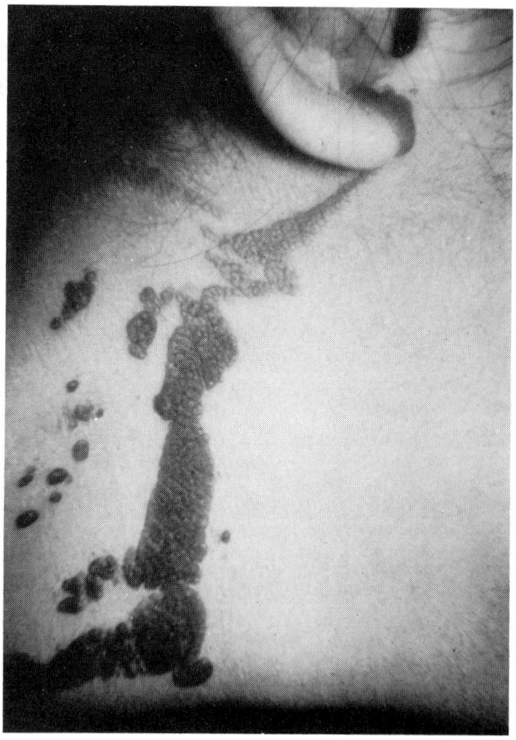

Figure 3-7. A verrucous pigmented linear lesion (epidermal nevus).

Figure 3-8. Iris lesions (erythema multiforme). (Courtesy of Dr. David Fretzin.)

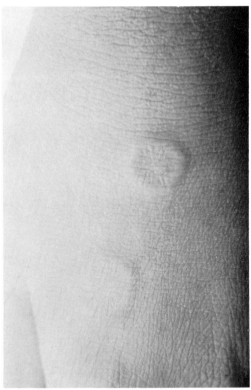

Figure 3-9. An annular lesion.

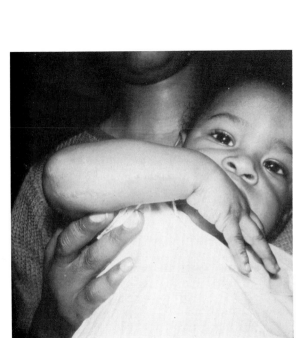

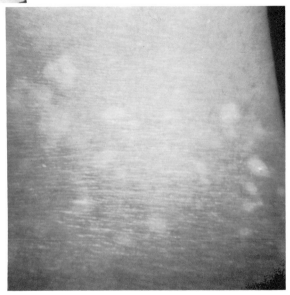

Figure 3-10. A papular linear lesion (lichen striatus).

Figure 3-11. Depigmented macules.

Light-exposed areas: face, arms, legs; Hartnup disease.

Extensor surfaces and cheeks: atopic dermatitis (the reasons for this distribution are unknown).

Central face: acne neonatorum (the site of abundant sebaceous glands), and milium.

Scalp: cradle cap; trichodysplastic diseases.

Unilaterality: harlequin color change (see Figure 6–4); developmental anomalies.

Flexures: intertrigo.

Palms and soles: hyperkeratosis palmaris et plantaris.

Some entities follow a ubiquitous distribution (e.g., cavernous hemangiomas) and criteria other than distribution must be applied to make the diagnosis.

Chapter Four

DIAGNOSTIC PROCEDURES

A variety of diagnostic procedures may help the physician support a clinical impression. Most of the commonly used procedures are simple to follow and, with a little practice, may be used successfully as valuable aids in solving the patient's problem. We will briefly discuss several of these procedures, give some indications for their use, detail the method and, where appropriate, describe their occasional complications and contraindications.

SKIN BIOPSY

The cutaneous biopsy for light or electron microscopic study is an invaluable aid in the diagnosis of bullous diseases, tumors, nevi, infiltrative diseases, scaling disorders, appendageal defects and certain hereditary disorders. It is less helpful for eczematous diseases and certain common infectious diseases.

PROCEDURE

Choice of Biopsy Site. This depends in part on the nature of the eruption. If the eruption is diffuse, then that site which can most readily bear a small scar and at the same time displays an early typical lesion is most desirable. For acute eruptions and bullous diseases an entire small early lesion should be removed. For large chronic lesions, a specimen from the periphery of the lesion, including an edge of normal skin, is most helpful. For certain melanocytic or keratinocytic nevi

the more mature areas provide optimal information. When malignancy is suspected multiple biopsies are indicated and should include early lesions as well as fully developed ones.

The Size of the Biopsy. The neonate necessarily imposes certain limitations on the size of the biopsy to be obtained. In general, a punch biopsy (see following section) 2 mm or less in diameter places an almost self-defeating circumscription on the pathologist's ability to be of help. A 3 mm punch biopsy frequently is large enough to provide adequate material, yet will still leave an acceptable scar. The size of an excisional biopsy is restricted only by considerations of closure and grafting. Shave biopsies also may leave scars, are very difficult to do with confidence regarding the depth of shave in an infant and often do not provide an adequate specimen. Shave biopsies have their place as a diagnostic tool in the newborn but must be reserved for expert hands.

THE PUNCH BIOPSY TECHNIQUE. It is advisable to have two individuals participate in this procedure: one to hold the infant on a flat surface, and the other to perform the biopsy. Biopsy should be avoided around the eyelids and their margins, the tip and bridge of the nose, the cupid's bow of the lips, the columella or the nipples. The skin requires little preparation prior to biopsy. Hairy areas should be shaved. The site should be washed with soap and water. Seventy per cent alcohol is acceptable but should not be used around the eyes or genitalia.

The area to be biopsied is infiltrated with

0.5 to 1.0 cc of 1 per cent lidocaine hydrochloride without epinephrine. A *sharp* 3 mm punch is firmly pressed against the lesion and gently rotated until a *slight* give is felt. The punch is then removed. Very little effort is required to penetrate newborn skin. The following precautions are especially applicable: (1) It is not good practice to vacillate by multiple applications of the punch to one area. Each time the punch is applied, a circular incision will be made. It is extremely difficult to outline the same area repeatedly. (2) Considerable gentleness is required so that the epidermis is not torn away from the dermis in performing the biopsy, particularly in the blistering diseases. Loss of the epidermis makes the interpretation of the pathological process less valid. (3) It is desirable to obtain some subcutaneous fat with each biopsy. Newborn fat will generally separate quite readily. One may cut the plug away from the underlying tissue with a sharp scissors if a gentle tug on the plug with a blunt forceps will not cause it to separate. The tissue should not be squeezed. (4) Usually no sutures are necessary, and a simple dressing will suffice for the healing period.

The specimen should be placed in a bottle containing 10 per cent aqueous buffered formalin, the cap closed and the bottle agitated to insure that the skin plug is immersed in the formalin. The bottle should then be labeled as to name, date and site of biopsy. Clinical information should be included with the specimen sent to the pathologist. It is often desirable in a general pathology laboratory to inform the pathologist that a skin biopsy from an infant is being forwarded so that special care may be taken in the processing. Tiny specimens are easily lost during the gross examination or in the automated tissue processing devices.

Excisional biopsies require no special discussion except that an aseptic technique is desirable since suturing is usually required. Shave biopsies heal by secondary intention so that asepsis is not necessary. The shave is made very superficially and parallel to the skin surface. It is difficult to perform and routine use is not recommended.

Biopsy for Electron Microscopy. A 2 to 3 mm biopsy specimen is usually sufficient for electron microscopic studies. The specimen should be supported on a hard surface and divided vertically (through dermis and epidermis) into three pieces using a fresh, sharp, single-edged razor blade. The pieces are then placed in 3 per cent glutaraldehyde buffered with Milonig's buffer pH 7.4 and can be stored in the refrigerator at 4° C or shipped to the appropriate laboratory where the specimen will be dehydrated and post-fixed in osmium tetroxide. Tissue for electron microscopy should not be frozen as cellular detail will be destroyed.

Complications

Complications arising from a punch biopsy procedure include excessive bleeding and infection. Keloid scarring in the neonate is rare. Bleeding in normal infants can be controlled by simple pressure. Electrodesiccation or chemical coagulation of the wound base is *not* recommended. Infection occasionally occurs in the wound but this may be treated as a superficial pyoderma and is easily controlled.

Tissue Stains

For most entities hematoxylin-eosin staining of the formalin fixed specimen will permit adequate examination of the tissue by light microscopy (Lever, 1967). Certain other staining methods are helpful in the diagnosis of a variety of disorders. Unfixed frozen sections treated with 0.1 per cent DOPA will permit demonstration of tyrosinase activity, a procedure useful in the discrimination of some pigmentary disorders (see Chap. 10). The frozen section technique may also be used in staining for acid mucopolysaccharides with toluidine blue. Formalin fixed frozen sections are used for lipid stains. Special stains may also be used on formalin fixed tissue to demonstrate collagen (Masson's trichrome), elastic fibers (Verhoeff's), nerves (Bodian), melanin (Fontana-Masson), mast cells (Giemsa), bacteria (Gram's; Ziel-Neelson), fungi (Gridley's methenamine silver), iron (Perls'), calcium (Von Kossa's), and mucopolysaccharides (Alcian blue, colloidal iron and Schiff periodic acid). It is advisable to inform the pathologist of the differential diagnosis so that the appropriate stains may be employed.

OTHER DIAGNOSTIC TECHNIQUES

POTASSIUM HYDROXIDE PREPARATION FOR THE DEMONSTRATION OF FUNGI (YEAST)

The affected area should be gently washed with water if the lesion is moist and left unwashed if it is scaly. The lesion is then firmly scraped with a dull edged scalpel and the scrapings are placed on a glass slide. One drop of 20 per cent KOH is added and mixed with the debris on the slide to make a suspension (Fig. 4–1). A coverslip is applied and the slide is gently heated over an alcohol burner until a bubble appears under the coverslip. The preparation should then be examined microscopically with a medium power objective (about 40×) under subdued light, with the condenser turned to its lowest position. Fungal elements will appear as linear branching structures *crossing the outline of the cell walls.* Yeast spores are of varying size, rounded and budding shape. The addition of lactolphenol blue to the preparation will help outline fungal elements, but it is not essential.

CULTURE OF TISSUE FOR FUNGI AND BACTERIA

Scrapings from a lesion should be collected from the active border and placed on Sabouraud's medium for initial culture and further identification of the fungus. Candida usually grows quickly (two to five days), producing creamy, moist colonies. The dermatophytes may take longer to grow and cultures should be maintained for a minimum of three weeks. If heavy bacterial contamination is likely, scrapings should be cultured on Mycosel agar (a combination of Sabouraud's media and antibiotics) to avoid bacterial overgrowth.

Bacterial cultures should be obtained as follows: The surrounding skin should be thoroughly cleaned with 70 per cent alcohol. If the lesion is crusted, the crust should be lifted off with a sterile needle and a sterile cotton applicator touched to the open area. Vesicles and pustules should be ruptured with a needle and the exudate collected on a sterile swab. Large bullae may be aspirated and the fluid cultured directly from the syringe. Occasionally lesions may be draining freely, in which case the exudate can be swabbed without prior cleaning of the skin.

If not plated directly, applicators should be transported to the laboratory in some kind of media and not be allowed to dry out. Specimens should be plated on blood agar for gram-positive organisms and desoxycholate agar for gram-negative organisms. Neisseria require chocolate agar incubated in a high CO_2 environment, and sheeps' blood agar is helpful if infection with β-hemolytic streptococci is suspected.

All specimens, bacterial and fungal, should be labeled properly, including the type of material collected, the site from which it was obtained and the suspected diagnosis, so that the proper media is used in identification of the organism.

Virus Isolation. The isolation of virus from a skin lesion for culture and identification is rarely successful in the common viral cutaneous diseases. Although the rare wart virus has been cultured, it is usually fruitless to attempt viral cultures, even in cases of herpes simplex and varicella. Viruses may be seen by electron microscopy in appropriately fixed specimens, and herpes simplex and

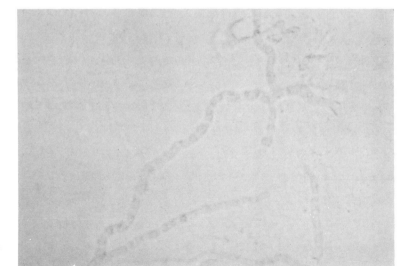

Figure 4–1. Hyphae. KOH preparation of skin scrapings.

herpes zoster (varicella) virus will grow on rabbit cornea snd chorioallantoic membrane, but these procedures remain primarily research tools and will rarely be required by the practicing physician. (The physician may employ the procedure, for example, when it becomes vital to separate the pox virus from the herpes virus groups.) Viral lesions can be identified in a crude manner by histological examination of the blister or by a touch smear of a blister base (see following section and Chap. 13).

Serological studies and viral cultures from throat and stool may be used to identify certain viral diseases involving the skin (i.e., Coxsackie virus causing hand, foot and mouth disease).

CYTODIAGNOSIS (TZANCK SMEAR)

The cytological changes occurring in blisters of herpes simplex, herpes zoster-varicella, vaccinia, smallpox and molluscum contagiosum can be seen by preparing a smear of cells from the base of a fresh blister or papule. Although the changes are not infallibly diagnostic, they can be a useful aid in separating some of these entities from a differential list of clinical possibilities (Plate III–A, page 83).

For the smear, a small, young, unruptured blister is chosen. The roof of the blister is removed with sharp scissors and the base is gently blotted with gauze. The base of the blister is firmly scraped with a blunt scalpel but bleeding should not be induced. The material on the scalpel is then spread thinly on a glass slide and stained with Giemsa or hematoxylin-eosin stains (Blank, 1952).

Certain viral infections cause a peculiar ballooning degeneration of the epidermal cells. Distorted eosinophilic mononuclear and multinuclear giant cells are frequently seen in lesions of herpes simplex and herpes zoster-varicella. These changes are less common in the pox virus group, for instance, in variola-vaccinia (see Chap. 13). The type of viral inclusion body (intracytoplasmic or intranuclear) may be further identified by the Feulgen reaction (for DNA), which is positive in variola but negative in the herpes-varicella group of diseases. The histological structure of the vesicle further helps to separate the variola group from the herpes group of diseases.

A smear of material expressed from a papule of molluscum contagiosum shows large round eosinophilic bodies. Frequently, the morphology stands out more clearly if the plug of material is compressed on a slide with 20 per cent KOH and heated gently as in the preparation for identification of fungal elements.

DARKFIELD EXAMINATION

The *Treponema pallidum* of syphilis is not easily stained in histological preparation and so closely resembles other spirochetes that, in order to make the diagnosis with certainty, the organism must be seen alive. The darkfield microscope (USPH pub. 1968) differs from the ordinary light microscope by having increased resolving power, permitting visualization of the extremely narrow treponeme. The darkfield condenser blocks out the central rays of light and realigns the peripheral light rays to focus on the object under study. The spirochete deflects the incident light rays through the objective and appears silver white on a black field, and moves back and forth with a spiral corkscrew motion. The spirochete of syphilis resembles the nonsyphilitic spirochetes found in the genitalia; therefore, some expertise is required to distinguish these organisms.

The skin of newborn infants may be contaminated with nonsyphilitic spirochetes from the mother's vagina. For this reason, if disease is suspected, the darkfield examination should be done carefully and only after the infant's skin has been washed. The examiner should wear rubber gloves for his protection. The affected area is carefully cleaned with water. If there are bullae, an intact lesion is aspirated with a sterile syringe and needle. If there are papular lesions, the moist perianal, axillary, inguinal or perinasal area is firmly abraded with a gauze square to the point of bleeding. The abraded area should then be squeezed until bleeding has stopped and a serous exudate is obtained. The exudate (or blister fluid) is touched to a clean, dry glass slide, normal saline is added and a coverslip is quickly applied. The darkfield condenser is adjusted and the fluid examined under oil. Syphilitic blisters usually teem with spirochetes and most papular lesions should also show *T. pallidum*. In contrast, a positive darkfield is rarely obtained from nonbullous palmar and plantar lesions. A rising serological titer, or one which is higher than the maternal titer, supports the diagnosis of active congenital syphilis (see Chap. 14).

WOOD'S LIGHT EXAMINATION

The Wood's lamp is helpful in the diagnosis of a variety of childhood and adult dermatologic problems (Fitzpatrick, 1971). Although it is used in older patients primarily to aid in the diagnosis of fungus infections, in the newborn a Wood's light examination is most helpful in differentiation of certain pigmentary disorders. The instrument is a mercury lamp fitted with a filter which mainly limits its emission to 3600 Å. When the light is reflected from the skin surface a white fluorescence can be seen which, by contrast, increases in areas of pigment loss. Lesions of vitiligo shine quite brightly. Areas of hypomelanosis, such as in the white macule of tuberous sclerosis, also appear whiter than the surrounding normal skin under the Wood's light. Hypermelanotic lesions, such as freckles, appear dark on a field of lighter normal skin. Urine from patients with erythropoietic porphyria will fluoresce orange-red or pink when exposed to the Wood's lamp.

TEST FOR WHITE DERMOGRAPHISM

This test is of limited usefulness in the newborn since vascular lability is an almost constant finding in the neonatal period. White dermographism is an abnormal reaction of the cutaneous blood vessels to stroking. It is most commonly found in patients with atopic dermatitis but is by no means a pathognomonic feature of that disease. It may, in fact, be found in a variety of acute and chronic eczematous conditions.

After stroking the skin with a blunt instrument (such as a tongue depressor) "the triple response of Lewis" should develop: that is, (1) a red line appears within 15 seconds as a result of capillary and arteriolar dilation; (2) an erythematous flare extends laterally beyond the stroked line in 15 to 45 seconds; and (3) one to three minutes later a wheal occurs in the central area of stroking. The first and third stages are caused by the release of histamine. The flare is mediated by an axon reflex and may be abolished by local anesthesia. In white (abnormal) dermographism, a white line develops instead of the usual red response; no flare or wheal is seen. The cause of white dermographism is unknown but it may be due to local vasoconstriction.

Test for Delayed Blanch

This test is an extension of the white dermographism phenomenon. Its indications, importance and limitations are similar to those of white dermographism.

To perform the test, 0.1 ml of a 1:1000 dilution of acetylcholine (or mecholyl) is injected superficially into the dermis with a #27 needle. Normally, within a few seconds erythema and sweating occur and contraction of the arrectores pilorum muscles (goose bumps) are apparent at the site of injection and last up to 30 minutes. In subjects with atopic dermatitis and in their unaffected relatives, this reaction is absent. In its place a pale area (a "blanch") appears in about three to five minutes ("delayed" reaction), possibly due to paradoxical vasoconstriction (although the pathogenetic mechanism remains a subject of controversy). This response lasts from about 15 to 45 minutes and may be preceded by an evanescent erythema.

It must be stressed that this test is particularly unreliable in the newborn infant. It has been shown that 30 per cent of apparently normal infants exhibit this paradoxical response (Hinrichs, 1966; Olive, 1970).

TEST FOR COLD SENSITIVITY

The application of a small ice cube to the thigh, deltoid region, buttock or back for two minutes may be useful in the diagnosis of familial cold urticaria or cold panniculitis (Solomon, 1963; Rotman, 1966). Under normal circumstances, when an ice cube is placed on the skin for two minutes, blanching occurs at the site of application and an axon reflex mediated flare—but no wheal—is seen around the area of blanching. Fifteen to 30 minutes after the test the skin should look normal. In cold urticaria the area to which the ice cube was applied will develop a large wheal with peripheral pseudopod formation. In cold panniculitis the immediate reaction is normal, but within three to 24 hours a painful, subcutaneous red nodule develops which may evolve into a plaque that may take several days to resolve.

Some care should be taken with ice cube tests. There is little danger from a localized area of cold urticaria, but if the physician suspects that the patient may suffer from hereditary angioneurotic edema (C'_1-esterase inhibitor deficiency), the local reaction to cold may trigger a severe systemic reaction so that it is best to omit the test. In cold urticaria the parents should be informed of the intention to induce a lesion and their permission should be obtained prior to implementation of the test.

O-PHTHALALDEHYDE SWEAT TEST

To determine the infant's ability to produce eccrine sweat, the following tests can be performed:

(1) Five per cent O-phthalaldehyde in xylene is painted on the questionable area of skin, as well as to a similar site on the contralateral side. Within one minute, in the presence of sweat, the area will be stained black (Juhlin, 1965).

(2) The above procedure may also be carried out on an area previously injected with 0.1 cc of 1:1000 dilution of acetylcholine. If the eccrine gland is capable of being stimulated by acetylcholine, the sweat pores and surrounding epidermis will be stained dark.

(3) In the absence of any reaction to the first two tests, a specimen of skin obtained by biopsy and stained with hematoxylin and eosin will demonstrate the presence or absence of sweat glands. An acetylcholinesterase stain (Hurley, 1953) will demonstrate whether innervation is intact.

It should be stressed that sweating during the first month may be sporadic, erratic and irregular.

EXAMINATION OF HAIR

The hair, an important cutaneous appendage, is grossly or microscopically defective in a large number of syndromes. Hair abnormalities are particularly significant in hereditarily determined diseases (Porter, 1970) and indeed may be the only manifestation of an abnormal gene (Solomon, 1971). In examining hair, a variety of procedures may be used which vary in complexity and sophistication.

Examination of scalp hair in the newborn infant may be deceptive. Because the hair cycles change from a synchronous to a dysynchronous pattern, one cannot draw conclusions readily at this time about the significance of diffuse alopecia. Most infants look "alopecic" during the first month. Since the hair is fine and the follicles are very close together, hair counts may also be misleading.

The *quality* of the hair as it appears to the eye and feels to the fingers is often an ex-

cellent index of hair shaft abnormalities. Hair which is matted, lusterless, brittle and cannot be combed is often abnormal hair. The *body* of the hair results from a combination of its fineness and stiffness. Hair which is fine (thin), round and very flexible results in poor body. This fineness is normal in the newborn. Hair which is flat, deformed, thick or brittle may feel like horse hair.

Examination of individual hairs can give a considerable amount of information. Using a small forceps or the fingers, a few hairs should be pulled out in a steady and gentle manner. A quick tug yields broken and deformed hairs unfit for examination.

The hairs are then examined under a loop or dissecting microscope for the following features: the follicular end of the shaft may contain a bulbous, less pigmented portion; the shaft should be examined for periodic disturbances in pigment; the medullary portion of the hair should be examined for pigment; and, the shaft's thickness should be uniform, without periodic thinning, breaks or nodularity. The cuticle should be smooth. The dissecting microscope is an invaluable aid to proper examination of the hair.

Additional information about the physical-chemical nature of hair can be gathered from a variety of more sophisticated tests including: stress-strain studies; chemical stressing; X-ray diffraction studies of the skeletal structure of keratin; amino acid analysis; and scanning, polarizing and electron microscopy.

DERMATOGLYPHICS

A variety of methods may be used to record the epidermal ridge patterns in adults but not all are appropriate for use on infants. A review of the commonly employed methods, materials, techniques and uses may be found in a publication by Smith (1970).

In the newborn infant, one of the most convenient methods of recording ridge patterns involves the use of a Hollister* printer set which gives satisfactory results in most instances. There are two types of Hollister footprinter pads available, both of which give a permanent record. The disposable pad yields smudgy prints when used for the fingers and palms and is not recommended. The regular footprinter dispenses less ink and is easier to manage.

---

*The kit is available from Hollister Incorporated, 211 East Chicago Avenue, Chicago, Ill. 60611.

The technique requires that the hands and feet be carefully washed and dried with soap and warm water. The baby's hand and foot, and the pad, must be warm. The pad may be warmed by breathing on it for a few seconds. The hands and feet are placed on the pad and then pressed on a special paper (also supplied by Hollister) which has a relatively hard and glossy surface. If finger patterns are needed each finger has to be rolled individually. Excess ink on the infant's hands and feet can be easily washed off with soap and warm water.

On occasion the dermal ridges are not developed enough in the newborn to permit adequate recording of the print. In such a case, direct observation with an otoscope of the fingertips and palms permits their inspection. Another (expensive) technique (Smith, 1971) employs the Norelco inkless fingerprint instrument*. The instrument uses Polaroid film and by the internal reflection of light from the print onto a glass prism extremely clear prints result. The instrument is not portable and does not allow rolling the finger to obtain prints of the lateral margins of the finger pad. The prints obtained should be classified using standard dermatoglyphic nomenclature.**

THE SKIN WINDOW

An examination of the cells participating in the inflammatory process may be helpful in studying some aspects of the cellular defense system in certain hereditary diseases or immune deficiency states. The normal newborn exhibits a diminished response to irritants and infection, but this improves with age (Adelsberger, 1927). The nonspecific normal cellular response to an inflammatory stimulus in this age group has been studied by Eitzman and Smith (1959) and by Bullock et al. (1969).

The skin window technique was first developed by Rebuck and Crowley (1955) and was predicated on the observation that leukocytes will migrate through an epidermis where the barrier layer has been removed and will adhere to a glass surface.

A skin window preparation may be performed in any nonhairy area but generally the forearm, upper arm, lower leg or back is used. The skin is thoroughly cleaned with hexachlorophene followed by 70 per cent alcohol, and dried with sterile cotton sponges. A half centimeter area is then *gently* abraded with a #15 scalpel blade. The blade is held perpendicular to the skin and any cutting motion avoided. The object is to remove just enough of the superficial cells of the epidermis (the stratum corneum) to produce a moist glistening surface. Frank bleeding renders the area unsuitable for study. A sterile, thin (preferably round) glass coverslip is placed over the abraded area; this is entirely covered by a one-inch-thick piece of styrofoam. A gauze square covers the entire area and the three layers, glass, styrofoam and gauze, hold the skin under mild pressure. The gauze is held in place by adhesive tape. The coverslips may be changed as often as desired during a 24-hour period, after which the wound will re-epithelialize. Upon removal the coverslip is air dried and stained with one of a variety of stains, such as Wright or Giemsa (Plate III–B, page 83).

The coverslip will contain a sampling of the leukocytes participating in the inflammatory response, and the relative number of various types of white cells can be tabulated for a given time period. Coverslips with less than 200 cells are inadequate for counting and should be discarded. Generally, 500 cells are counted for each time interval. The shift from early polymorphonuclear cell predominance (two to four hours), to mononuclear cell predominancy (six to 12 hours) seen in children and adults occurs later in the cycle and to a lesser degree in newborn infants (Bullock, 1969). In addition, some infants manifest a relatively marked eosinophilic response after 24 hours of age (Eitzman, 1959).

CHROMOSOMAL STUDIES

Many syndromes are associated with an abnormality in the structure or number of chromosomes. A clinician who sees a patient with multiple malformations and suspects an associated chromosomal abnormality may wish to refer his patient to the nearest genetic center offering diagnostic service. The National Foundation-March of Dimes* issues an International Directory of Genetic Services which is updated every two years.

---

*North American Philips Co., Inc. 100 East 42nd St., New York, N.Y.

**Memorandum on Dermatoglyphic Nomenclature, June 1968, Vol. IV, No. 3. Birth Defects, Original Article Series. The National Foundation-March of Dimes.

---

*International Directory of Genetic Services, 3rd ed., (Sept. 1971). Daniel Bergsma, M.D., The National Foundation-March of Dimes, 1275 Mamaroneck Ave., White Plains, N.Y. 10605.

If an abnormal number of X chromosomes is suspected, the preliminary screening test provided by a buccal smear may be requested. It should be stressed, however, that a buccal smear, although faster and easier than culturing white blood cells for chromosomes, does not supply data adequate for a definitive diagnosis.

The most informative test for chromosomal abnormalities is done by culturing leukocytes. Approximately 10 cc of venous blood is needed. Sometimes, in the more complex diagnostic problems, bone marrow or fibroblasts cultured from a skin biopsy may be required. In all of these situations the collection of samples (buccal smear, venous blood, bone marrow or skin) preferably is done at the genetic center to which the patient is referred.

The referring physician should explain to the parents or patient the procedures which may be done. The buccal smear involves scraping the buccal mucosa with a narrow, blunt metal scapula. The scrapings are spread on a clean slide and immediately fixed in alcohol. The smear is then stained and read. The values are reported as the per cent of chromatin-positive cells. The range for a normal female varies, but most laboratories consider 15 per cent chromatin-positive cells as an acceptable lower limit.

For leukocyte culture and karyotyping, 10 cc of venous blood is used. A few centers use a microtechnique where five drops of blood (obtained by pricking the finger) are immediately added to freshly thawed culture medium. The sample obtained is then immediately incubated at 37° C.

Bone marrow and skin biopsies are obtained in the usual manner. The bone marrow sample must be added to the culture medium immediately. The skin must be taken and cultured under strictly aseptic conditions.

The results of the buccal smear may be available in two to 10 days, depending on the laboratory. A minimum of four to six weeks is required to obtain the results of leukocyte cultures, bone marrow cultures and so forth. The code used to describe the chromosomal arrangements has been standardized and may be interpreted with the aid of a publication issued by the National Foundation-March of Dimes, 800 Second Avenue, New York, 10017.*

---

*Guide to Human Chromosome Defects, Sept. 1968, Vol. IV, No. 4. Birth Defects, Original Article.

IMMUNOFLUORESCENT EXAMINATION

The immunofluorescent technique has been shown to be of value in the diagnosis of two blistering skin diseases, bullous pemphigoid and pemphigus vulgaris. Tissue sections from biopsies of skin lesions taken from these patients, when stained with fluorescein-conjugated antiserum to human gamma globulin (FAHG), show a linear staining pattern at the dermo-epidermal junction in bullous pemphigoid (Jordan, 1967), and an intercellular pattern in the epidermis in pemphigus (Beutner, 1965). Patients with these two diseases also have circulating serum antibodies to components of the dermo-epidermal junction in bullous pemphigoid and to the intercellular substance in pemphigus. Patients with blistering disorders such as dermatitis herpetiformis, erythema multiforme and epidermolysis bullosa show no specific epidermal staining patterns. Although neither pemphigoid nor pemphigus occurs in the newborn, the technique is gaining in usefulness and, for this reason, a description of it is included here.

The technique is also of value in the diagnosis and follow-up evaluation of patients with lupus erythematosus. Approximately 90 per cent of examined skin lesions of patients with systemic lupus erythematosus (SLE) and chronic discoid LE, and 60 per cent of examined sections from uninvolved sun-exposed skin in SLE, show a diffuse or stippled staining pattern at the dermo-epidermal junction (Burnham, 1969; Tuffanelli, 1969). Patients with SLE do not have circulating antibodies to the dermo-epidermal junction but do have serum antinuclear antibodies detectable by the indirect immunofluorescent technique.

To detect *in vivo* bound tissue immunoglobulins, the direct immunofluorescent technique is employed. A fresh skin biopsy is snap-frozen in liquid nitrogen or solid carbon dioxide. The specimen is mailed or transported in dry ice if it must be sent any distance. Thin, cryostat-cut sections are placed on a glass slide and air dried. The slides are incubated with FAHG. Additional sections, when indicated, can be incubated with fluorescein-conjugated antihuman IgG, IgM, IgA, IgD, IgE and B_1C. After washing, the slide should be examined immediately with a microscope appropriately fitted with filters and utilizing an ultraviolet light source. Although the fluorescent pattern is most discernible immediately after staining, it will remain visible for about a week if the slides are kept in covered boxes at 4° C.

To detect circulating immunoglobulins, the indirect technique is used. Five ml of serum may be sent thawed or frozen at 5° C. to the appropriate laboratory. In this method the serum is first incubated with thin cryostat-cut sections of normal epithelial tissue to allow binding of circulating immunoglobulins (antibodies) to the tissue. The most commonly used tissues are human or primate skin, guinea pig lip and guinea pig or rabbit esophagus. The FAGH (or fluorescein-labeled anti-human globulin fraction) is then incubated with the tissue to tag the serum immunoglobulin that has been fixed to tissue components during the initial incubation. Finally, the slide is examined with the fluorescent microscope and the specific staining noted.

REFERENCES

Adelsberger, L.: Das Verhalten der kindlichen Haut gegenüber verschiedenen Reizen. Stschr. Kinderh. 43:373, 1927.

Beutner, E. H., Lever, W. F., Witebsky, E., Jordan, R. E. and Chertock, B.: Autoantibodies in pemphigus vulgaris. JAMA 192:682–688, 1965.

Blank, H. and Burgoon, C.: Abnormal cytology of epithelial cells in pemphigus vulgaris: A diagnostic aid. J. Invest. Derm. 18:213, 1952.

Bullock, J. D., Robertson, A. F., Bodenbender, J. G., Kontras, S. B. and Miller, C. E.: Inflammatory response in the neonate re-examined. Pediatrics 44: 58, 1969.

Burnham, T. K. and Fine, G.: The immunofluorescent "band" test for lupus erythematosus. Arch. Derm. 99:413, 1969.

Clinical Diagnosis of Syphilis. In Syphilis, A Synopsis. U.S. Public Health Service Publication No. 1660. U.S. Government Printing Office, Washington, D.C., 1968.

Eitzman, D. V. and Smith, R. T.: The nonspecific inflammatory cycle in the neonatal infant. AMA J. Dis. Child. 97:326, 1959.

Fitzpatrick, T. B. and Johnson, D. P.: Fundamentals of dermatologic diagnosis. In Fitzpatrick, T. B., Arndt, K. A., Clark, W. H., Eisen, A. Z., Van Scott, E. J. and Vaughan, J. H. (eds.): Dermatology in General Medicine. New York, McGraw Hill, 1971, p. 10.

Hinrichs, W. L., Logan, G. B. and Winklemann, R. K.: Delayed blanch phenomenon as an indication of atopy in newborn infants. J. Invest. Derm. 46:189, 1966.

Hurley, H. J., Jr., Shelley, W. B. and Koelle, G. B.: The distribution of cholinesterases in human skin, with special reference to eccrine and apocrine sweat glands. J. Invest. Derm. 21:139, 1953.

Jordan, R. E., Beutner, E. H., Witebsky, E. et al.: Basement zone antibodies in bullous pemphigoid. JAMA 200:751–756, 1967.

Juhlin, L. and Shelley, W. B.: A stain for sweat pores. Nature 213:408, 1967.

Lever, W. F.: Laboratory methods. In Histopathology of the Skin. 4th ed. Philadelphia, J. B. Lippincott Co., 1967, p. 43.

Olive, J. T., O'Connell, E. J., Winkelmann, R. K. and Logan, G. B.: Delayed blanch phenomenon in children: Re-evaluation of 5 year old children originally tested as newborns. J. Invest. Derm. 54:256, 1970.

Porter, P. S., and Lobitz, W. C. Jr.: Human hair: A genetic marker. Brit. J. Derm. 83:225, 1970.

Rebuck, J. and Crowley, J.: A method of studying leukocytic functions in vivo. Ann. N.Y. Acad. Sci. 59:757, 1955.

Rotman, H.: Cold panniculitis in children. Arch. Derm. 94:720, 1966.

Smith, D. W.: Methods of recording dermatoglyphics. In Recognizable Patterns of Human Malformation. Philadelphia, W. B. Saunders Co., 1970, p. 361.

Solomon, L. M. and Beerman, H.: Cold panniculitis. Arch. Derm. 88:897, 1963.

Solomon, L. M., Esterly, N. B. and Medenica, M.: Hereditary trichodysplasia: Marie Unna's hypotrichosis. J. Invest. Derm. 57:389, 1972.

Tuffanelli, L., Kay, D. and Fukuyama, K.: Dermal-epidermal junction in lupus erythematosus. Arch. Derm. 99:652, 1969.

Chapter Five

PRINCIPLES OF THERAPY

GENERAL PRINCIPLES

The skin of the newborn infant exhibits certain characteristics requiring special consideration in applying topical therapy. This principle is simply an extension of the fact that most systemic medications require an adjustment of dosage when given to infants.

The following list attempts to correct some of the common misconceptions in the therapeutic management of skin disease in the neonatal infant:

(1) Newborn infants, for reasons that are not known with certainty but are probably related to vascular lability, frequently develop minor, fleeting erythematous macular or nondescript papular eruptions at the end of the first month. For these nonspecific lesions it may be wise to apply dollops of delay prior to use of extensive investigative or therapeutic modalities.

(2) It is important not to further injure an already damaged skin, particularly the vulnerable skin of the newborn infant. Unfortunately, the more severe the dermatitis, the greater the tendency to use "powerful"* therapy when, in fact, the reverse attitude should prevail.

(3) In order to treat with a sense of security it is important to know the natural course of a disease, as well as the expected course of an optimally treated disease. Not only should the physician be aware of what is most likely to take place, but parents should also be so advised.

*This term can be translated into "complicated and concentrated."

(4) It is difficult to treat localized areas differently on the same tiny body. Therefore, one should treat the most acute areas first. When these resolve, the treatment may be changed. In contrast to the adult, where treatment can be both spatial and temporal, treatment in the infant must be primarily temporal.

(5) Systemic manifestations of cutaneous disease occur more readily in infants than in the young adult, so complications should be anticipated and treated early.

(6) It is better to know a few topical remedies well than to experiment with a broad list of different drugs reputed to do the same thing.

(7) Pruritus in the infant is more aggravating to the parent than to the infant. Heavy sedation or tying the infant's hands is never necessary or desirable. Properly applied topical therapy, mild sedation and environmental control of temperature and humidity usually do the trick.

(8) Patience, reassurance, careful observation and the passage of time are probably the best treatment for small, uncomplicated cavernous hemangiomas.

(9) Little harm and much good can be achieved by using water compresses for any erosive, weeping and acute dermatitis.

(10) The infant's skin adjusts relatively poorly to changes in environmental temperature. For this reason, widespread application of cool water compresses to lesions may result in excessively lowering body temperature, causing shivering and discomfort. Unless a rapid drop in skin temperature is desirable (i.e., for fever), compress water should be

tepid (slightly warm to the touch) rather than hot or cold. Wet dressings (except for treatment of furuncles) should never be occluded.

(11) Potassium permanganate and aluminum acetate added to compresses probably contribute little to the effect of water alone.

(12) A hexachlorophene wash should not be used on extensively denuded areas since it may be absorbed, and it should never be used for this purpose at full concentration. *Compressing* with hexachlorophene may be dangerous (Curley, 1971). It should not be used except under extraordinary circumstances, and then only in localized areas in premature infants (FDA bulletin). The use of hexachlorophene in nursery populations to prevent staphylococcal infections has benefits not to be overlooked; therefore, its continued and cautious use must remain a decision of the supervising physician.

(13) Boric acid has been widely used in the past in wet dressing solutions. It is toxic when absorbed. Since boric acid has negligible pharmacologic activity, and because the hazards are significant, it has no place in modern pediatric dermatologic therapy.

(14) Corn starch powder mixed with sweat constitutes a suitable medium for proliferation of Candida. Talc and zinc oxide are therefore preferable for routine use.

(15) The normal skin of an infant does not require extensive lubrication. If a lubricant is desired it is probably better to use a cream (i.e., hydrophilic ointment USP) in preference to oils such as olive oil, corn oil or butter. These may become rancid and sticky and have little effect on normal skin.

(16) Pastes or ointments used for protecting the diaper area are not an adequate answer to diaper dermatitis if impermeable panties are also being used. Paste is protective rather than curative. Cultures should be made from the lesions of an erosive diaper dermatitis and appropriate antimicrobials used. Impermeable diapers should be left off as much as possible.

(17) Scrubbing of the anal and perianal areas with soap and water is useless if residual paste has not previously been removed by wiping it away *gently* with mineral oil.

(18) Generally, calamine lotion, talc or paste should not be used on weeping lesions.

(19) Topical vitamins contained in pastes probably add nothing to the effectiveness of the paste-base itself.

(20) Tar ointments have little place in the treatment of the newborn infant, although they are quite useful for the treatment of eczematous lesions after three months of age.

(21) Topically applied hydrocortisone for treatment of limited areas of dermatitis is very useful and, if used in rational concentration for the proper indications, is not harmful.

(22) Occlusive dressings (i.e., Saran wrap) should not be used in this age group. First, they are not necessary since skin permeability is already quite adequate; second, they rarely stay in place on an active infant; and third, they constitute a hazard which may lead to suffocation.

(23) A daily shampoo for seborrheic dermatitis of the scalp (cradle cap) is not harmful.

(24) Exposure to sunlight should be very gradual and in small doses.

(25) Topical proteolytic enzymes have little or no use in pediatric dermatologic therapy. There is no condition discussed in this book in which these enzymes have proved to be of value.

(26) Topical anesthetics may be helpful in alleviating the pain of erosive lesions on mucous membranes, but they have little usefulness on skin. Anesthetics either do not penetrate the intact stratum corneum or, if the barrier layer is breeched, merely suppress symptoms. For acute dermatitis, cool compresses *both* suppress symptoms and treat the underlying inflammatory reaction.

TOPICAL THERAPY

Wet Dressings

Open wet dressings are primarily used in dermatitis in the early stages of the acute inflammatory reaction where epidermal integrity has been breeched (for example, erosions and blisters). Their purpose is to cool the skin by evaporation, thereby causing mild vasoconstriction and decreasing vascular permeability. Water also cleans and removes an exudate.

Tepid tap water is the medium of choice in most cases. Physiological saline is acceptable but most laymen either over- or underestimate the amount of salt to be added, and more harm than benefit can come from this mistake. For erosive or ulcerative lesions, 0.25 per cent silver nitrate may be added to the compressing solution. Boric acid should not be used.

The dressing should be made of cotton or

old soft linen. Wool, silk, satin, gauze and cotton fluff should be avoided. The dressing, two or three layers thick, may be soaked and applied to the lesion *without occlusion*. The dressing should be kept in place by the parent's hand or with a light wrapping of gauze and be remoistened every 20 to 30 minutes by dripping fresh water onto it. For most acute conditions, four to five treatments of this type each day for one or two days suffices. Adhesive tape has no place on dermatitic skin.

Lubricants (Bases): Ointments, Creams, and Oils

There are a multitude of compounded substances whose main purpose is to act as a lubricant or as a vehicle for delivering a pharmacologically active substance to the skin. In general, it probably is desirable to be familiar with a few such compounds, including at least one of each class, to know how they behave, what they accomplish, and what drugs they can carry.

Ointments. These are generally oleaginous bases consisting of hydrophobic oils or greases. They are anhydrous, insoluble in water and take up little or no water. *Petrolatum*, derived from petroleum, is the most important agent in this group. It varies in color from white to amber, it is an excellent vehicle for topical medicaments and provides protection and lubrication.

Absorbent Ointment Bases. These bases contain no water, but the mixture of oleaginous materials with emulsifying agents permits them to take up water. An example of such a base is *hydrophilic petrolatum USP*. This substance is less greasy than petrolatum. *Cold cream USP* is somewhat less greasy than hydrophilic petrolatum, containing a water-in-oil emulsion. Cold cream lubricates, provides water for hydration of the epidermis, makes an excellent vehicle for the incorporation of many medicaments and has cooling properties. The least greasy creams are water washable and feel as if they are incorporated into the skin quickly. They are oil-in-water emulsions. *Hydrophilic ointment USP* is useful as such a mixture.

Oils. Finally, *oils* are liquid fats of mineral, vegetable or animal origin. *Mineral oil* is useful for lubrication and the removal of pastes. It is difficult to wash off. Occasionally, it may be desirable to add an oil to a water bath. Since oils are not soluble in water, they form a film on the surface of the water and make the bath a messy affair. Many *commercial bath oils* have been developed containing emulsifiers. This leads to dispersion of the oil in the form of tiny globules in the water. When the infant has been removed from the bath (slippery and hard to hold) a fine layer of oil remains on the skin for lubrication and hydration of the epidermis. Bath oils are most useful for dry eczematous skin.

Powders

Zinc oxide and *talc* (mainly hydrous magnesium silicate) are dusting powders frequently applied to the skin. They reduce friction, increase evaporation and provide a cooling, antipruritic sensation. Dusting powders may be applied directly or in a vehicle such as lotion or paste. Starch, another powder, should not be used on the infant because it may provide a medium for candidal proliferation. Powder should not be applied to any weeping or open skin lesion because, if it penetrates the dermis, it may give rise to foreign body granulomas. The main function of a powder is in the treatment and prevention of miliaria and diaper dermatitis.

Lotions

The term "lotion" (synonymous with "shake lotion") is used here to refer to any unstable suspension of powder in a suitable liquid—which for infants is usually water. A lotion requires shaking prior to application. Lotions function much like dusting powders, but the water and water-dispersible oils provide some lubrication for the skin and may add to the cooling effect. A most useful preparation is as follows:

zinc oxide	20 gm
talc	20 gm
glycerine	20 gm
Alpha Keri	5 gm
water	to make 120 gm

The parent should be directed to shake and apply the lotion sparingly as often as necessary. The lotion is not used near the eyes, scalp or in the vulva. This preparation is useful for mosquito bites, mild sunburn, mild diaper dermatitis and miliaria. The addition of small quantities of calamine renders the lotion pink, and for unknown reasons this is preferable to some people.

Pastes

Pastes are made by incorporation of a fine powder (in a concentration of 20 to 60 per cent) into an ointment base. Pastes are protective against external irritants, such as urine, and also act as an effective sunscreen. If an adequate amount of paste has been applied, almost total screening of the sun's rays can be achieved. Simple pastes are quite inert and nonsensitizing. They make poor vehicles for the delivery of active pharmacologic agents to the skin. A useful, very thick and simple paste for prevention and treatment of diaper dermatitis contains:

zinc oxide	300 gm
talc	300 gm
petrolatum	400 gm

The instructions are to apply the paste at each diaper change. Soiled paste is removed with mineral oil.

Antiseptics

A wide variety of antiseptic substances are available that are reputed to destroy microorganisms or inhibit their growth. Most of them are too limited in their antimicrobial activity, injurious to the delicate skin of the newborn if used in adequate concentrations, pain producing, may cause injury on absorption or may be sensitizers. For these reasons, extreme caution must be employed, even with the few agents which are useful in the newborn period. A 70 per cent aqueous solution of *ethyl* or *isopropyl alcohol* is effective for cleaning small areas of *normal* skin (i.e., prior to venipuncture or injection) but should not be used on dermatitic skin. Hexachlorophene 3 per cent in a detergent emulsion (pHisoHex) may be used to clean a *small* abraded area but should not be used for compresses or bathing. *Soap and water* are probably adequate for small, minor abrasions. *Silver nitrate* 0.25 per cent is useful for treatment of burns and small denuded areas.

Substances to be Avoided

These substances include chlorine compounds, mercurial compounds, quaternary ammonium compounds, other phenolic compounds, boric acid and gentian violet. One per cent aqueous or alcoholic tincture of iodine may be useful as a prep for venipuncture but should not be used to treat abnormal skin.

Antibiotics

A wide choice of antibiotic substances for topical application are available in various vehicles from ointments to sprays. In general, the following rules are applicable:

(1) Antibiotics should not be used unless an organism has been identified and sensitivities established.

(2) Streptococcal and *Staphylococcus aureus* infections should be treated systemically in this age group.

(3) The perineum is prone to gram-negative bacterial and candidal infections, and this should be considered prior to the application of an antibiotic.

(4) Ointment bases are preferable to all others for the application of antibiotics to the skin.

(5) Topically applied antibiotics should not be those one may wish to use systemically at a later date (i.e., gentamicin, tetracycline).

(6) Debilitated infants are more likely to develop septicemia from a cutaneous infection than normal infants, so any infection on the skin should be carefully observed and treated early with systemic therapy.

(7) Vigorous treatment of a bacterial infection may assist the growth of opportunistic fungi. Transformation from one type of infection to another may be difficult to perceive, so frequent cultures on media suitable for bacteria and fungi are informative.

(8) Viral infections of the skin rarely need an antibiotic if simple cleanliness is observed and excessive scratching avoided.

(9) An eroded skin permits absorption of topically applied antibiotics; therefore, systemic toxicity may result.

Topical Corticosteroids

Numerous glucocorticoids for topical application are available in several bases. Two types of glucocorticoids are used: Non-fluorinated (hydrocortisone); and fluorinated (for example, triamcinolone and fluocinolone). The latter are far more potent than the former. In the first few weeks of life, if a topical glucocorticoid is indicated for a mild benign condition, hydrocortisone (0.5 per cent) is usually quite adequate. Where potent local therapy is indicated (i.e., localized lesions of epidermolysis bullosa), a fluorinated steroid will be more effective. Where lesions are widespread and threaten the infant's general well-being, systemic therapy should be administered. Two types of bases are employed: an ointment and a cream. Both have their proper places in therapy. If the lesions are chronic, an ointment should be used unless there is weeping. Ointments and creams containing a mixture of steroid, antibiotics and antifungal agents are also available. The only condition in which such a combination may be useful is a diaper dermatitis where both gram-negative organisms and candida may play a role.

Antihistamines

Topically applied antihistamines have not proved effective on the skin. We mention them to condemn their use. The judicious use of systemic antihistamines may provide a degree of sedation which reduces pruritic stimuli.

Soaps and Shampoos

Soaps in bar and liquid form (shampoo) have acquired certain properties by the addition of detergents, antiseptics, tars, abrasives and keratolytics that carry their function beyond simple cleaning. In general, medicated soaps and shampoos may be injurious to the newborn's skin and should be avoided. Detergents in bubble bath are particularly irritating. Plain soaps (sodium or potassium salts of fatty acids) are probably adequate for the purpose. For those concerned about a soap with a pH closer to 7.5, a superfatted soap such as Basis or Oilatum may be used, but other neutral soaps or soap substitutes (Acidolate, Dove, Lowila, Neutrogena) may be preferable.

For cradle cap, frequent shampooing is desirable. A shampoo containing a detergent and minimal amounts of salicylic acid and sulphur may be helpful. The shampoo is accomplished by diluting a half cup of shampoo (e.g., Sebulex) in a cup of lukewarm water. The scalp is *gently* shampooed with a wash cloth, keeping the soapy material out of the eyes. This procedure is repeated twice for each shampoo. Three shampoos a week for one or two weeks usually suffice. The shampoo may be followed by application of a mild keratolytic agent to the affected area on the scalp (see following section). Fostex cream, used as a shampoo, serves the same function and may avoid the hazard of shampoo running into the eyes.

Keratolytics

Although traditionally, numerous substances have been used to loosen scales in the adult, it is wise to restrict oneself to a single preparation and to know it well. One such substance is salicylic acid. A 1 to 2 per cent concentration in hydrophilic ointment USP, applied following a shampoo to scaly areas on the scalp, is effective in the treatment of cradle cap. If used over large areas, salicylic acid may be absorbed and cause salycilism; therefore, application should be restricted to small areas for limited periods of time.

Sunscreens

Totally opaque substances will block most of the sun's spectrum. In a highly sensitive infant, this form of protection may be required. In fair infants, gradual exposure to the sun and use of a partial sunscreen may be necessary. Oils inadequately block the sun's burning spectrum, but a host of effective partial sunscreens (blocking rays of 2900 to 3150 Å units) are available. None of them has a proven advantage over the others. In general, they contain p-aminobenzoic acid, o-aminobenzoates, certain salicylates, cinnamates and oxy-, dioxy- and sulisobenzone.

REFERENCES

Curley, A., Kimbrough, R. D., Hawk, R. E., Nathenson, G. and Finberg, L. Dermal absorption of hexachlorophene in infants. Lancet 2:296, 1971.

Hexachlorophene and Newborns. FDA Drug Bulletin, December, 1971.

Chapter Six

TRANSIENT CUTANEOUS LESIONS

A number of benign and transient lesions are commonly observed in a normal nursery population. Some of these lesions, such as erythema toxicum and harlequin color change, are fleeting phenomena limited to the first few days of life. Others, such as Mongolian spot and macular hemangiomas, usually persist for at least several months. The significance of these lesions is that once alternative diagnoses have been excluded, none of them require special therapeutic consideration.

MILIA

Approximately 40 per cent of full-term infants have multiple yellow or pearly white 1 mm papules scattered over the cheeks, forehead, nose, naso-labial folds and rarely, on the penis (Gordon, 1949). They may be few or numerous but are frequently grouped (Fig. 17–15). Histologically, milia are tiny epidermal cysts containing laminated keratinous material and developing in connection with the pilosebaceous follicle (Plate III–C, page 83).

All of these lesions exfoliate spontaneously during the first few weeks of life. Persistence of milia or an unusually widespread distribution, particularly in association with other defects, may be a manifestation of the oral-facial-digital syndrome (type I) or hereditary trichodysplasia (Marie Unna hypotrichosis; see Chap. 17).

Epstein's pearls (Fig. 6–1) are clinically and histologically the intraoral counterpart of facial milia and occur in about 85 per cent of newborn infants (Bhaskar, 1966). These lesions are recognizable as discrete, round, pearly and freely moveable cystic structures located on the midline of the palate or on the alveolar ridges. Like milia, these cysts rupture spontaneously and disappear shortly after birth. They should be differentiated from intraoral *mucinous cysts* (Fig. 6–2).

SEBACEOUS GLAND HYPERPLASIA

In addition to epidermal inclusion cysts or milia, many infants have a profusion of tiny white or yellow lesions visible at the opening of each pilosebaceous follicle. The lesions are most prominent on the nose, upper lip and over the malar regions, and probably represent hyperplastic sebaceous glands. They usually are not seen in the preterm infant. The presence of these lesions seems to correlate positively with cytologic studies of amniotic fluid which, as gestation reaches completion, contains mature sebaceous cells that are identifiable by staining with Nile blue sulfate (Andrews, 1970). These glands spontaneously diminish in size after birth and are no longer visible after the first few weeks of life. (See Plate III–D, page 83.)

MONGOLIAN SPOT

Mongolian spot, the most frequently encountered pigmented lesion at birth, is present in more than 90 per cent of Negro, Oriental and American Indian infants and in 1 to 5 per cent of Caucasian infants (Pratt, 1953). Although the majority of these lesions

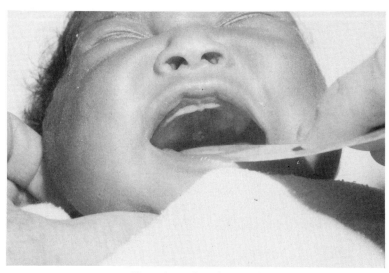

Figure 6–1. Epstein's pearls.

are found in the lumbosacral area, involvement of the buttocks, flanks and shoulders is not uncommon (Plate X–B). The lesions are macular with irregular borders, may be single or multiple, and may cover an area as large as 10 cm in diameter. The pigmentation is a slate blue or gray color resulting from an infiltrate of melanocytes deep in the dermis. Biopsy shows collections of spindle-shaped melanocytes, containing fine melanin granules, dispersed between the collagen fibers with no disruption of dermal organization. Melanophages are absent. The lesion is said to result from the failure of some melanocytes to cross the dermo-epidermal junction in their migration from the neural crest during fetal life, but may in fact represent the localization of mesodermal melanocytes.

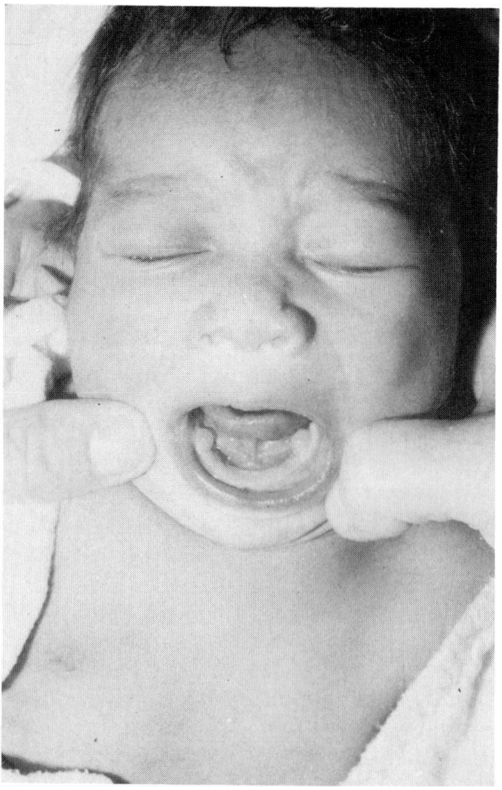

Mongolian spots usually fade within the first year or two but persistence during childhood and even into adulthood has been noted occasionally. A gray patch which is similar to Mongolian spot histologically, occurring over and in the eye or on the shoulder, may be present as a lifelong nevus. Such lesions are particularly common in Oriental individuals (see Chap. 10).

MACULAR HEMANGIOMA
(Salmon patch)

Macular hemangiomas are present in 30 to 50 per cent of infants in a normal nursery population. The most frequent sites of involvement are the nape, the eyelids and the glabella (Plate IV–A page 84). These hemangiomas are pale pink in color, have diffuse borders and may become more prominent when the infant is crying. Salmon patches are smaller in size and less intense in color than the true nevus flammeus (port-wine stain) and do not carry the same prognosis (see Chap. 9). In a prospective study of

Figure 6–2. Mucoid inclusion cyst of lower gingiva.

affected infants (Smith, 1962), most of the eyelid lesions had faded by one year of age. Glabellar lesions were slower to fade and those on the neck were the most persistent, with more than half still visible at one year of age (Plate IV–B). Surveys of school children and adults (Oster, 1970) confirm the chronicity of nuchal lesions in 25 to 50 per cent of the population. These persistent lesions are also referred to as erythema nuchae or Unna's nevus.

HARLEQUIN COLOR CHANGE

Harlequin color change (Plate IV–C) is a phenomenon observed in the immediate neonatal period and seems to be more common in the low birth weight infant (Mortensen, 1959). When the infant is placed on his side, a sharp longitudinal midline demarcation bisects the body into a pale superior half and a deep red dependent half (Neligan, 1952). The intensity of color varies considerably in individual infants and, in some, the line of demarcation may be incomplete, sparing the face and genitalia. The mucous membranes are not involved. The length of an attack may vary from approximately 30 seconds to 20 minutes.

This physical finding occurs only when the infant is lying on his side; the difference in color will disappear almost immediately if his position is altered by turning him onto his back or abdomen. If his position is changed from one side to the other during an attack a reversal of the color pattern is observed; the formerly pale upper half, which is now dependent, becomes suffused, while the previously dark, dependent half lightens in color. Intense muscular activity and crying will cause generalized flushing and obliterate the color difference entirely.

The peak frequency of attacks of harlequin color change in one series occurred on days two, three, and four (Mortensen, 1959), and, in another, on the third, fourth and fifth days of life (Neligan, 1952). An occasional infant may experience an attack up to three weeks of age. Affected infants may have single or multiple episodes. The phenomenon appears with equal frequency among healthy and sick infants and is probably of no pathological significance. Because of the sharp longitudinal demarcation in the midline, these episodes have been attributed to a temporary imbalance in the autonomic regulatory mechanism

of the cutaneous vessels. There are no accompanying changes in respiratory rate, papillary reflexes, muscle tone or response to external stimuli.

CUTIS MARMORATA

This term describes the familiar cutaneous marbling effect most pronounced when the infant has been chilled or exposed to low environmental temperature (Plate IV–D). The mottling has a pattern resembling a net or a branching configuration that is due to dilatation of the capillaries and venules in the darker areas. The marbling usually disappears when the infant is rewarmed, although some infants display a faint pattern even in a neutral thermal range. The reaction is a physiological one in some infants and may be evoked in certain instances until early childhood. Persistent cutis marmorata is a frequent finding in the Cornelia de Lange syndrome, Down's syndrome and Trisomy 18. It has also been observed in a new syndrome with the features of low birth weight, dwarfism, congenital anomalies and dysgammaglobulinemia (Christian, 1971). This physiologic response should not be confused with a nevoid vascular defect having the forbidding name of cutis marmorata telangiectatica congenita (see Chap. 9).

ERYTHEMA TOXICUM

This benign and self-limited eruption usually occurs within the first two days of life and has a peak incidence between 24 and 48 hours, although it may appear up until the 14th day of life (Plate V–A, page 85). Rarely, lesions have been observed immediately after delivery of the infant (Carr, 1966). The recorded incidence of affected term-weight newborns in a normal nursery population has varied from 30 to 70 per cent (Taylor, 1957; Harris, 1956), but figures as low as 4 per cent (Levy, 1951) have been reported. The disorder is less common with decreasing birth weight and gestational age. In a prospective study of the relationship of infant maturity to the development of erythema toxicum (Carr, 1966), the frequency of affected infants progressed from 0 per cent to 55 per cent as the birth weight increased from less than 1500 gm to 2500 gm or more, and from 0 per cent to 59 per cent as the gestational age increased from less than 30 weeks to 42 weeks. No sexual or racial predisposition to the condition has been noted.

The lesions are firm, shotty, 1 to 3 mm pale yellow or white papules and pustules on an erythematous base. Some infants display only erythematous macules or a splotchy erythema. Typical macules are large (up to 3 cm) and irregular; the redness contrasts sharply with the sourrounding normal skin. Occasionally the macules may become confluent. The erythema blanches with pressure and involved tissues may appear to be slightly thickened. Sites of predilection are the anterior and posterior trunk, but any body surface may be involved except for the palms and soles. The lesions may be widely scattered and few in number, or extensive and numerous. Total duration of the eruption varies from a few hours to a few days. Recurrences are uncommon but several episodes have been documented within the first two weeks of life. Signs of systemic involvement are absent.

Biopsy of a lesion in any of its stages demonstrates a characteristic infiltrate of eosinophils (Luders, 1960; Freeman, 1960). Macular erythematous areas show mild dermal edema with a sparse perivascular infiltrate of eosinophils and a few neutrophils and mononuclear cells. Papular lesions have more pronounced edema and an intense cellular infiltrate with eosinophils predominating. Involvement is most marked about the superficial half of the pilosebaceous follicle. The pustules are subcorneal or intraepidermal and are associated with a pilosebaceous orifice. The intraepidermal spaces are filled with massive collections of eosinophils and a few neutrophils and mononuclear cells.

Diagnosis depends on recognition of the eruption. A smear of the intralesional contents prepared with Wright or Giemsa stain may support the clinical diagnosis by demonstrating the characteristic concentration of eosinophils. A gram stain of the pustular contents should be negative for bacteria. Peripheral eosinophilia has been noted by some investigators in affected infants and is said to correlate positively with the severity of the eruption (Harris, 1956). Staphylococcal pyoderma may be considered in the differential diagnosis, but can be excluded by demonstrating the absence of neutrophils on smear and by the sterility of the exudate on culture. Occasionally the lesions may also be confused with miliaria or candidiasis.

Although the eruption has been attributed to an immediate hypersensitivity reaction, specific allergens have never been implicated nor has the placental transfer of allergens been proved to be a significant factor in these cases. Mechanical irritation or extrauterine contactants have also been invoked as etiologic factors. Since some infants over 24 hours of age develop an eosinophilic exudate, demonstrated by the skin window technique (Eitzman, 1959), it has been suggested that these lesions may simply represent a cutaneous reponse to nonspecific stimuli. In a more recent study of the neonatal inflammatory response using the skin window technique (Bullock, 1969), eosinophilia was not striking and seemed instead to correlate with a family history of an allergic diathesis. Treatment is unnecessary since the disorder is self-limited.

SUCKING BLISTERS

An occasional healthy infant may present at birth with a few intact or ruptured bullae localized to the upper extremity (Murphy, 1963). The bullae tend to be small (from 0.5 to 1.5 cm) and are commonly found on the radial surface of the forearm, the dorsum of the thumb or index finger or central upper lip. These lesions are presumed to occur in utero as a result of vigorous sucking, a tenable supposition since infant skin is known to blister easily and affected infants usually fail to develop further lesions after birth. Sucking blisters contain serous fluid which should be sterile on culture. Rapid resolution is the usual outcome and no therapy is required.

MILIARIA

Since the advent of the air-conditioned nursery this eruption is probably a less frequent occurrence in the immediate neonatal period than the textbooks suggest (Rook, 1968). Nevertheless, it may be troublesome if the infant is maintained in an excessively warm, humid environment. The lesions result from obstruction of the eccrine gland ducts and are of two principal types: clear, superficial vesicles without inflammation (miliaria crystallina) and small, erythematous, grouped papules (miliaria rubra). The former appear as thin-walled vesicles because the retained sweat is localized just beneath the stratum corneum (Plate V–B). The lesions of miliaria rubra are more deeply situated in the epidermis and result from rupture of the intraepidermal portion of the sweat duct with formation of an intraepidermal vesicle in the area of the basal layer (Fig. 6–3; Plate II–D, page 82). If a marked inflammatory reaction is present, the lesion may appear pustular.

Sites of predilection for the eruption are the intertriginous areas, but lesions may also be numerous over the face and scalp. During the first week of life these lesions are most frequently confused with erythema toxicum; occasionally a profuse eruption confined to the neck and diaper area may suggest candidal infection. The vesicular lesions of miliaria crystallina may be distinguished from other vesicular disorders by their grouping, the superficial nature of the vesicle, the absence of bacteria and yeasts on culture of their contents, the absence of inflammation and the lack of systemic findings. Rapid resolution of the eruption helps to differentiate it from an incipient pyoderma. Removal to a cooler environment is the only treatment necessary.

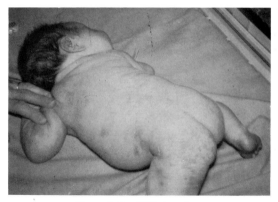

Figure 6–3. Miliaria rubra.

LESIONS DUE TO OBSTETRICAL COMPLICATIONS

The circumstances of labor and delivery may predispose the infant to cetain traumatic lesions which have visible cutaneous manifestations. *Caput succedaneum* is a diffuse edematous swelling of the presenting portion of the scalp (or scrotum in scrotum succedaneum, see Fig. 6–4), usually resulting from the combined factors of a large head and prolonged labor. The boggy, swollen skin may also display a few ecchymoses, and molding of the head with overriding sutures is an additional common finding. The edema recedes during the first week of life, whereas the molding usually requires several weeks to disappear.

Cephalhematoma, the result of a subperiosteal hemorrhage, is limited to the surface of one cranial bone because the affected periosteum adheres to the margin of the bone. If two bones are involved the hematomas are always sharply localized and separated by a depression corresponding to the intervening suture. In one study (Kendall, 1952) an underlying skull fracture was documented in about 25 per cent of the cases. Cephalhematomas present as tense or somewhat compressible tumors, often with a palpable rim of

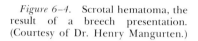

Figure 6–4. Scrotal hematoma, the result of a breech presentation. (Courtesy of Dr. Henry Mangurten.)

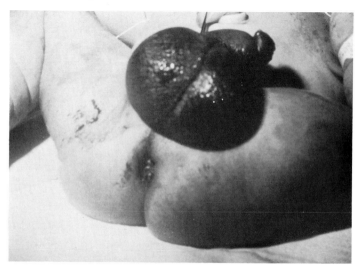

periosteum which is elevated because of the underlying accumulation of blood. By the end of the second week the periosteal rim becomes calcified and is more easily felt.

Most cephalhematomas are resorbed during the first six weeks of life. Occasionally they may calcify and persist as bony protuberances, disappearing slowly over several months or years. Treatment is unnecessary, and aspiration is contraindicated. Infection of the mass or anemia from massive bleeding into the tumor are rare complications.

SKIN TRAUMA

Cutaneous abrasions and ecchymoses may result from birth trauma particularly during a forceps delivery. Sites of involvement depend on the obstetrical presentation of the infant. Subconjunctival hemorrhage and petechiae are also commonly seen. These lesions are of no consequence and disappear gradually during the first week or two after birth. If extensive areas of skin are involved, hyperbilirubinemia may result from breakdown of large numbers of red blood cells. Rarely, subcutaneous fat necrosis may occur in the buccal fat pads if forceps have been applied to that area (see Chap. 9).

REFERENCES

Andrews, B. F.: Amniotic fluid studies to determine maturity. Pediat. Clin. N. Amer 17:49, 1970.

Bhaskar, S. N.: Oral lesions in infants and newborn. Dent. Clin. N. Amer. pp. 421–435, July, 1966.

Bullock, J. D., Roberston, A. F., Bodenbender, J. G.,

Kontras, S. B. and Miller, C. E.: Inflammatory response in the neonate re-examined. Pediatrics 44:58, 1969.

Carr, J. A., Hodgman, J. E., Freedman, R. J. and Levan, N. E.: Relationship between toxic erythema and infant maturity. Amer. J. Dis. Child. 112:129, 1966.

Christian, J. C., Johnson, V. P., Biegel, A. A., Gresham, E. L. and Rosenberg, G. J.: Sisters with low birth weight, dwarfism, congenital anomalies, and dysgammaglobulinemia. Amer. J. Dis. Child. 122:529, 1971.

Eitzman, D. V. and Smith, R. T.: The nonspecific inflammatory cycle in the neonatal infant. A.M.A. J. Dis. Child. 97:326, 1959.

Freeman, R. G., Spiller, R. and Knox, J. M.: Histopathology of erythema toxicum neonatorum. Arch. Derm. 82:586, 1960.

Gordon, J.: Miliary sebaceous cysts and blisters in the healthy newborn. Arch. Dis Child. 24:286, 1949.

Harris, J. R. and Schick, B.: Erythema neonatorum. A.M.A. J. Dis. Child. 92:27, 1956.

Kendall, N. and Woloshin, H.: Cephalhematoma associated with fracture of the skull. J. Pediat. 41:125, 1952.

Levy, H. and Bagner, A. B.: The effect of an antihistamine substance (Pyribenzamine) on erythema neonatorum. Arch. Pediat. 68:413, 1951.

Luders, D.: Histologic observations in erythema toxicum neonatorum. Pediatrics 26:219, 1960.

Mortensen, O. and Stougård-Andresen, P.: Harlequin color change in the newborn. Acta Obstet. Gynec. Scand. 38:352, 1959.

Murphy, W. F. and Langley, A. L.: Common bullous lesions presumably self-inflicted occurring in utero in the newborn infant. Pediatrics 32:1099, 1963.

Neligan, G. A. and Strang, L. B.: A "harlequin" colour change in the newborn. Lancet 2:1005, 1952.

Øster, J. and Nielsen, A.: Nuchal naevi and interscapular telangiectasis. Acta Paediat. Scand. 59:416, 1970.

Pratt, A. G.: Birthmarks in infants. Arch. Derm. 67:302, 1953.

Rook, A., Wilkinson, D. S. and Ebling, F. J. G.: Textbook of Dermatology. Philadelphia, F. A. Davis Co. 1968. p. 112.

Smith, M. A. and Manfield, P. A.: Salmon patches in the first year of life. Brit. J. Derm. 74:31, 1962.

Taylor, W. B. and Bondurant, C. P.: Erythema neonatorum allergicum. Arch. Derm. 76:591, 1957.

Chapter Seven

DEVELOPMENTAL ABNORMALITIES

A number of abnormalities discussed here, such as skin dimples, supernumerary nipples, ear tags, lip pits and thyroglossal cysts, are characterized by relatively conspicuous and localized changes due to a minor defect in embryonic development. Other localized defects may result in anomalies with more serious repercussions such as urachal cysts, sacrococcygeal sinuses and cysts. Still other abnormalities occurring at an extremely early stage of development, that is, during meiosis or soon thereafter, may give rise to widespread changes reflecting the resultant gross chromosomal aberrations (e.g., the trisomy syndromes).

Several conditions are included in this chapter whose cause is unknown or genetic in nature but which may be confused, because of their phenotypic picture, with a minor localized defect.

CUTANEOUS ABNORMALITIES

SKIN DIMPLES

Some infants are born with deep dimples localized to the bony prominences and occasionally associated with subsidiary pits and creases, particularly in the sacral area. These are usually of no pathological significance and tend to disappear as the child grows. Sharply circumscribed skin dimples have also been reported in infants with the congenital rubella syndrome (Hammond, 1967) and the long arm 18 deletion syndrome (Smith, 1970). Deep sacral dimples are seen in occasional patients with Bloom's syndrome and cerebro-hepato-renal syndrome. H-shaped

dimpling on the chin is characteristic of the Freeman-Sheldon (Whistling face) syndrome (Smith, 1970). (See Fig. 7–1.)

REDUNDANT SKIN

Loose folds of skin over the posterior neck (Pterygium colli) are a frequent finding in Turner's syndrome, Down's syndrome and Trisomy 13. Redundant skin in a more generalized distribution has been observed in infants with Trisomy 18 and combined im-

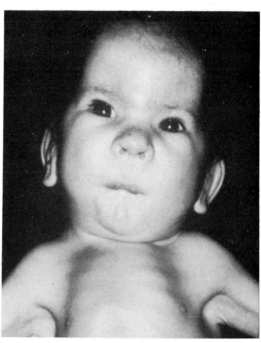

Figure 7–1. Whistling face syndrome. (Courtesy of Dr. Hermine Pashayan.)

munodeficiency disease with short-limbed dwarfism (see Chap. 17). A syndrome consisting of micrognathia with an incomplete mandibular ramus, redundant skin, malformed tracheal cartilages and a defect between the posterior osseous portion and the cartilaginous ventral portion of the ribs, has also been described (Smith, 1967). Redundant skin must be differentiated from cutis laxa, in which there is a histologically demonstrable deficiency of elastic tissue in the papillary dermis (see Chap. 16).

CONGENITAL LIP PITS AND FISTULAS

Congenital fistulas of the lower lip may be unilateral or bilateral and are occasionally combined with other anomalies of the face and extremities. Cleft lip or palate is the most frequently associated defect, occurring in approximately 70 per cent of cases (Gorlin, 1964). The condition is inherited as an autosomal dominant trait with variable expressivity. Females are more often affected than males.

The lesions may range from small, flat, circular or cleft-like depressions which do not admit a probe, to deep sinuses with prominent elevated orifices. They are located on the vermilion portion of the lip on each side of the midline. When the sinuses, which are lined by a stratified squamous epithelium, communicate with an underlying mucous gland, the secretion of mucus onto the lip surface becomes an annoying cosmetic problem. The treatment of choice is surgical excision of the complete sinus tract and its glandular tissue or transposition of the sinus tract orifice onto a buccal site (Soricelli, 1966).

AMNIOTIC CONSTRICTION BANDS
(Pseudo-ainhum)

Partial or complete ring-like constrictions in the skin are a rare developmental anomaly, and when they involve the extremities, amputation of one or more digits may result (Fig. 7–2). On examination of fetal material, fibrous bands have been observed at the site of constrictions, occasionally with a strand connected to the amnion. The formation of amniotic strands is believed to be secondary to amniotic rupture during gestation (Torpin, 1965). The strands are probably derived from both amnionic and chorionic tissue and may encircle the various fetal parts, depending on their length (Fig. 7–3). It has been suggested that the strands have a tendency to constrict at the smallest diameter of the enmeshed part, that is, between the joints, rather than across them. These malformations can be seen in otherwise normal infants (Raque, 1972).

CUTIS VERTICIS GYRATA

This rare skin abnormality may be congenital or acquired. The term refers to a corrugated appearance or deep furrowing of the scalp resembling the convolutions of the brain. The vertex is most often involved; however, transverse furrows may be found on the forehead and occiput. Hair growth is usually normal. In a large series of affected patients (Polan, 1953), 85 per cent were male. In approximately 25 per cent of the males and 50 per cent of the females the lesions were present at birth. In some families the anomaly appears to be inherited, and pat-

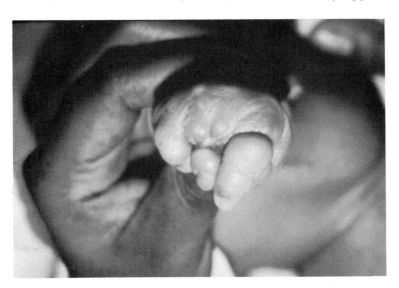

Figure 7–2. Pseudo-ainhum. Partial amputation due to intrauterine constriction bands. (Courtesy of Drs. David Fisher and John Paton.)

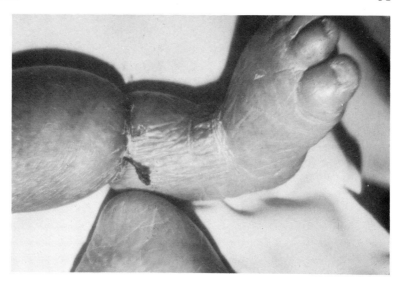

Figure 7–3. Intrauterine constriction bands. (Courtesy of Drs. David Fisher and John Paton.)

terns suggestive of both dominant and recessive types of inheritance have been documented.

Cutis verticis gyrata has also been described in association with disorders of the central nervous system, most commonly mental retardation, epilepsy, cranial deformities, cerebral palsy, tuberous sclerosis and ocular defects. In these instances the onset of the scalp lesion is usually at puberty and, for this reason, an endocrinologic etiology has been suspected. Nevertheless, no evidence for endocrine dysfunction has been demonstrated (Palo, 1970). All of the patients studied by pneumoencephalography have had pathologic findings, most frequently in the posterior cranial fossa or cerebellum (Palo, 1970).

CONGENITAL AURICULAR FISTULAS

Auricular fistulas are narrow sinus tracts or pits that are most often located at the anterior margin of the ascending limb of the helix. Other, less common sites are along a curve passing from the temple to the anterior margin of the helix, in the interspace between the tragus and the helix, in the interspace between the tragus and the antitragus, in the external auditory meatus and in the center of the lobule. Rarely, a fistula may extend from the floor of the external meatus to the angle of the mandible (Warkany, 1971). Generally these lesions are benign and considered an incidental physical finding. Occasionally, however, they may become chronically infected and form retention cysts which drain intermittently. These complications may require surgical intervention.

Auricular fistulas are a common developmental defect and may be associated with multiple anomalies of the ear and face, including microtia, auricular appendages, bronchiogenic fistulas and facial clefts. Most cases appear to be sporadic, although transmission by an autosomal dominant gene is suggested by the distribution of affected individuals within some kindreds. Hereditary aural fistulas have also been described in combination with deafness and bronchial fistulas (Fourman, 1955).

AURICULAR APPENDAGES

Cutaneous skin tags on or anterior to the pinna are another common minor developmental malformation (Fig. 7–4). They may be unilateral or bilateral, sessile or pedunculated, solitary or multiple and can vary greatly in size. They can be soft or cartilaginous in consistency, and are usually skin-colored. Like auricular fistulas, they are most often an isolated anomaly, but may occur in conjunction with more serious anomalies of the ears and face.

The site of predilection is the line of junction of the mandibular and hyoid arches; less commonly they occur on the cheek between the auricle and the angle of the mouth (the line of junction of the mandibular and maxillary processes). In the latter location they are more often associated with other defects (Warkany, 1971). Histological examination permits differentiation from ordinary skin tags or papillomas; auricular tags contain numerous telogen follicles, sebaceous and eccrine glands, abundant lobules of fat, and

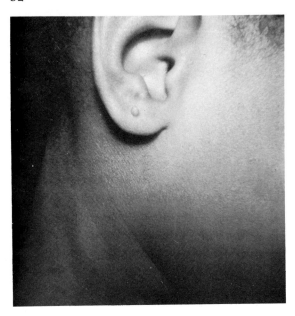

Figure 7–4. Ear tag.

frequently, a central core of cartilage (Brownstein, 1971). The treatment of choice is simple surgical excision.

TREACHER-COLLINS' SYNDROME
(Mandibulofacial dysostosis)

This syndrome consists of down-sloping palpebral fissures, underdeveloped malar bones, a prominent nose with hypoplastic cartilages, a large fish-like mouth, colobomas of the lower lid and iris, deformed or misplaced auricles and a poorly developed external auditory canal and middle ear. The cutaneous features include a tongue-shaped process of hair extending from the scalp onto the cheek (present in about 25 per cent of cases), the absence of eyelashes medial to a coloboma (about 50 per cent of cases) and auricular tags and fistulas that may be located at any point between the tragus and the angle of the mouth. Skeletal anomalies, heart malformations and mental deficiency may also exist. The Treacher Collins' syndrome is inherited as an autosomal dominant trait with incomplete penetrance and variable expressivity (Gorlin, 1964).

GOLDENHAR'S SYNDROME
(Oculoauriculovertebral dysplasia)

Goldenhar's syndrome includes epibulbar dermoids, auricular appendages and fistulas, vertebral anomalies and a characteristic facies with malar hypoplasia, receding chin and, in some instances, hemifacial microsomia (Gorlin, 1964). This syndrome is not inherited nor is there any evidence for a chromosomal defect.

The epibulbar dermoids or lipodermoids are solid, yellow or white, smooth or granular plaque-like growths which may be covered with fine hairs. The dermoids usually occur at the corneal limbus in the lower outer quadrants of the eye, whereas lipodermoids are more often located in the upper outer quadrant. They may be unilateral or bilateral. A unilateral coloboma of the upper lid is another common finding.

The ears are small and the external auditory meatus may be defective. Bilateral ear tags are a constant feature and may be single or multiple, sessile or pedunculated. They are located anterior to the tragus or in a line from tragus to the corner of the mouth. Blind-ended fistulas may be found in the same regions.

BRANCHIOGENIC FISTULAS AND CYSTS

External branchial *fistulas* are usually detectable at birth, and are located in the lower part of the neck at the anterior border of the sternomastoid muscle (Fig. 7–5). The fistulas may be incomplete, terminating blindly in the tissues of the neck, or may complete their course, opening internally on the pharyngeal wall. If portions of the sinus tract are closed off, cysts may be formed along its course. Most of these fistulas are derived from the

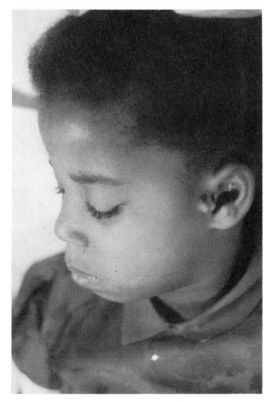

Figure 7-5. Branchial cleft cyst.

second branchial cleft and are lined by a stratified squamous epithelium. The external opening may be inconspicuous or may exude a mucous secretion. Secondary infection is frequent and may require multiple courses of antibiotics administered systemically and, ultimately, surgical extirpation of the fistulous tract.

Fistulous anomalies appear to have a hereditary basis with an autosomal dominant gene being the usual mode of transmission. Approximately one-third of affected patients have bilateral lesions; periauricular pits may be an associated finding. Internal branchial fistulas with no cutaneous orifices can also occur in the neck region. Fistulas with an open communication between the pharynx and the surface of the neck are rare (Warkany, 1971).

Branchial *cysts* are found anterior to the sternomastoid muscle in the upper third of the neck, but occasionally occur in other locations. They may vary in size and usually are unilocular and lined with a squamous epithelium. Most of these cysts are not apparent during the neonatal period. A familial predisposition has not been noted in most instances although, in some kindreds, the anomaly

does seem to have a genetic basis. Infection, as with fistulas, is a common complication.

Thyroglossal cysts and fistulas are similar malformations located in or near the midline of the neck close to the hyoid bone. On surgical removal the cysts are found to be filled with a mucoid material (Guimaraes, 1972).

UMBILICAL ANOMALIES

Granulomas

These rather common umbilical lesions become apparent after the cord has separated from the abdominal wall. Generally, the umbilical skin heals in approximately two weeks. Occasionally a nubbin of dull red granulation tissue of varying size remains within the umbilicus. If uninfected these lesions have a dry velvety appearance, but more often they exude a purulent secretion due to secondary infection by surface pathogens. Umbilical granulomas must be differentiated from umbilical polyps which are much less common, representing persistent remnants of the omphalomesenteric duct or urachus. Umbilical granulomas will usually recede if cauterized with silver nitrate every few days until the base is dry. The silver nitrate must be applied with care in order to avoid burns of the contiguous skin.

Polyps

A remnant of the distal portion of the omphalomesenteric duct may persist in the form of a bright red, firm umbilical polyp. A sinus tract of variable depth or a subcutaneous cyst may also be found. These lesions are usually moist and sticky, owing to a tenacious secretion which is particularly abundant if gastric glands are present in the overlying mucosa. The polypal mucosa may contain glandular elements resembling those of the small intestine, large bowel or ectopic pancreas. Occasionally, a condylomatous fibroepithelial polyp may be present in addition to the omphalomesenteric remnant (Steck, 1964). The type of tissue present in the polyp can be identified by histological examination of a biopsy specimen.

A urachal remnant may provoke a similar lesion. In this case the overlying mucosa histologically resembles bladder transitional epithelium rather than gastrointestinal tissue, and the discharge is clear, water and yellow, and has the odor of urine. These lesions are usually resistant to conservative therapy. The treatment of choice is excision of the entire remnant.

SUPERNUMERARY NIPPLES
(Accessory nipples)

Extra nipples in an otherwise healthy infant are a not infrequent occurrence. The nipples may be unilateral or bilateral and rarely number more than one or two. Appearing as a small pink or brown papule, frequently surrounded by a pigmented areola, they are located above or just below the breast in a line stretching from the mid-axilla through the inguinal area to the inner thigh. It is not unusual to mistake them for a melanocytic nevus. On tickling the papule the skin around it may pucker because it contains erectile tissue. Histologically, accessory nipples contain mammary ductile tissue. Since, rarely, they may develop malignant changes, and often induce feelings of inferiority in the self-conscious adult, they should be excised in childhood.

The nipples may be widely spaced and small in Turner's and Cornelia de Lange's syndromes, and supernumerary nipples may be found in hemihypertrophy (see next section). Inverted nipples and asymmetry in nipple and breast size are frequent anomalous findings in normal individuals.

HEMIHYPERTROPHY

Hemihypertrophy is a developmental defect in which one side of the body is larger than the other; it may be congenital or acquired, limited or total, involving all the organ systems on the affected side (Fig. 7–6). It can occur on either side but is more frequent on the right than on the left side. Differences in the symmetry of these patients are often detectable during the newborn period, although they usually become more striking with the growth of the child (Fig. 7–7). The birth weight is always normal for the gestational age (Warkany, 1971).

The involved skin appears thickened and may show increased warmth and sweating. Approximately 50 per cent of affected patients have other skin lesions, most commonly pigmentary abnormalities, hypertrichosis and nail defects. Nevi, lymphatic and vascular malformations, ichthyosis and alteration in hair color have also been observed (see the epidermal nevus syndrome in Chap. 8).

Noticeable facial asymmetry can be the sole manifestation of the defect, or it may accompany more extensive forms of the disorder. In hemihypertrophy the cheeks and lips are enlarged, the angle of the mouth is depressed, the palpebral fissure is widened and the bony structures are asymmetrical. Heterochromia iridum and eccentric pupil may be present (Warkany, 1971). Oral changes include enlargement of the tongue with hypertrophied fungiform papillae, thickening of the alveolar ridges and uvula, widening of the palate and differences in tooth size (Gorlin, 1964).

Unilateral enlargement of the skeletal system may be accompanied by other developmental defects including polydactyly, syndactyly, lobster claw deformity, clubfoot and scoliosis. The breast on the affected side may

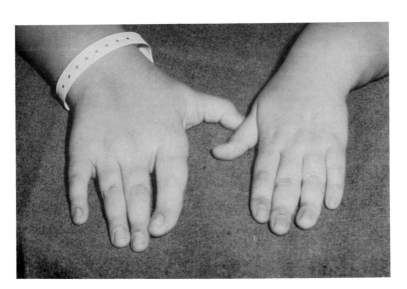

Figure 7–6. Hemihypertrophy.

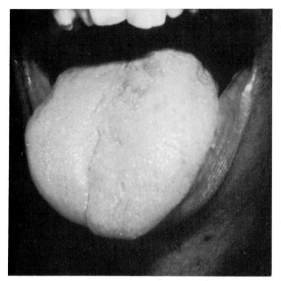

Figure 7-7. Hemihypertrophy of tongue.

be enlarged and supernumerary nipples can occur. Internally, the kidney and adrenal glands are the most frequently involved viscera. Approximately 25 per cent of patients with hemihypertrophy are mentally retarded; alteration in brain size, convulsions, abnormal cerebral cysternae, sciatica and intermittent attacks of pain can also be associated with the disorder. Hemihypertrophy has also been observed in the phakomatoses, Silver's syndrome and the visceral cytomegaly syndrome.

An increased incidence of embryonal tumors affecting the liver, kidney and adrenal cortex, particularly Wilms' tumor, has been noted in patients with hemihypertrophy (Fraumeni, 1967). The reason for this association is obscure; however, it has recently been suggested that the syndromes involving aniridia, Wilms' tumor and disorders of growth control may be interrelated, possibly on the basis of common teratogenic and oncogenic mechanisms (Haicken, 1971).

CONGENITAL ABSENCE OF SKIN
(Aplasia cutis congenita)

Localized congenital absence of skin is a relatively rare developmental anomaly. The site of predilection is the midline area of the posterior scalp, although lesions can occur elsewhere on the scalp, face, trunk and extremities. Typical lesions are 1 to 2 cm in diameter, circular or oval, sharply marginated

and hairless. At birth the surface may be covered by a smooth membrane or it may be ulcerated and crusted. Generally these lesions heal slowly by re-epithelialization, leaving a hypertrophic or atrophic scar. Although most lesions heal without incident, hemorrhage and infection are infrequent complicating factors. Congenital absence of skin can be associated with other malformations, including cleft lip and palate, syndactyly, lack of digits, clubbing of hands and feet, congenital heart disease and vascular malformations (Resnick, 1965).

Congenital scalp defects may occur sporadically or in several members of a family; in the latter instances the anomaly appears to be inherited as an autosomal dominant trait with variable penetrance and expressivity (Deeken, 1970). Sex distribution is equal. The midline scalp defect has been attributed to an embryonic error, possibly defective closure of the neural tube; however, this explanation is not tenable for lesions in other locations.

More extensive congenital defects of the skin have been described in some affected infants. These lesions are usually multiple with a symmetrical distribution and heal by epithelial growth from the borders, leaving a depressed area of scar tissue. Bart (1966, 1970) has reported several patients with a more extensive form of aplasia cutis who were also afflicted with recurrent bullous lesions of the skin and mucous membranes, and aplasia and dystrophy of the nails. These patients may, in fact, represent atypical cases of epidermolysis bullosa.

Histological examination of biopsy material from an area of aplasia cutis shows an absence of epidermis, a paucity of appendageal structures and a variable decrease in dermal elastic tissue. Biopsy findings help exclude other diagnostic possibilities, should confusion arise. Although most of the smaller lesions do not require treatment, surgical excision of an unsightly scar or punch-graft hair transplants into scalp defects (Deeken, 1970) may be utilized for cosmetic management.

SINUS DEFECTS

Congenital Dermal Sinuses

Dermal sinus tracts are channels lined with stratified squamous epithelium that connect from the skin to the central nervous system. They may be located in the occipital region, or at any point along the dorsal midline from the cervical to the sacrococcygeal region. Dermal sinuses differ from pilonidal sinuses in that they penetrate the spine to make contact with the meninges or spinal cord. The anomaly has been attributed to incomplete separation of the neural ectoderm from the epithelial ectoderm (Warkany, 1971).

Dermal sinus openings may be difficult to visualize, particularly in the occipital region where they may be hidden by hair. A localized thickening of the scalp or a vascular nevus may provide a clue to the presence of a dermal sinus; likewise, hypertrichosis, dimpling or other cutaneous abnormalities in the midline of the neck and back should alert the physician to the possibility of such an anomaly. Roentgenograms of suspicious areas should be obtained and carefully scrutinized for evidence of a bony abnormality. The path taken by radiopaque material injected into the ostium of the sinus is sometimes helpful in demonstrating the defect. These lesions are much more serious than other types of sinus tracts because of the predisposition of affected patients to meningitis. Once recognized, immediate surgical excision is the treatment of choice.

Pilonidal Sinus

The congenital pilonidal sinus is a not uncommon anomaly in the newborn infant. In a series of 38 patients diagnosed while under one year of age (Lewin, 1965), two-thirds were noted to have the defect at birth. In this series, clues to the presence of a sinus tract included coccygeal dimples in approximately one-third of the infants, cystic swellings in half of the cases and visible midline sinus in almost two-thirds. There were associated congenital anomalies in 40 per cent of the infants. Although infection of these sinus tracts is rare in infancy and childhood, some authors recommended early surgical excision and primary closure as the treatment of choice. Eighty per cent of the infants in Lewin's series were so treated and none had postoperative complications.

DIASTEMATOMYELIA

Localized cutaneous anomalies in the lumbosacral area may be evidence for diastematomyelia, a condition in which the spinal cord is split in the midline and separated in the lumbar region by a bony septum. The cutaneous markers include patches of hypertrichosis, pigmented nevi, hemangiomas, li-

pomas, dimples, dermoid sinuses or dermoid cysts overlying the skeletal abnormality. Such lesions should suggest the possibility of an anatomical defect of the spine and indicate the need for careful examination and roentgenographic studies of such infants.

CHROMOSOMAL ABNORMALITY SYNDROMES

TRISOMY 13-15 (TRISOMY D₁) SYNDROME

The salient features of Trisomy 13-15 are cerebral malformations, ocular defects, cleft lip and palate, capillary hemangiomas, congenital heart disease, polydactyly and simian creases. The defect usually is due to the presence of a large supernumerary acrocentric chromosome in the D (13-15) group, although cytogenetic variations do exist. The prevalence of the disease is extremely low since almost all these infants die within the first year of life.

Systemic and Cutaneous Manifestations

The most common anomalies of the brain are arhinencephaly, defects of the cerebellum and corpus collosum and microcephaly. Ocular defects include anophthalmia, microphthalmia, colobomas of the iris and retinal dysplasia. Cleft lip or palate is a consistent finding. Capillary hemangiomas on the forehead, eyelids, nasal bridge, nape and lower back occur in a high percentage of these infants. Other cutaneous stigmata include localized scalp defects in the parieto-occipital area, redundant skin of the posterior neck and hypoplastic nails. The ears are abnormal and hearing is deficient. The hands show polydactyly, trigger thumbs, flexion of the fingers with or without overlapping and camptodactyly, simian creases and distal palmar axial triradii. The feet are frequently normal but may have prominent heels or polydactyly. Cardiac defects occur with high frequency and include ventricular and auricular septal defects, patent ductus arteriosus and dextroposition. Cystic kidneys are the most common renal anomaly. Male infants are often cryptorchid, and females may have a bicornuate uterus. The neutrophils in the peripheral blood are typically abnormal with nuclear projections. Persistence of embryonic or fetal hemoglobin in the erythrocytes also has been noted (Warkany, 1966, 1971).

TRISOMY 18 (TRISOMY E) SYNDROME

The distinctive constellation of findings in the Trisomy 18 syndrome includes low set abnormal ears, micrognathia and microstomia, flexion of the fingers with overlapping of the index and fifth finger over the third and fourth fingers, congenital heart disease, usually ventricular septal defect, horseshoe kidney (in a small percentage of cases), short sternum, rocker-bottom feet, mental retardation, hypertonicity, inguinal and umbilical hernias.

The characteristic cutaneous features are hypoplasia of the nails, especially on the fifth fingers and toes, low arch dermal ridge patterning on the fingertips, redundant skin, hirsutism of the forehead and back, cutis marmorata and hypoplasia of the subcutaneous tissue. A wide spectrum of other abnormalities in all organ systems has also been reported (Warkany, 1966).

The infants are usually of low birth weight and may be born preterm (approximately one-third of the cases) or postterm (about one-third of the cases) (Smith, 1970). Polyhydramnios, a small placenta and a single umbilical artery are frequent findings. The disorder is associated with an extra chromosome in the E group. Nondisjunction appears to account for most of these cases, but translocations and mosaicisms have also been identified. The mean maternal age is increased as it is in Trisomy 21.

Infants with Trisomy 18 do poorly at birth and often require resuscitation. Poor feeding and apneic episodes characterize the neonatal period. Few such infants survive the first year of life.

TRISOMY 21 (DOWN'S SYNDROME; MONGOLISM; TRISOMY G)

Down's syndrome usually is readily recognized even in the newborn infant because of the characteristic appearance and resemblance of these patients one to another. This disorder is the most frequent of the trisomy syndromes with an incidence of 1 to 2 per 1,000 live births. The most common cause of mongolism is an extra chromosome in group G due to nondisjunction during meiosis. A few of these individuals have a translocation (D/G or G/G) or 21 Trisomy/normal mosaicism (Smith, 1970). Faulty chromosome distribution resulting in Down's syndrome is more likely to occur with increasing maternal age. Since a parent may be a translocation carrier and thus have a relatively high risk of recurrence, chromosome studies of the parents are indicated where this genetic situation might obtain.

Systemic and Cutaneous Manifestations

A sufficient number of characteristic signs are almost always present at birth so that correct diagnosis can be made in the newborn nursery. Affected infants may be undersized and hypotonic. The head is brachycephalic with a flattened occiput. The ears are small, the eyes slant upward with prominent epicanthal folds and the nose is small with a depressed nasal bridge. Speckling of the iris (Brushfield's spots), peripheral hypoplasia of the iris and lenticular opacities detectable by slit lamp examination are common. The mouth remains open, the tongue protrudes and the palate is short and narrow.

The cutaneous findings are prominent cutis marmorata, redundant skin of the posterior neck and sparse fine hair. The hands are short and square with low set thumbs, a simian crease and a short, incurved fifth finger, with hypoplasia of the mid-phalanx of the finger demonstrable by X-ray. A distal position of the palmar axial triradius and, less frequently, an ulnar loop dermal ridge pattern on all digits are typical dermatoglyphic abnormalities. The feet show a wide gap with a plantar crease between the first and second toes. Umbilical hernias are common. As the infant grows the following cutaneous features develop in a significant number of patients with Down's syndrome: The skin remains dry and at times appears ichthyotic; obese children may develop pseudoacanthosis nigricans in the fleshy folds; cheilitis (Butterworth, 1960) is an almost constant finding and angular stomatitis may become granulomatous and very bothersome; syringomas—papular lesions around the eyes—occur in about 20 per cent of patients (Butterworth, 1964); and elastosis perforans serpiginosum also has an increased incidence. The authors have seen psoriasis, patchy eczematous lichenified lesions, dermatophytic and bacterial infections of the skin and pityriasis rubra pilaris in these patients, but no special relationship is suggested between these skin lesions and Trisomy 21.

A cardiac anomaly is present in about 40 per cent of patients with mongolism (Smith,

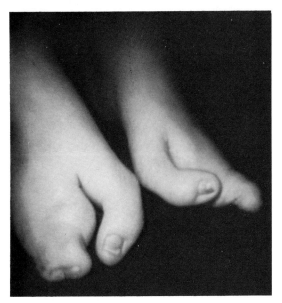

Figure 7–8. Syndactyly. "Lobster claw" deformity of the feet (EEC syndrome). (Courtesy of Dr. Samuel Pruzansky.)

1970); ventricular septal defect and persistent ostium primum are the most frequent defects. Roentgenograms of the pelvis dem-

onstrate hypoplasia and an outward flaring of the iliac wings and a shallow acetabular angle. Associated duodenal atresia, imperforate anus and an annular pancreas may constitute surgical emergencies.

With increasing age, developmental retardation rapidly becomes apparent. Other characteristic findings include hyperextensibility of the joints, hypoplasia or aplasia of the frontal sinuses, late closure of the fontanelles and anomalous dentition. Numerous other abnormalities have been documented but occur with less frequency (Smith, 1971).

Mental and motor progress is slow and an IQ of more than 50 is rarely achieved. Osseous maturation may also be delayed, but hypotonia tends to improve with age. The prognosis for survival to adulthood is best for those children without cardiac defects or gastrointestinal anomalies. Respiratory infections constitute a chronic management problem.

Other Anomalies. There are other developmental anomalies associated with a variety of syndromes, such as the EEC syndrome (Fig. 7–8), acrocephaly and Apert's syndrome (Figs. 7–9 and 7–10). These are discussed elsewhere in this book.

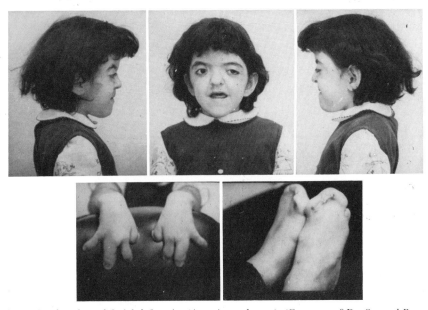

Figure 7–9. Syndactyly and facial deformity (Apert's syndrome). (Courtesy of Dr. Samuel Pruzansky.)

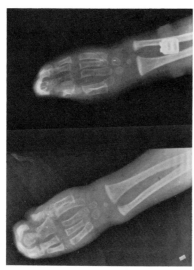

Figure 7–10. Syndactyly (Apert's syndrome).

REFERENCES

Bart, B. J.: Congenital absence of skin and associated abnormalities resembling epidermolysis bullosa. Arch. Derm. 93:296, 1966.

Bart, B. J.: Epidermolysis bullosa and congenital localized absence of skin. Arch. Derm. 101:78, 1970.

Brownstein, M. H., Wanger, N. and Helwig, E. B.: Accessory tragi. Arch. Derm. 104:625, 1971.

Butterworth, T., Leoni, E., Beerman, H. and Wood, M. G.: Cheilitis of mongolism. J. Invest. Derm. 35:347, 1960.

Butterworth, T., Strean, L. P., Beerman, H. and Wood, M. G.: Syringoma and mongolism. Arch. Derm. 90:483, 1964.

Deeken, J. H. and Caplan, R. M.: Aplasia cutis congenita. Arch. Derm. 102:386, 1970.

Fourman, P. and Fourman, J.: Hereditary deafness in family with ear-pits. Brit. Med. J. 2:1354, 1955.

Fraumeni, J. F., Geiser, C. F. and Manning, M. D.: Wilms' tumor and congenital hemihypertrophy: Report of five new cases and review of literature. Pediatrics 40:886, 1967.

Gorlin, R. J. and Pindborg, J. J.: Syndromes of the Head and Neck. New York, McGraw-Hill, 1964.

Guimaraes, S. B., Uceda, J. E. and Lynn, H. B.: Thyroglossal duct remnants in infants and children. Mayo Clin. Proc. 47:117. 1972.

Hacken, B. N. and Miller, D. R.: Simultaneous occurrence of congenital aniridia, hamartoma, and Wilms' tumor. J. Pediat. 78:497, 1971.

Hammond, K.: Skin dimples and rubella. Pediatrics 39:291, 1967.

Lewin, R. A.: Pilonidal sinus in infancy. Pediatrics 35:795, 1965.

Palo, J., Iivanainen, M., Blomqvist, K. and Pesonen, S.: Aetiological aspects of the cutis verticis gyrata and mental retardation syndrome. J. Ment. Defic. Res. 14:33, 1970.

Polan, S. and Butterworth, T.: Cutis verticis gyrata: A review with report of seven new cases. Amer. J. Ment. Defic. 57:613, 1953.

Raque, C. S., Stein, K. M., Lane, J. M. and Reese, E. D., Jr.: Pseudoainhum constricting bands of the extremities. Arch. Derm. 105:434, 1972.

Resnick, S. S., Koblenzer, P. J. and Pitts, F. W.: Congenital absence of the scalp with associated vascular anomaly. Clin. Pediat. 4:322, 1965.

Ringrose, R. G., Jabbour, J. T. and Keele, D. K.: Hemihypertrophy. Pediatrics 36:434, 1965.

Smith, D. W., Theiler, K. and Schachenman, G.: Rib-gap defect with micrognathia, malformed tracheal cartilages and redundant skin: A new pattern of defective development. J. Pediat. 69:799, 1966.

Soricelli, D. A., Bell, L. and Alexander, W. A.: Congenital fistulas of the lower lip. A family case report. Oral Surg. 21:511, 1966.

Steck, W. D. and Helwig, E. B.: Cutaneous remnants of the omphalomesenteric duct. Arch. Derm. 90:463, 1964.

Torpin, R.: Fetal Malformations Caused by Amnion Rupture During Gestation. Springfield, Charles C Thomas, 1965.

Warkany, J.: Congenital Malformations. Chicago, Year Book Medical Publishers, 1971.

Warkany, J., Passarge, E. and Smith, L. B.: Congenital malformations in autosomal trisomy syndromes. Amer. J. Dis. Child. 112:502, 1966.

Chapter Eight

MISCELLANEOUS NEVI AND TUMORS

TERMINOLOGY

The skin is frequently the site of minor localized developmental disorders, or tumors (Lever, 1967). In order to appreciate fully the array and complexity of these tumors, as well as understand their classification, it may be helpful to consider their embryologic origins. Table 8–1 summarizes the spectrum of nevi to be covered in this chapter.

Development of Nevi and Tumors. The skin is populated by melanocytes derived from the neural crest. These are found in the epidermis and dermis and, as a result, melanocytic nevi may occupy either or both sites. Proliferation of keratinocytes may result in localized areas of hyperplasia consisting of mature cells that are either normal in appearance or somewhat altered. The hair follicles and the sebaceous, apocrine and eccrine glands derive from epithelial germ buds; these buds may give rise to localized collections of cells whose differentiation achieves varying degrees of completion. A highly differentiated collection of cells, or their formation into organized tissue, is called a nevus. The term "nevus" is not an entirely satisfactory one but it is concise, and its meaning is fleshed out by common understanding.

A nevus is a hamartoma* in which the cells

---

*Pinkus (1969a) makes a distinction between a malformation, which he equates with nevus, and hamartoma, which indicates a cellular lesion. This concept does not reflect the common clinical understanding of the word "nevus," although it may have merit for the histopathologist.

Table 8–1. Spectrum of Nevi

EPIDERMAL
Keratinocytic (Epidermal) Nevi

Nevus unius lateris
Systematized verrucous nevi
Small verrucous nevi
Ichthyosis hystrix
Unilateral congenital ichthyosiform erythroderma
Epidermal nevus syndrome
Benign congenital acanthosis nigricans
Porokeratosis of Mibelli

Appendageal (Organoid) Nevi

Sebaceous nevi ⎫
Hair follicle nevi ⎬ Comedo Nevi
Apocrine duct nevi ⎭
  (nevus syringocystadenoma papilliferus)

Melanocytic Nevi

DERMAL NEVI
Melanocytic Nevi
Vascular Nevi
Connective Tissue Nevi

Collagen
Elastic tissue
Digital fibroma
Juvenile fibromatosis
Osteoma cutis

Nervous Tissue Nevi

Nasal glioma
Meningioma

FAT TISSUE

Lipoma
Nevus lipomatosis superficialis
Michelin tire baby

MIXED

Benign teratomas (Dermoids)

60

are highly differentiated, may function (i.e., produce pigment), and are organized into a semblance of their intended organs (such as hair follicles, sebaceous or eccrine glands). When cell differentiation is less complete they may form gland-like structures (adenomas), nonmetastasizing cancer-like tumors (epitheliomas), or frank cancer. The mysterious way in which nevi arise after the period of embryonic development may be explained by Pinkus' theory (1969b) that benign neoformations may arise from the adult basal layer within pluripotential cells functioning as not-quite-perfect epithelial germ buds. This hypothesis is highly regarded, but the evidence does not permit the issue to be considered as settled. A more perfect taxonomy of benign congenital skin tumors awaits greater knowledge of cellular differentiation, induction, growth and development. Since nevi are ubiquitous, the skin offers exciting prospects for research.

From the foregoing discussion it may be clear that the term "nevus" does not specify the tissue involved; therefore, it is necessary, to use a qualifying adjective to further define the lesion. Thus, we can appreciate the origin of the terms *melanocytic nevus, keratinocytic nevus, sebaceous nevus,* and so on. It is useful to remember that qualifying adjectives, and other names applied to these developmental anomalies, simply reflect the gross or microscopic morphological characteristics of the tumors, and nothing more. It is possible, for example, that the verrucous changes which occur in keratinocytic nevi may reflect a metabolic abnormality in the underlying dermis or its vessels. But if tissue-specific, metabolically active inducers exist they have not yet been identified. What is visible, however, is the thickened stratum corneum, so the term "epidermal nevus" is applicable.

KERATINOCYTIC TUMORS

EPIDERMAL NEVI (Verrucous nevi)

Epidermal nevi are a group of keratinocytic tumors which have the following features in common: They are primarily composed of keratinocytes; they may be congenital but are not clearly hereditarily transmitted; they are all more or less verrucous; and they differ somewhat in their clinical appearance, distribution, rate of development and histopathological features. Some nevi have a low potential for malignant transformation. In a

highly significant number of cases, more extensive lesions are associated with skeletal, vascular and central nervous system anomalies (see following section).

Epidermal nevi may be present at birth or appear within the first month or they may develop later. The cutaneous changes in the newborn may be barely visible. Usually, what is noticed is a streaky area of hyperpigmentation that is not palpable but that may be scraped off with the fingernail. It is not uncommon for the inexperienced observer to consider it adherent extraneous material. As the infant grows the streak becomes more persistent and raised, perhaps extending linearly or laterally to involve a larger area (Plate V–D, page 85). Clinically, epidermal nevi may take several forms:

(1) Small, warty papillomatous or velvety pigmented lesions occurring in a string a few centimeters in length (Fig. 8–1).

(2) Long unilateral streaks involving a limb or two, or part of the thorax or pelvic area (*nevus unius lateris,* Fig. 8–2). These lesions commonly become very verrucous and can cause severe deformity of the nails if the matrices are involved. They may become pruritic, inflamed (Altman, 1971), or associated with an underlying hemangioma (Imperial, 1969). (See Plate VI–A, page 86).

(3) Very widespread linear verrucous lesions which may involve the oral mucosa or ocular conjunctiva, and possibly associated

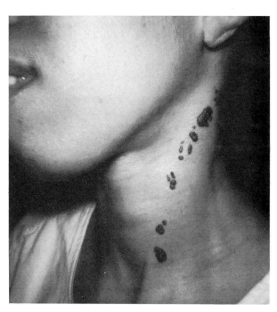

Figure 8–1. Epidermal nevus: a string of pigmented papillomas.

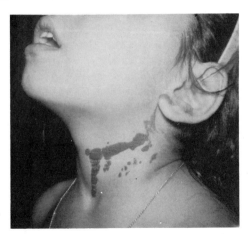

Figure 8-2. Epidermal nevus: long pigmented streak. This lesion entered the ear and traversed the tympanic membrane (nevus unius lateris).

with a large cerebriform lesion on the scalp. Hypo- and hyperpigmentation, or small vascular anomalies, frequently accompany this type of nevus (Fig. 8–3).

(4) A scaly, diffuse eruption often involving both sides of the body. The resulting feathered or marbled pattern forms streaks and whorls of hyperkeratosis (*ichthyosis hystrix*, Fig. 8–4).

(5) Poorly circumscribed, velvety pigmented hyperkeratotic areas over the extensor surfaces of the hands and feet (especially the knuckle areas), the axillae, neck, and other skin folds (*benign congenital acanthosis nigricans*) and associated with profound mental retardation (Plate VI–B). In a case described by Beane (1969) there were other abnormalities including cleft palate, hypertelorism, anodontia, retarded bone growth and corrugation of the skin (cutis gyratum).

(6) A diffuse, unilateral scaly eruption, involving exactly half the body and identical to congenital ichthyosiform erythroderma (Cullen, 1969).

These clinical pictures often are not clearly separable. Intermediate forms are seen, especially among types 1, 2, and 3. Furthermore, epidermal hypertrophy may form a minor part of a lesion whose cardinal histologic feature is sebaceous gland, apocrine duct or vascular hyperplasia.

Histopathology

The histological features of epidermal nevi result in two distinctive patterns:

(1) Hyperkeratosis of varying severity, papillomatosis, acanthosis and elongation of the rete ridges. The granular layer may be diminished or increased.

(2) Hyperkeratosis and vacuolization (ballooning) of the cells may be found in a thickened granular layer and in the mid-epidermis. The vacuolized cells may give rise to microvesicles (epidermolytic hyperkeratosis).

Thickened localized lesions tend to show the first pattern, whereas widespread scaly lesions tend to show the second pattern. However, the reverse may be seen as well.

Epidermal nevi frequently have an associated overgrowth of dermal elements, such as sebaceous glands, apocrine glands, vessels and localized accumulations of melanocytic nevus cells. These findings suggest that hyperplasia of all the affected tissues, epidermal, appendageal, and vascular, may be due to some common inducer localized in the dermis. The fact that these lesions cannot be removed permanently without also removing the underlying dermis further supports this notion.

The Epidermal Nevus Syndrome

Solomon, Fretzin, and Dewald (1968) reviewed the associated findings in 23 patients with epidermal nevi, including all the types described previously. In more than two-thirds of these patients they found associated skeletal defects, vascular anomalies and serious central nervous system disease (Plate VI–C). The anomalies found included kyphoscoliosis, vertebral defects, short limbs, phocomelia, osseous hypertrophy, angiomas

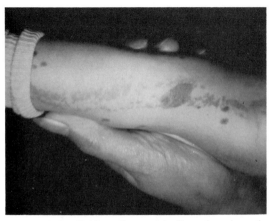

Figure 8-3. Epidermal nevus: the linear keratinocytic nevus is traversing an oval café-au-lait patch.

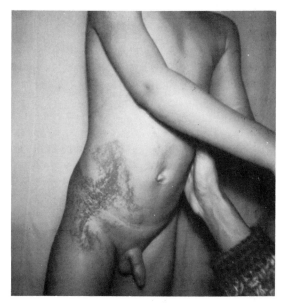

Figure 8–4. Epidermal nevus: marbled and feathered superficial scales (ichthyosis hystris).

POROKERATOSIS OF MIBELLI

This localized disorder of keratinization results in a clinical picture very similar to that of a linear epidermal nevus (Goldner, 1972). The lesions may occur in several members of a family, suggesting an autosomal dominant type of inheritance. The lesions are crateriform, scaly papules that tend to have a linear or circular arrangement. The edge of each small crater forms a horny ledge. The center of the craters are atrophic. Once seen closely the individual lesions are not difficult to recognize, but at a distance the eruption resembles an epidermal nevus. Histologically, the central atrophy is surrounded by a collarette of hyperkeratosis. The central portion is occupied by a parakeratotic plaque, the coronoid lamella.

APPENDAGEAL TUMORS

Benign appendageal tumors are localized lesions which may be found in the newborn. They undergo three phases of evolution: (1) Absence of hair; (2) tumor formation; and (3) possible malignant transformation (Mehregan, 1965). Although the tumors have been considered separate entities because of their characteristic clinical and histological appearance, they may, as a group, result from common inductive process. Therefore, these lesions, together with epidermal nevi, verrucous hemangiomas and certain pigmented

of skin and central nervous system, mental retardation and convulsive disorders (Plate VI–D). A greater likelihood of associated anomalies existed if the lesions were large.

On discovering the existence of an epidermal nevus (Plate VII–A, page 87) it is necessary to take a careful family history and perform a thorough physical examination (Fig. 8–5). Particular emphasis should be placed on the musculoskeletal and nervous systems, as well as on the skin. Periodic electroencephalograms, psychologic testing and radiographic examination of the long bones, pelvis and vertebral column should be made, if indicated.

Treatment. The treatment of verrucous epidermal nevi is, at best, unsatisfactory. The only effective treatment is removal of the lesion, together with its underlying dermis. In localized lesions this may be accomplished by electrodesiccation or plastic repair. This treatment is not recommended in the one month old infant since lesions may develop over a period of years. The scars resulting from surgery may be as cosmetically unsatisfactory as the original lesions, and an extension of the nevus may appear beyond the repaired area. In the older child, salicylic acid (3 per cent in cold cream) may keep the lesions soft, and water-dispersible bath oils provide some palliative relief. When the nails are involved no treatment is effective; and, aside from filing or avulsion of the affected nails, none is suggested (Solomon, 1970).

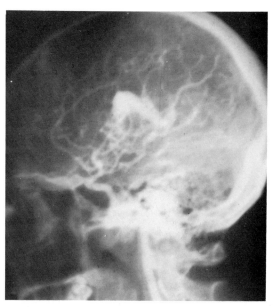

Figure 8–5. The epidermal nevus syndrome: intracerebral arteriovenous malformation.

tumors, may represent different manifestations of a common etiologic mechanism. For this reason they have been called organoid (containing multiple tissue elements) nevi.

SEBACEOUS NEVI

These lesions are sharply demarcated, hairless, yellow-orange, verrucous nodules or plaques which are present at birth (Plate VII–B). They are most often found on the scalp, ears, forehead and face, but may occur on the neck. If left untreated they remain localized, enlarging only slightly, if at all, and occasionally undergoing transformation into basal cell epitheliomas (Wilson Jones, 1970; Mehregan, 1965). On occasion, large lesions involving half the scalp and face may be associated with ocular dermoids, mental retardation, pigmentary disorder and skeletal abnormalities. Taken together the aspects of the defect resemble the epidermal nevus syndrome to a great extent, and we consider this to be a variant of the epidermal nevus syndrome, although characterized by a predominance of sebaceous gland elements in the skin lesions (Feuerstein, 1962; Solomon, 1968). Histologically, sebaceous nevi show hyperkeratosis of the papillary type, an increase in immature hair follicles and large numbers of sebaceous glands of varying maturity. Effective treatment of smaller lesions can be achieved by surgical excision.

Figure 8–6.   Nevus comedonicus.

NEVUS COMEDONICUS
(Comedo nevi)

A linear verrucous lesion consisting of comedones may be present at birth and represents a defect in the formation of pilosebaceous follicles (Fig. 8–6) (Beerman, 1959). The punctate lesions are dilated, shallow hair follicles filled with keratin. There is no hair in the lesion, but some rudimentary sebaceous glands may be found at its base. Several cases have been reported in association with basal cell epitheliomas and vertebral column defects (Bleiberg, 1969), again underscoring the need to study patients with localized nevi of epidermal origin for bony anomalies.

NEVUS SYRINGOCYSTADENOMA PAPILLIFERUS

The inconspicuous lesion bearing this imposing name is frequently mistaken for a sebaceous nevus, since, in the newborn, they look identical. This lesion deserves a special appelation, however, because histologically it contains structures resembling apocrine ducts, as well as sebaceous glands (in about one-third of cases), and hair. About 10 per cent of these lesions eventuate in basal cell epitheliomas (Helwig, 1955). They should be excised during childhood.

OTHER APPENDAGEAL DISORDERS

Hair Follicle Tumors.   Hair follicle nevi, such as trichofolliculoma and trichoepithelioma, generally do not appear until after the first month of life.

Eccrine Gland Nevi.   This disorder and other sweat gland tumors are extremely rare and usually are not evident until after the first years of life.

Melanocytic Nevi.   The melanocytic nevi are discussed in the chapter on pigmentary disorders (see Chap. 10).

DERMAL NEVI AND TUMORS

(*Vascular Nevi* are discussed in Chapter 9, Vascular Disorders.)

CONNECTIVE TISSUE NEVI

These rare lesions are generally found in the lumbosacral region. They usually occur in the three to five year old child, but are occasionally present at birth. The lesions appear as yellow or flesh-colored plaques several centimeters in diameter. The surface is often pebbled and the lesion feels rubbery. A disseminated nodular form has also been seen. The connective tissue nevus may occur as an isolated phenomenon, in association with tuberous sclerosis (in which case it is called "shagreen patch"), or as part of a syndrome which includes skeletal anomalies and pheochromocytomas (Plate VII–C).

The same clinical picture is produced by a great increase in elastic tissue in the mid and lower dermis *(nevus elasticus)* or results from dermal sclerosis. Connective tissue nevi tend to remain unchanged or grow with the infant. Surgical removal does little to improve the appearance since grafting is often required, and the graft looks no better than the original lesion.

DIGITAL FIBROMA

A rare congenital lesion, digital fibroma is found on the distal phalanges of fingers and toes and may mimic sarcoma (Shapiro, 1969). This aggressive, fibroblastic neoplasm is manifested as smooth, red, fleshy nodules (Fig. 8–7). The etiology is unknown, but virus-like inclusion bodies found in the dermis suggest an infectious source. Hematoxylin-eosin staining of the specimen shows an impressive infiltrate of fibroblasts and collagen bundles,

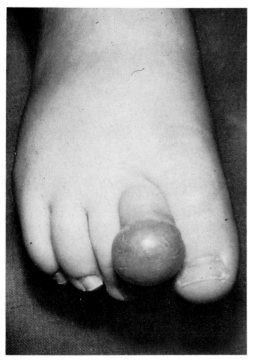

Figure 8–7. Digital fibroma. (Courtesy of Dr. Lewis Shapiro).

as well as 3 to 10 micron, red, intracellular inclusions. Surgical excision of the lesions is the treatment of choice but recurrences are common.

JUVENILE FIBROMATOSIS

This tumor, like digital fibroma, is another pseudo-cancer detectable at birth (Pinol-Aguade, 1969). The lesions are rubbery, flesh-colored or pale nodules that vary in number and location, although the limbs are a favored site.

Disseminated fibrous nodules are also a manifestation of the rare disorder *dermatofibrosis lenticularis disseminata*, or *Buschke-Ollendorf syndrome* (Curth, 1934). Features of the disorder include a familial occurrence and characteristic osseous lesions (osteopoikilosis) consisting of minute radiodense areas in the skull, spine, clavicle, patella and scapula.

PRIMARY OSTEOMA CUTIS

Primary osteoma cutis usually is present at birth (O'Donnell, 1971). These extremely rare lesions may occur in several areas on the same patient. The initial lesion is a firm or fleshy mass which becomes stony hard. The osseous tissue, presumably derived from primordial pluripotential mesenchymal cells, develops in the subcutis. Osteoma cutis may also be a cutaneous feature of *Albright's hereditary osteodystrophy* (Brook, 1971).

NEURAL TUMORS

Neural tumors are found in von Recklinghausen's neurofibromatosis (this condition is discussed in Chapter 10); however, these neural tumors usually do not arise during the neonatal period. An unusual benign neural tumor, *nasal glioma,* may be found in the nose, nasopharynx or extranasally (Christianson, 1966). The tumor is a fleshy, purple, rubbery mass found on the bridge of the nose near its root and can be confused with a hemangioma. The lesion may be connected to, and traverse, the skull. Biopsy is *not* recommended prior to radiographic examination of the area, and neurosurgical consultation should be sought. The tumor consists of glial tissue, giant cells, blood vessels and fibrous tissue.

MENINGIOMAS

These lesions may appear in the newborn as a rubbery mass adhering to the skin overlying the scalp or spine (Bain, 1956). The histologic pattern of these lesions is identical to that of intracranial meningiomas.

FAT TUMORS

Soft fatty tumors, *lipomas*, very rarely are seen in the newborn infant (Perlman, 1960). Their appearance is similar to that of the ubiquitous lipoma found in the adult. Histologically, lipomas are composed of apparently normal fat cells arranged in lobules that are traversed by connective tissue and vessels. The entire anomaly is encapsulated. When the connective tissue component is very prominent the tumor is called a *fibrolipoma;* however, when the vasculature is most prominent, it is called an *angiolipoma.*

NEVUS LIPOMATOSIS SUPERFICIALIS

Another extremely rare cutaneous nevus is manifested in the newborn infant as localized groups of soft papules or nodules (Lynch, 1958). The lesions are usually slightly yellow or of normal skin color, and are found on the buttocks, or occasionally, on the upper thorax. Histologically, the dermis is infiltrated by groups of fat cells that localize around the vessels. Melanocytic nevus cells are sometimes found associated with the fatty infiltrate.

"MICHELIN TIRE BABY"
(Nevus lipomatosis diffusa)

A case of diffuse lipomatosis described by Ross (1969) was associated with severe transverse folding of the skin, resulting in a gyrate pattern (similar to that of the manikin in French advertisements for Michelin Tires). Rh incompatibility and hemitrophy were also present. The increase in fat was found in the deeper dermis and subcutis.

DERMOIDS

Tumors containing embryonic nests, resulting in the mixture of elements described previously, may occasionally occur, particularly on the forehead or along lines of embryonic closure. Dermoids have a capsule and contain sebaceous material and hair (Warkany, 1971).

MALIGNANT CONGENITAL TUMORS

The skin is very rarely the primary or secondary site of involvement in congenital malignancies (Table 8–2). In fact, Wells (1940) found only four congenital malignant tumors in 3000 autopsies of newborn infants, several of whom had secondary manifestations in the skin.

A massive tumor on the face may result from an *adenocarcinoma* of the *parotid gland* (Tefft, 1965). *Teratomas* may present as large facial tumors, but also occur in the sacrococcygeal and retroperitoneal areas. Congenital *malignant melanoma* has been described in one infant (Wells, 1940). Sarcomas are among the more common malignant tumors and include *leiomyosarcoma* (tumor of the scalp [Heieck, 1970]), *fibrosarcoma, myxosarcoma* and *neuroblastoma.* Less differentiated *sarcomas* may also contain vascular, round cell, spindle cell and myxomatous elements.

Neuroblastoma is the most common cancer found at birth (Hawthorne, 1970; Shown, 1970). One-third of these patients have metastatic nodules in the skin which are small, blue and nontender on palpation. For this reason these infants have been called "Blueberry Muffin Babies." (The same name is also given to infants with congenital *rubella syndrome*). The lesions can exhibit a peculiar blanching, due to release of catecholamine from the tumor cells. The skin findings are accompanied by the systemic manifestations of neuroblastoma, including hepatomegaly, anemia, intra-abdominal masses and failure

Table 8–2. Miscellaneous Malignant Tumors

Parotid tumors—adenocarcinomas
Teratomas (sacrococcygeal, oral and retroperitoneal)
Malignant melanoma
Leiomyosarcoma of scalp
Fibrosarcomas
Myxosarcoma
Neuroblastoma—ischiorectal
　　　　　　　adrenal
　　　　　　　other locations
Undifferentiated sarcoma—vascular
　　　　　　　　　round cell   ⎱ Elements
　　　　　　　　　spindle cell   ⎰ may be
　　　　　　　　　myxomatous   present
Leukemia

to thrive. The diagnosis may be established by cutaneous biopsy and catecholamine determinations in the urine. The prognosis in patients with metastases is grave, but a palliative response may be achieved by surgery and cancer chemotherapy.

Congenital leukemia has been described in a few infants. The cutaneous features include purpura, ecchymoses, pallor, and papular, plaque-like and nodular infiltrates of leukemic cells.

REFERENCES

Altman, J. and Mehregan, A. H.: Inflammatory linear verrucose epidermal nevus. Arch. Derm. *104*:385, 1971.

Bain, G. O. and Shnitka, E. K.: Cutaneous meningioma. Arch. Derm. *74*:590, 1956.

Beane, J. M., Dodge, J. A. and Nevin, N. C.: Cutis gyratum, acanthosis nigricans, and other congenital anomalies. Brit. J. Derm. *81*:241, 1969.

Beerman, H. and Homan, J. B.: Naevus comedonicus. Arch. klin. exp. Derm. *208*:325, 1959.

Bleiberg, G. and Brodkin, R. H.: Linear unilateral basal cell nevus with comedones. Arch. Derm. *100*:187, 1969.

Brook, C. G. D. and Valman, H. B.: Osteoma cutis and Albright's hereditary osteodystrophy. Brit. J. Derm. *85*:471, 1971.

Christianson, H. B.: Nasal glioma. Arch. Derm. *93*:68, 1966.

Cullen, S. I., Harris, D. E., Carter, C. H. and Reed, W. B.: Congenital unilateral ichthyosiform erythroderma. Arch. Derm. *99*:724, 1969.

Curth, H. O.: Dermatofibrosis lenticularis disseminata and osteopoikilosis. Arch. Derm. *30*:552, 1934.

Dabska, M.: Malignant endovascular papillary angioendothelioma of skin in childhood. Cancer *24*:503, 1969.

Feuerstein, R. C. and Mims, L. C.: Linear nevus sebaceous with convulsions and mental retardation. Amer. J. Dis. Child. *104*:675, 1962.

Goldner, R.: Zosteriform parakeratosis of Mibelli: *In* Bergsma, D. (ed.): Clinical delineation of birth defects. Vol. 12. The Skin. Baltimore, Williams and Wilkins Co., 1972, p. 251.

Hawthorne, H. C., Jr., Nelson, G. S., Witzleben, C. L. and Giangiacoma, J.: Blanching subcutaneous nodules in neonatal neuroblastoma. J. Pediat. *77*:297, 1970.

Helwig, E. G. and Hackney, V. C.: Syringadenoma papilliferus. Arch. Derm. *71*:361, 1955.

Imperial, R. and Helwig, E. G.: Verrucous hemangioma. Arch. Derm. *96*:247, 1967.

Lever, W. F.: Tumors of the epidermal appendages. *In* Histopathology of the Skin. 4th ed. Philadelphia, J. B. Lippincott Co., 1967, pp. 482, 695.

Lynch, F. W. and Goltz, R. W.: Nevus lipomatosus cutaneous superficialis. Arch. Derm. *78*:479, 1958.

Mehregan, A. H. and Pinkus, H.: Life history of organoid nevi. Arch. Derm. *91*:574, 1965.

O'Donnell, T. F. and Geller, S. A.: Primary osteoma cutis. Arch. Derm. *104*:325, 1971.

Perlman, H. H.: Tumors of the Skin. *In* Pediatric Dermatology. Chicago, Year Book Publishers, 1960, p. 421.

Pinkus, H. and Mehregan, A. H.: A Guide to Dermatohistopathology. New York, Appleton-Century-Crofts Inc., 1969, pp. 352, 354.

Piñol-Aguade, G. M., Mascaro, G. A., Rubio, J. and Roselo-Ochoa, E.: Benign juvenile fibromatosis. Med. Cutanea. *3*:475, 1969.

Ross, C. M.: Generalized folded skin with an underlying lipomatous nevus. Arch. Derm. *100*:32, 1969.

Shapiro, L.: Infantile digital fibromatosis and aponeurotic fibroma. Arch. Derm. *99*:37, 1969.

Shown, T. E. and Durfee, M. F.: Blueberry muffin baby: Neonatal neuroblastoma with subcutaneous metastases and thrombocytopenia. J. Urol. *104*:193, 1970.

Solomon, L. M.: Epidermal nevi. *In* Madden, S. and Brown, T. H. (eds.): Current Dermatologic Management. St. Louis, C. V. Mosby Co., 1970, p. 171.

Solomon, L. M., Fretzin, D. F. and DeWald, R. L.: The epidermal nevus syndrome. Arch. Derm. *97*:273, 1968.

Tefft, M., Vawter, F. and Neuhauser, E. B. D.: Unusual facial tumors in the newborn. Arch. Derm. *102*:213, 1970.

Warkany, J.: Congenital malformations. Chicago, Year Book Medical Publishers, 1971, pp. 1216–1217.

Wells, H. G.: Occurrence and significance of congenital malignant neoplasms. Arch. Path. *30*:535, 1940.

Wilson-Jones, E. and Heyl, T.: Naevus sebaceus. Brit. J. Derm. *82*:99, 1970.

Chapter Nine

VASCULAR DISORDERS AND MALFORMATIONS

Cutaneous hemangiomas are exceedingly common developmental malformations involving the dermal and subcutaneous vasculature (Donsky, 1968). Although these nevi have been observed in several members of one family, there is no evidence that, as an isolated finding, they are genetically determined. Hemangiomas can be superficial (approximately 63 to 68 per cent), subcutaneous (15 per cent), or mixed (22 per cent) (Lampe, 1959; Rook, 1968). The terms "capillary" and "cavernous," often applied as qualifying adjectives to hemangiomas, refer to their histopathologic pattern. Capillary hemangiomas show only dilated vessels with or without endothelial proliferation, while cavernous hemangiomas have large, dilated, blood filled cavities with a compressed, single layer endothelial lining.

NEVUS FLAMMEUS

The port-wine stain, or telangiectatic nevus, is present at birth and should be considered a relatively permanent developmental defect (Plate VII–D, page 87). These lesions may be only a few millimeters in diameter or they may cover extensive areas, occasionally involving up to one-half of the body surface (Plate VIII–A, page 88). They do not proliferate after birth, so their apparent increase in size is due to growth of the child.

A nevus flammeus may be localized to any body surface, but facial lesions are probably the most common. Some lesions are distributed unilaterally and may involve mucous membranes as well as skin. Port-wine nevi are usually sharply demarcated and flat, but a pebbly or slightly thickened surface can occur. Variation in color ranges from pale pink to a deep red or purple; in black skin they appear jet black. Lighter lesions may involute spontaneously, although most are unlikely to fade appreciably. On histologic examination numerous dilated capillaries without endothelial proliferation are found in the dermis.

Treatment of a port-wine nevus is generally unsatisfactory; however, if treatment is contemplated, it should be deferred until school age or older. Among the procedures used are excision and grafting for small lesions, and tattooing for larger lesions. In many instances, the most successful modality is the use of a cosmetic cream, such as Covermark, which is carefully matched to blend with the surrounding skin. Most port-wine nevi occur as an isolated defect and do not indicate involvement of other organs; however, occasionally a nevus flammeus may be a clue to the presence of certain vascular syndromes.

Sturge-Weber Syndrome
(Encephalofacial or trigeminal angiomatosis)

This syndrome consists of a facial port-wine nevus (Fig. 9–1), convulsions, hemiparesis contralateral to the facial lesion and ipsilateral intracranial calcification (Chao, 1959; Peterman, 1958). Although the disorder is often considered to be inherited as an autosomal dominant trait, there is no sound evidence for genetic transmission. The characteristic nevus is most often unilateral, but may be bilateral, and is usually localized to the trigeminal region of the face. Lesions may also be present on the scalp, neck, trunk and extremities. Intraoral manifestations include vascular hyperplasia of the lips, maxillary gingiva, tongue and buccal mucosa. The mandibular gingiva and palate are rarely affected (Royle, 1966). Neurologic findings are due to atrophy of the cerebral cortex or irritation by calcification secondary to angiomatous involvement of the meninges (usually over the posterior parietal and occipital lobes) on the same side as the facial lesion.

Convulsions are a frequent manifestation of the syndrome and focal motor seizures are the most common type. Hemiparesis and hemiatrophy are less frequent findings, occurring contralateral to the facial lesion. Behavior disturbances and deficient mentality are variable and do not always correlate with the severity of the vascular anomaly. Ocular manifestations are frequent, and include buphthalmos, glaucoma, angioma of the choroid, hemianoptic defects and optic atrophy. A careful ophthalmologic examination is essential since untreated glaucoma will result in blindness.

In a few cases the vascular defect may affect other organs. Roentgenograms of the skull show pathognomonic "tram-line" double contoured calcification in the cerebral cortex on the same side as the nevus flammeus and, occasionally, cerebral hemiatrophy. Calcification is progressive, but it is not seen in the neonatal period. Electroencephalography shows unilateral depression of cortical activity with or without spike discharges. Cerebral angiography may be useful in delineating the extent and distribution of the intracranial angioma.

The prognosis depends on the extent of cerebral involvement, rapidity of progression and response to treatment. Anticonvulsant therapy and neurosurgical procedures have been of value in some patients (Chao, 1957; Peterman, 1958). The modalities used for palliation of gingival overgrowth have included surgical excision of excess tissue, injection of sclerosing solutions and irradiation therapy (Royle, 1966).

Klippel-Trenaunay-Weber Syndrome

Cutaneous vascular nevi, venous varicosities and overgrowth of bony structures and soft tissues of the involved limb constitute this syndrome (Mullins, 1962) (Fig. 9-2). The vascular lesions are usually apparent at birth, and boys are more frequently affected than girls. The hemangioma may be either capil-

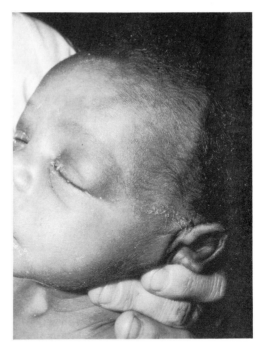

Figure 9–1. Sturge-Weber syndrome. (Courtesy of Dr. Ruth Seeler.)

lary or cavernous and is often complicated by arteriovenous shunts and lymphangiomatous anomalies. The hemangiomas may be macular and pale to deep red in color with considerable thickening and deformity of the involved tissue. The lesions vary in size from relatively inconspicuous occurrences to involvement of an entire limb. The defect is usually unilateral, but occasional cases with bilateral involvement have been reported. The upper extremity is involved more frequently than the lower. Affected limbs may be large at birth or show increased growth during childhood, and bony hypertrophy may be demonstrable roentgenographically. Occasionally, atrophy of the bones and involved soft tissues occurs instead.

Polydactyly, syndactyly and oligodactyly have been associated findings. Complications include severe edema, phlebitis, thrombosis, ulceration and hyperhidrosis of the affected area. The prognosis depends on the extent of involvement, which should be carefully assessed by complete peripheral vascular studies. A surgical approach may be effective in preventing severe limb hypertrophy in occasional patients.

Miscellaneous Conditions with Nevus Flammeus

Macular capillary hemangiomata also occur with moderate frequency in *Trisomy 13, Rubenstein-Taybi syndrome* (broad thumbs and

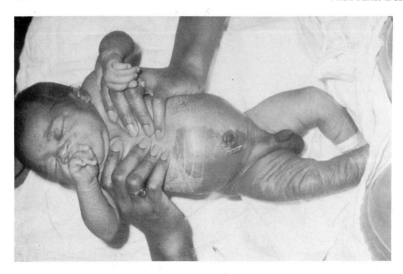

Figure 9–2. Kippel-Trenaunay syndrome. (Courtesy of Dr. Ruth Seeler.)

toes, slanted palpebral fissures and hypoplastic maxilla) and the *Wiedemann-Beckwith syndrome* (macroglossia, omphalocoele, macrostomia and cytomegaly of the fetal adrenal) (Smith, 1970). In the *"SC"* or *pseudothalidomide syndrome*, probably inherited in an autosomal recessive fashion, a nevus flammeus of the face is associated with limb malformations resembling phocomelia, flexion contractures of the joints, hypoplastic cartilages of the ears and nose, micrognathia, sparse silvery-blond hair, cloudy corneas, growth retardation and possible mental retardation (Hermann, 1969).

Telangiectatic nevi are also an inconstant feature of the *epidermal nevus syndrome* (see Chap. 13) and of several rare neurocutaneous syndromes. *Bonnet-Dechaume-Blanc* syndrome consists of facial vascular nevi and retinal and intracranial angiomatosis (Paillas, 1959). Facial nevi in a trigeminal distribution, arteriovenous aneurysm of the mid-brain and anomalies of the retinal vessels ipsilateral to the facial nevus constitute the *Wyburn-Mason syndrome.* Vascular accidents, increased intracranial pressure and retinal hemorrhage are common complications.

CAPILLARY AND CAVERNOUS HEMANGIOMA
(Strawberry nevus)

The term strawberry nevus, although commonly used to describe a simple capillary hemangioma, has been applied to all types of raised hemangiomas present in infancy. Some authors restrict the term to elevated capillary nevi with and without endothelial proliferation, but others include cavernous and mixed types. As a general rule, differentiation of the type of hemangioma by biopsy is of little value prognostically, nor is such a procedure always practical. It is helpful, however, to gauge the depth of the nevus clinically (i.e., whether the lesion is solely dermal or has a subcutaneous component), particularly if there is concern about involvement of underlying structures.

The classic strawberry hemangioma is a raised, circumscribed, soft and bright red tumor which is lobulated and compressible. When a subcutaneous component is present, the hemangioma consists of a bluish-red mass with less distinct borders. If the entire nevus is deeply situated the overlying skin may appear normal or show only a blue discoloration. The histologic pattern will depend on whether the angioma is purely capillary, cavernous or mixed in type.

Approximately 20 to 30 per cent of raised angiomatous nevi are present at birth, and roughly 90 per cent are evident by the second month of age (Simpson, 1959; Rook, 1968). The remainder have their onset between the second and ninth months of life. Girls are affected more often than boys. The developing hemangioma is preceded by a sharply demarcated pale area which is frequently recognizable in the newborn infant (Payne, 1966). These areas develop telangiectases that evolve into strawberry hemangiomas. The most common site of involvement is the face (Fig. 9–3); the back, scalp and anterior chest are the next most frequently affected areas (Simpson, 1959; Bowers 1966). The majority of infants have a single lesion; however, multiple tumors are not unusual.

Virtually all of these lesions show some increase in size during the first six months of

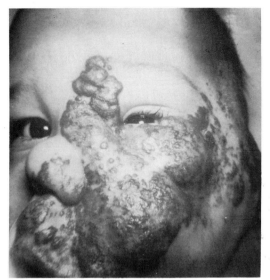

Figure 9–3. Massive cavernous hemangioma of the face. (Courtesy of Dr. Alan Lasser.)

life, often with initial rapid growth (Fig. 9–4). The phase of active expansion, particularly in larger nevi, may result in ulceration which is usually of little consequence unless complicated by severe secondary infection or hemorrhage.

If left untreated most hemangiomas in this group will involute spontaneously. Regression may be anticipated when pale gray areas appear on the previously bright red surface of the lesion (Fig. 9–5). This change is followed by further blanching and fibrosis, as well as flattening and softening of the entire area (Plate VIII–B). Hemangiomas may involute in infancy or take up to seven years to regress completely; rarely, resolution has been noted even in adolescence. Approximately 50 per cent disappear by age five and

70 per cent by age seven (Simpson, 1959; Bowers, 1960). Rapidity and completeness of resolution seem unrelated to the size of the lesion or age of appearance. In some patients there are no residual skin changes; others show redundant skin and variable degrees of atrophy and telangiectasia following involution of the hemangioma. Lesions that ulcerate tend to scar, and may therefore eventuate in a poorer cosmetic result. Plastic procedures can be performed to correct residual deformity.

Profuse hemorrhage is rare unless there is an accompanying thrombocytopenia or coagulation defect. Minor degrees of hemorrhage can usually be managed by compression bandages, and secondary infection controlled by application of warm wet compresses, followed by a topical antibiotic preparation. Severe or extensive infection may require systemic antibiotic therapy; choice of antibiotic should be determined by the organism obtained on bacterial culture.

Knowledge of the course of these lesions has led most physicians to follow an expectant rather than an aggressive approach to therapy. The vast majority of patients with strawberry hemangiomas require no treatment other than careful follow-up to detect possible complications. Routine measurements of lesions and documentation by serial photographs help to provide much needed reassurance to parents. Under certain circumstances, however, intervention may be indicated. Such circumstances include rapid growth of a lesion which compromises a vital structure or results in marked tissue destruction and associated symptomatic thrombocytopenia.

Figure 9–4. Cavernous hemangioma. (Courtesy of Dr. Alan Lasser.)

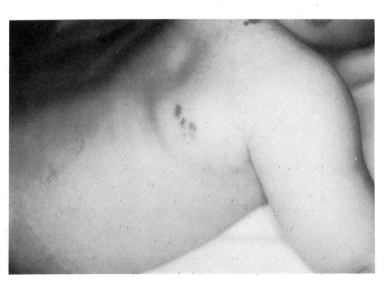

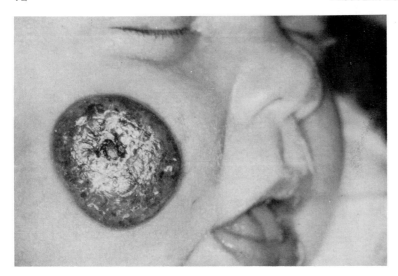

Figure 9–5. Cavernous hemangioma with central necrosis.

Therapeutic modalities include irradiation, injection of sclerosing solutions, application of solid carbon dioxide, surgical excision and systemically administered corticosteroids. All types of therapy have disadvantages. Small doses of X–ray will reduce the size of rapidly expanding lesions but may cause damage to epiphyses, breasts, gonads, eyes, skin and thyroid (Lampe, 1959). Sclerosing solutions and solid carbon dioxide may cause considerable scarring and atrophy, and the method of administration is painful. Surgical excision may offer the best means of approach in selected cases with well-circumscribed lesions, but an acceptable cosmetic result is not always achieved.

A short, intensive course of orally administered corticosteroids may be effective in young infants if radical therapy seems warranted (Fost, 1968; Zarem, 1967; Hiles, 1971; Brown, 1972). Dosages of up to 30 mg. daily of prednisone may be required to effect a response, but reduction in the size of the lesion should be evident after two to four weeks of therapy. The drug should be continued until the desired reduction in size is achieved. Rebound growth may occur after cessation of therapy and some infants have required more than one course (Fost, 1968; Hiles, 1971; Brown, 1972). Indications for trial of corticosteroid therapy include rapidly expanding lesions that interfere with vision, obstruct the nasal airway or ear canals, or involve the lips, parotid gland, breasts, perineal area of the vital structures in the neck. Because of the hazards of corticosteroid therapy such infants should be carefully selected, thoroughly evaluated for contraindications to steroid therapy and closely followed in a pediatric setting.

Kasabach-Merritt Syndrome

The association of thrombocytopenia with hemangiomas is a phenomenon most frequently seen in early infancy (Fig. 9–6). In one author's series of 72 cases culled from the literature and two of his own (Shim, 1968), the median age of hospital admission for this problem was five weeks. Most of the hemangiomas associated with thrombocytopenia are exceedingly large; however, it should be stressed that enormity of size is not an invariable requirement since several children with lesions as small as 5 to 6 cm have had confirmed thrombocytopenia (Shim, 1968; Kontras, 1963). Infants with rapidly expanding lesions should be checked frequently for incipient thrombocytopenia. When thrombocytopenia is present bleeding becomes a problem and the resultant anemia may be severe. Splenomegaly has also been noted in some patients.

The etiology of the thrombocytopenia is not unequivocally established. Most investigators favor sequestration of platelets in the hemangioma as the most important factor. In the Kasabach-Merritt syndrome, bone marrow preparations show increased megakaryocytes, so the low platelet counts may be a manifestation of increased platelet destruction. In studies with radioactively tagged platelets, Kontras and associates (1963) demonstrated trapping of platelets in the hemangioma and decreased platelet survival. Although absence of platelet thrombi in some extirpated hemangiomas has been interpreted as evidence against the platelet sequestration theory, it has been suggested that damaged and clumped platelets may be

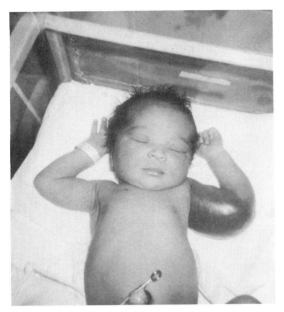

Figure 9–6. Kasabach-Merritt syndrome. (Courtesy of Dr. Ruth Seeler.)

rapidly removed from the hemangioma and phagocytosed in the reticuloendothelial system. An increased production of fibrinolytic enzymes within the hemangioma has also been postulated.

Multiple coagulation defects, in addition to thrombocytopenia, have also been reported in association with hemangiomas (Wacksman, 1966). These defects include deficiency of Factors II, V, and VII and hypofibrinogenemia.

In contrast to the infant with a hemangioma and normal hematologic findings, the infant with Kasabach-Merritt syndrome should be hospitalized and treated promptly. The emergence of petechiae or ecchymoses in the adjacent skin or overt bleeding is an indication for fresh blood or platelet-rich transfusions. Surgical extirpation of the lesion or a course of irradiation to the hemangioma usually results in alleviation of the thrombocytopenia. Splenectomy is not indicated and corticosteroid therapy has produced equivocal results (Dargeon, 1959; Shim, 1968). A few of these infants have recovered without treatment following spontaneous involution of the hemangioma.

Miscellaneous Syndromes

Capillary and cavernous hemangiomas also occur in the following uncommon syndromes:

Diffuse Neonatal Hemangiomatosis. (Dis-seminated hemangiomatosis; visceral hemangiomatosis). A number of infants have been reported with multiple hemangiomas in several visceral organs (Plates VIII–C and D). Some have had a myriad of small cutaneous lesions, most commonly in association with lesions of the gastrointestinal tract, liver, central nervous system and lungs, but others have had involvement of fewer organ systems. Nomenclature in this area has been confused, but *miliary hemangiomatosis* (Burman, 1967) has been the term most commonly used. However, as pointed out by Holden and Alexander (1970), *diffuse neonatal hemangiomatosis* may be a more accurate name since these infants may have only a few hemangiomas several centimeters in size. Although these authors suggest excluding infants with less than three affected organ systems from this group, it is important to realize that variability in both size of lesions and number of affected organs can occur.

An occasional infant with visceral hemangiomatosis (Fig. 9–8) has had no cutaneous involvement (Touloukian, 1970), a single lesion or a few large cutaneous lesions (Raphan, 1966), but most infants have had widely disseminated, small, red to blue-black papular cutaneous hemangiomas numbering in the hundreds (Fig. 9–7). These lesions are usually apparent at birth or develop during the first few weeks of life. A profusion of cutaneous angiomas should therefore alert the physician to the possible existence of visceral lesions. In a few infants with this pattern of cutaneous hemangiomatosis, involvement of internal organs has not been detected by either physical examination or laboratory studies.

Despite supportive therapy, affected infants often die early in life from intractable high output cardiac failure, gastrointestinal hemorrhage, respiratory tract obstruction or severe central neurological deficit due to extensive compression of neural tissue (Holden, 1970). Corticosteroid therapy may be effective in these patients (Brown, 1972) and should be given an adequate trial. A few have survived to experience spontaneous regression of the hemangiomas (Burke, 1964), but these infants seem to have had involvement of fewer organ systems.

Blue Rubber Bleb Nevus Syndrome. This rare disorder consists of multiple cavernous hemangiomas of the skin and bowel (Bean, 1958; Fretzin, 1965). In this syndrome, cutaneous lesions are sometimes present at birth, and their appearance is char-

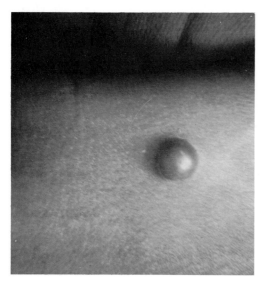

Figure 9–7. Visceral hemangiomatosis. One of the dome-shaped cutaneous hemangiomas. (Courtesy of Dr. Ruth Seeler.)

acteristic, as the name strikingly suggests. The lesions are blue to purple, rubbery, compressible protuberances varying in size from a few millimeters to 3 to 4 centimeters in diameter. Some lie deep in the skin, appearing as irregular blue marks, while others are thin-walled sacs filled with liquid (blood and thrombi) which may be partially emptied on pressure. A few lesions may be pedunculated. The lesions are diffusely spread over the body surface and mucous membranes, and may be sparse or number in the hundreds. The lesions are often spontaneously painful

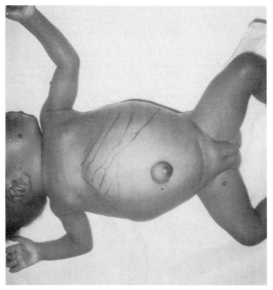

Figure 9–8. Visceral hemangiomatosis. The hepatosplenomegaly is outlined. (Courtesy of Dr. Ruth Seeler.)

or tender to palpation and may sweat excessively.

Angiomas are commonly found in the small bowel but the colon may also be involved. Occasional ectasias have been found in the liver, spleen and central nervous system. Neither the skin nor bowel lesions regress spontaneously. Severe anemia may result from recurrent episodes of gastrointestinal bleeding. Surgery is sometimes palliative, but it may be impossible to resect all the affected bowel.

Riley-Smith Syndrome. Macrocephaly, pseudopapilledema and multiple cavernous hemangiomas, presumably of autosomal dominant transmission, were documented by Riley (1960) in a mother and four of her seven children. The nodules, initially skin-colored, were noted at birth or up to five years of age. These lesions gradually increased in size and became bluish in color. The hemangiomas were troublesome because they bled following trauma or caused disability due to their large size.

Cavernous hemangiomas have been reported as a variable feature of *Leroy's syndrome,* or I-cell disease (Smith, 1970). *Maffucci's syndrome* (cavernous hemangiomas and dyschondroplasia) and *Gorham's disease* (cavernous hemangiomas and disappearing bones) are not usually apparent in the neonatal period (Bean, 1958; Frost, 1965).

CUTIS MARMORATA TELANGIECTATICA CONGENITA

(Congenital generalized phlebectasia)

This disorder is apparent at birth and characterized by the presence of a reddish-blue cutaneous reticulation (Plate IX–A, page 89). Superficially, the lesions resemble the physiologic cutis marmorata seen in normal infants (see Chap. 6), but are much more vivid and often restricted to a single extremity or limited portions of the trunk. Involvement may be segmental with a sharp midline demarcation between normal and abnormal skin. Marbling becomes particularly intense with crying or change in environmental temperature. In some infants the subcutaneous tissue appears to be underdeveloped, and ulcerations over the reticulated bands are a prominent feature in the neonatal period (Mayer, 1966). Telangiectatic capillary nevi may also be present (Petrozzi, 1970), and a rare patient has had defective growth of the long bones and soft tissues underlying a lesion (Fitzsimmons, 1970). Usually no other abnormalities are associated, although congenital glaucoma and mental retardation were noted in one case (Petrozzi, 1970).

The histopathologic features of the reported cases have varied. Some of the cutaneous sections have shown normal architecture, others had dilated, mature-looking vessels in the dermis and subcutaneous tissue and one ultrastructural study demonstrated dilatation of the normal capillary system of the skin (Lynch, 1967). The disorder is usually regarded as a vascular ectasia involving both capillaries and veins. The usual course is one of steady improvement, although a few patients have persistence of the cutaneous marbling into adulthood.

FAMILIAL ANNULAR ERYTHEMA

This rare syndrome, described in three generations of an Irish family (Beare, 1966), appears to be inherited in an autosomal dominant fashion. The affected patients developed an eruption on the skin and oral mucous membranes in the neonatal period (Plate IX–B). The initial lesion was a pruritic urticarial wheal which enlarged, cleared centrally and resolved, leaving a transient brown discoloration (Fig. 9–9). Vesiculation and scaling were absent but dermographism was a prominent feature. A single lesion evolved over four to five days. Lesions were ubiquitous in distribution and showed no cyclical character or periodicity. Remissions occasionally lasted for several weeks. The patients were found to be otherwise healthy and had no consistent abnormal laboratory findings, although alterations in serum globulin levels had been noted on occasion. His-

topathological examination of the skin showed perivascular inflammation in the dermis, possibly related to changes in the small vessels. No treatment is known to be effective in altering the condition.

ERYTHEMA GYRATUM PERSTANS

This disorder, another uncommon figurate erythema, has rarely been observed in early infancy. Lesions are symmetrical, confined mainly to the trunk, and are severely pruritic. Initially an erythematous papule, the typical lesion rapidly evolves to form gyrate erythematous rings with a ragged, scaly cuticular fringe. Vesiculation is an inconstant feature. The eruption is apparently aggravated by stressful stimuli. The course is chronic with rare remissions. Biopsy shows hyperkeratosis, focal parakeratosis, hypertrophy of the epidermis with intracellular edema and vacuolization of the epidermal cells, marked edema of the papillary dermis and a mixed cellular infiltrate. Differential diagnosis includes familial annular erythema, erythema annulare centrifugum and erythrokeratoderma variabilis (see Chap. 11). The etiology of erythema gyratum perstans is unknown and no treatment is suggested.

ERYTHEMA ANNULARE CENTRIFUGUM

Although not uncommon in the adult, erythema annulare centrifugum has been reported in only one newborn infant (Fried, 1957). The lesions were generalized, except for the palms and soles, and consisted of nonpruritic, raised red rings with minimally

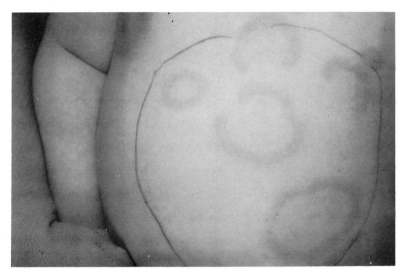

Figure 9–9. Familial annular erythema. (Courtesy of Dr. J. Martin Beare)

scaling borders that became scalloped and gyrate as the lesions migrated, broke up and reformed. The etiology is unknown.

PERIARTERITIS NODOSA
(Polyarteritis nodosa)

Vasculitis is a rare occurrence in early infancy but a few such patients have been reported (Wilmer, 1945; Fager, 1951). The clinical signs and symptoms are determined by the location and size of the arterial lesions and by the particular organ systems involved. Skin lesions occur in 25 to 50 per cent of cases and are quite variable in morphology. Diffuse erythema, urticaria, Raynaud's phenomenon, purpura and focal gangrene are common manifestations, but macules, papules, vesico-pustules and even bullous lesions have been described. Hemorrhagic blisters may become necrotic and eventuate in punched-out ulcers.

The classic cutaneous lesions of periarteritis nodosa are subcutaneous nodules that occur in crops along the course of the superficial arteries of the trunk and extremities. They vary in size from 0.5 to 1.5 cm, are tender on palpation and are usually red to purple in color. Nodules persist for days or months, may ulcerate and scar or disappear

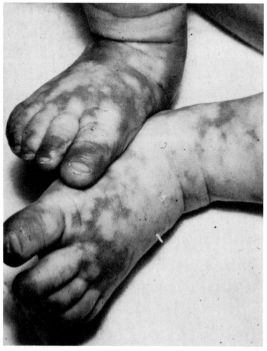

Figure 9–10. Vasculitis. (Courtesy of Dr. Mark A. Everett)

spontaneously leaving normal skin, depending on the degree of necrosis produced. Livido reticularis is also commonly associated with periarteritis nodosa, both the systemic type and the benign variety known as cutaneous polyarteritis nodosa. Boren (1965) described an affected infant of a mother with cutaneous periarteritis nodosa. Reticulated erythema, ecchymoses and gangrene of the infant's digits were noted in the first week of life, but all these lesions gradually resolved (Fig. 9–10).

Histologically, the cutaneous lesions are characterized by a necrotizing arteritis with fibrinoid necrosis of the media, endothelial proliferation and infiltration of the vessel wall, predominantly with polymorphonuclear leukocytes. Systemic symptoms and alteration of laboratory values directly relate to involvement of specific organ systems such as kidney, lungs, central nervous system, cardiovascular system, muscle, joints, gastrointestinal tract, eye and bone. Extensive investigations are usually required if periarteritis is suspected. Systemic corticosteroids are the treatment of choice.

Multiple Glomus Tumors. Glomus tumors are encapsulated tumors of the glomus tissue (neurovascular shunt organ) which surrounds many small blood vessels. Two types of tumors are recognized: Single, painful lesions appearing sporadically in adults; and multiple, painless lesions occurring in several members of a family.

The second type may be found in the newborn infant, particularly on the plantar surface. The lesions gradually increase in number, resulting in racemose hemangiomata which may involve the limbs, chest and back. The condition is probably inherited as an autosomal dominant gene (Conant, 1971). Histologically, the lesions consist of vascular spaces lined by a double layer of polygonal endothelial cells. Conspicuous or troublesome lesions may be excised.

Juvenile Benign Hemangioendothelioma. This very rare lesion appears at birth or very soon thereafter, and usually is located on the scalp. It looks and feels like a hard nodular hemangioma several centimeters in diameter. The tumor tends to grow and become highly invasive, involving subcutaneous tissue. Radiotherapy or excision is the treatment of choice. The benign nature of the lesion is due to its orderly histologic features and its positive response to therapy. The tumor has a relatively good prognosis (Domonkos, 1971).

DISORDERS OF THE LYMPHATIC VESSELS

Lymphangiomas (Kittredge, 1965) are hamartomatous malformations composed of dilated lymph channels that are lined by a flat or cuboidal lymphatic endothelium. They may be superficial or subcutaneous and are often associated with anomalies of the regional lymphatic vessels. Involvement of underlying muscle can occur. The tumors are generally slow growing and their appearance is often a reflection of the size, depth and site of involvement. The following types of tumors may occur in the neonatal period.

LYMPHANGIOMA CIRCUMSCRIPTUM

This is probably the most common type of lymphangioma and may be present at birth or appear in early childhood (Peachey, 1970). Areas of predilection are the oral mucosa, the proximal limbs, the axillary folds and the perineum. The tumor consists of small, clustered, thick-walled vesicles resembling frog spawn; the lesions are often skin-colored but, in some instances, have a blue cast due to a hemangiomatous component (Plate IX–C). At times the surface may become verrucous. Usually these lesions are located superficially, but some are associated with anomalies of the larger regional lymphatic vessels. On biopsy, dilated cystic lymph vessels lined by a single layer of endothelium are seen in the dermis. The lesions may be excised; however, the removal of large lesions may leave defects requiring full-thickness skin grafts, and even within the grafted area the lymphangioma may recur.

SIMPLE LYMPHANGIOMAS

The simple lymphangioma occurs in infancy as a solitary, circumscribed and skin-colored dermal or subcutaneous nodule. Such tumors may also occur in the mucous membranes. Occasionally, extensive deep lymphatic involvement has been found in association. These tumors either remain inactive or slowly increase in size. Following trauma a chronic serous exudate may ensue. Uncomplicated lesions can be removed by simple excision.

CAVERNOUS LYMPHANGIOMA

The cavernous lymphangioma is a diffuse, soft tissue mass consisting of large cystic dilatations of lymphatic vessels in the dermis, subcutaneous tissue and intermuscular septa (Fig. 9–11). Clinically, these lesions are ill-defined and often involve large areas of the face, trunk and extremities (Raphan, 1966). Macroglossia and macrocheilia result from involvement of the oral structures. Treatment is unsatisfactory since surgery is impractical in most cases.

CYSTIC HYGROMA

Cystic hygroma (Fig. 9–12) is a benign, multiloculated tumor usually found in the neck region (Fig. 9–13), but also occasionally seen in the axilla, groin or popliteal fossa. These tumors tend to increase in size rapidly and should be treated by surgical excision, even though extirpation may necessarily be incomplete.

LYMPHEDEMA

Primary, noninflammatory lymphedema can be congenital or of late onset. Females are more frequently affected than males, and the lower limbs are the sites of predilection, although the upper extremities, genitalia and face may also be involved (Kinmouth, 1957). Associated anomalies of the vascular system are occasionally present and, rarely, chylothorax and chylous ascites result from abnormalities of the parietal and visceral lymphatics in the chest and abdomen (McKendry, 1957). The most frequent complication is sec-

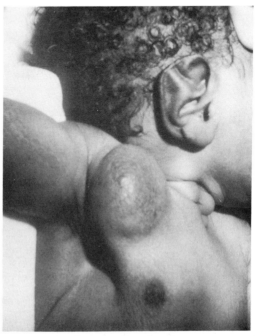

Figure 9–11. Cavernous lymphangioma. (Courtesy of Drs. David Fisher and John Paton.)

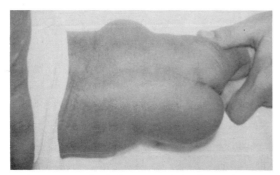

Figure 9–12. Cystic hygroma of the flank. (Courtesy of Dr. Ruth Seeler.)

ondary infection usually due to streptococci or *Staphylococcus aureus*.

The affected patients have a brawny edema of the involved tissues that will, at first, partially respond to elevation, pressure bandages and diuretics. Lymphatic dysfunction is progressive and becomes permanent as fibrosis of the tissues becomes more marked. Lymphangiography and dye screening tests demonstrate either hypoplasia, dilatation and tortuosity of the lymphatics, or less commonly, aplasia of the lymphatic vessels (Kinmouth, 1957). Some of the symptoms may be palliated by reconstructive surgery. Occasionally, lymphedema may be a manifestation of a congenital arteriovenous fistula, probably as the result of combined high venous pressure and external vascular pressure on the terminal lymph channels (O Beirn, 1965).

MILROY'S DISEASE
(Congenital hereditary lymphedema)

Milroy's disease, in contrast to sporadic congenital lymphedema, is a familial disorder with autosomal dominant transmission and is

almost always confined to the legs and feet (Schroeder, 1950). Rarely, the genitalia or hands may be involved (Esterly, 1965). The edema is apparent at birth and, although it becomes more persistent and severe with aging, it remains compatible with good health and normal activity. Affected limbs are firm, but easily pitted, and are covered by a relatively normal looking integument; verrucous changes, most commonly seen on the dorsum of the feet and toes, are a phenomenon of long standing edema and are virtually never seen in early childhood (Fig. 9–14). Skin temperature in the areas of edema is elevated (Schroeder, 1950). These patients have normal serum proteins and renal function studies.

The pathogenesis of Milroy's disease is unclear since studies of the lymphatics have not been performed routinely in these patients. The results of the few investigations which have been attempted are suggestive of hypoplasia or aplasia of the lymphatic vessels because they cannot be seen after injection with dye. Increased numbers of grouped arteriolar structures have been observed in the deep dermis on biopsy, but this vascular proliferation may represent a secondary, rather than primary event. Treatment is relatively ineffective.

HEREDITARY LYMPHEDEMA AND OBSTRUCTIVE JAUNDICE

A familial disorder characterized by chronic recurrent obstructive jaundice, anomalies of the lymphatic system and cutaneous hemangiomas has been described (Sharp, 1971; Cassady, 1964). Affected patients present in the neonatal period with severe

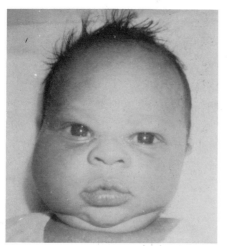

Figure 9–13. Cystic hygroma. (Courtesy of Dr. Ruth Seeler.)

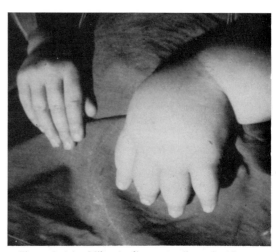

Figure 9–14. Milroy's disease (unilateral). (Courtesy of Dr. Hermine Pashayan.)

pruritus, jaundice and edema of the lower extremities. Giant cell transformation, bile stasis, minimal bile duct proliferation and portal fibrosis are apparent on liver biopsy. Lymphangiograms and dye screening tests of the lower extremities show hypoplasia of the lymphatics, abnormal tortuosity of the larger vessels, dermal backflow and delayed clearing of the contrast material (Sharp, 1971). In some families the edema does not develop until early childhood (Aagenaes, 1970). The lymphedema is progressive and may ascend to involve the genitalia. In the early stages elevation of the legs and diuretics may provide some relief, but surgical procedures may be required for more effective management.

PURPURA

At almost any age the appearance of purpuric lesions is a worrisome event and a diagnostic challenge. In the adult, and particularly in the aged, bleeding into the skin is characteristic of several primary skin disorders which may remain benign and self-limited. This is not true in the neonatal period. Apart from petechiae and ecchymoses due to vascular damage from trauma, the presence of purpura constitutes an emergent situation and should alert the physician to begin an immediate search for the underlying disorder.

Some possible causes of purpura in the immediate newborn period are listed in Table 9–1 (Oski, 1966). It is important to recognize that purpura in the newborn infant is a nonspecific cutaneous finding attributable to numerous pathogenetic mechanisms. Unless it is nonprogressive and directly related to trauma, a careful physical examination and laboratory investigations are always warranted. It should also be noted that a history of birth trauma does not preclude the presence of a coagulation defect or platelet disorder.

The investigation of any infant with purpura requires an evaluation of the mother, including a history of maternal bleeding, a family history of bleeding disorders, drug ingestion, exposure to or symptoms of infectious diseases, hematologic and serologic evaluation. On examination of the infant the presence of organomegaly and congenital anomalies should be carefully noted, as they may be a clue to the etiology of the bleeding. Hematologic studies should include a hemoglobin, hematocrit, white blood count, platelet count, smear and bone marrow examination. Coagulation tests and serologic tests for

Table 9–1. Some Causes of Neonatal Purpura*

1. *Infections:*
    Syphilis
    Cytomegalic inclusion disease
    Rubella syndrome
    Disseminated herpes simplex
    Congenital toxoplasmosis
    Septicemia, particularly from gram-negative
      bacillary organisms
2. *Giant hemangioma with thrombocytopenia*
   (Kasabach-Merrit syndrome)
3. *Congenital leukemia*
4. *Congenital Letterer-Siwe disease*
5. *Immune disorders*
    Passively transferred from mothers
      Idiopathic thrombocytopenic purpura
      Drug-induced thrombocytopenia
      Systemic lupus erythematosus with thrombocytopenia
    Active
      Isoimmune thrombocytopenic purpura
      Erythroblastosis fetalis
6. *Maternal drug ingestion pre-partum — thiazide diuretics*
7. *Congenital megakaryocytic hypoplasia*
    Congenital hypoplastic thrombocytopenia
    Amegakaryocytic thrombocytopenia with
      bilateral absence of the radii
8. *Inherited thrombocytopenias*
    Wiskott-Aldrich syndrome
    Autosomal thrombocytopenia
9. *Coagulation defects*
    Hereditary coagulation disorders
    Hemorrhagic disease of the newborn
      (vitamin K deficiency)
    Secondary hemorrhagic disease

*Adapted from Oski and Naiman, *Hematologic Problems in the Newborn.* 1st Ed., W. B. Saunders Co., 1966.

platelet antibodies and syphilis are indicated. The laboratory studies useful in the diagnosis of infectious diseases are considered in Chapter 14. A skin biopsy is helpful in confirming a possible diagnosis of Letterer-Siwe disease.

REFERENCES

Aagenaes, O., Sigstad, H. and Bjørn-Hansen, R.: Lymphedema in hereditary recurrent cholestasis from birth. Arch. Dis. Child. *45*:690, 1970.

Bean, W. B.: Vascular Disorders and Related Lesions of the Skin. Springfield, Ill., Charles C Thomas, 1958.

Beare, J. M., Froggatt, P., Jones, J. H. and Neill, D. W.: Familial annular erythema. Brit. J. Derm. *78*:59, 1966.

Boren, R. J. and Everett, M. A.: Cutaneous vasculitis in mother and infant. Arch. Derm. *92*:568, 1965.

Bowers, R. E., Graham, E. A. and Tomlinson, K. M.: The natural history of the strawberry nevus. Arch. Derm. *82*:667, 1960.

Brown, S. H., Jr., Neerhout, R. C., and Fonkalsrud, E. W.: Prednisone therapy in the management of large hemangiomas in infants and children. Surgery, *71*:168, 1972.

Burke, E. C., Winkelmann, R. K. and Strickland, M. K.: Disseminated hemangiomatosis. Amer. J. Dis. Child. *108*:418, 1964.

Burman, D., Mansell, P. W. A. and Warin, R. P.: Miliary haemangiomata in the newborn. Arch. Dis. Child. *42*:193, 1967.

Cassady, G., Morrison, A. B. and Cohen, M. M.: Familial "giant-cell hepatitis" in infancy. Amer. J. Dis. Child. *107*:456, 1964.

Chao, D. H.-C.: Congenital neurocutaneous syndromes of childhood. III. Sturge-Weber disease. J. Pediat. *56*:635, 1959.

Conant, M. A. and Wiesenfeld, S. L.: Multiple glomus tumors of the skin. Arch. Derm. *103*:481, 1971.

Dargeon, H. W., Adino, A. C. and Pack, G. T.: Hemangioma with thrombocytopenia. J. Pediat. *54*:285, 1959.

Domonkos, A. N.: Andrews' Diseases of the Skin. 6th Ed. Philadelphia, W. B. Saunders Co., 1971, pp. 708–709.

Donsky, H.: Vascular tumours of the skin. Canad. Med. Ass. J. *99*:993, 1968.

Esterly, J. R.: Congenital hereditary lymphoedema. J. Med. Genet. *2*:93, 1965.

Fager, D. B., Bigler, J. A. and Simonds, J. P.: Polyarteritis nodosa in infancy and childhood. J. Pediat. *39*:65, 1951.

Fitzsimmons, J. S. and Starks, M.: Cutis marmorata telangiectatica congenita or congenital generalized phlebectasia. Arch. Dis. Child. *45*:724, 1970.

Fost, N. C. and Esterly, N. B.: Successful treatment of juvenile hemangiomas with prednisone. J. Pediat. *72*:351, 1968.

Fretzin, D. F. and Potter, B.: Blue rubber bleb nevus. Arch. Intern. Med. *116*:924, 1965.

Fried, R., Schonberg, I. L. and Litt, J. Z.: Erythema annulare centrifugum (Darier) in a newborn infant. J. Pediat. *50*:66, 1957.

Frost, J. F. and Caplan, R. M.: Cutaneous hemangioma and disappearing bones. Arch. Derm. *92*:501, 1965.

Hermann, J., Feingold, M., Tuffli, G. A. and Opitz, J. M.: A familial dysmorphogenetic syndrome of limb deformities, characteristic facial appearance and associated anomalies: The "pseudothalidomide or SC-syndrome." *In* Birth Defects. Original Article Series. Vol. 5, No. 3, 1969, p. 81.

Hiles, D. A. and Pilchard, W. A.: Corticosteroid control of neonatal hemangiomas of the orbit and ocular adnexa. Amer. J. Ophthal. *71*:1003, 1971.

Holden, K. R. and Alexander, F.: Diffuse neonatal hemangiomatosis. Pediat. *46*:411, 1970.

Kinmouth, J. B., Taylor, G. W., Tracy, G. D. and Marsh, J. P.: Primary lymphoedema: Clinical and lymphangiographic studies of a series of 107 patients in which the lower limbs were affected. Brit. J. Surg. *45*:1, 1957.

Kittredge, R. D. and Finby, N.: The many facets of lymphangiomas. Amer. J. Roent. *95*:56, 1965.

Klaber, R.: Erythema gyratum perstans (Colcott Fox): A case report with discussion on relations with erythema centrifugum annulare (Darier) and dermatitis herpetiformis. Brit. J. Derm. *58*:111, 1946.

Kontras, S. B., Green, O. C., King, L. and Duran, R. J.: Giant hemangioma with thrombocytopenia. Amer. J. Dis. Child. *105*:188, 1963.

Lampe, I. and Latourette, H. B.: Management of cavernous hemangiomas in infants. Pediat. Clin. N. Amer. *6*:511, 1959.

Lynch, P. J. and Zelickson, A. S.: Congenital phlebectasia. Arch. Derm. *95*:98, 1967.

Mayer, D. G.: Cutis marmorata telangiectatica congenita. Arch. Derm. *93*:583, 1966.

McKendry, J. B. J., Lindsay, W. K. and Gerstein, M. C.: Congenital defects of the lymphatics in infancy. Pediatrics *19*:21, 1957.

Mullins, J. F., Naylor, D. and Redetski, J.: The Klippel-Trenaunay-Weber syndrome. Arch. Derm. *86*:202, 1962.

O Beirn, S. F.: A large solitary congenital arteriovenous fistula presenting as lymphoedema. Brit. J. Surg. *52*:358, 1965.

Oski, F. A. and Naiman, J. L.: Hematologic Problems in the Newborn. 1st ed. Philadelphia, W. B. Saunders Co., 1966.

Paillas, J. E. et al.: Encephalo-retinal facial angioma. Rev. Neurol. *101*:698, 1959.

Payne, M. M., Moyer, F., Marcks, K. M. and Trevaskis, A. E.: The precursor to the hemangioma. Plast. and Reconstr. Surg. *38*:64, 1966.

Peachy, R. D. G., Lim, C. C. and Whimster, J. W.: Lymphangioma of skin. A review of 65 cases. Brit. J. Derm. *83*:519, 1970.

Peterman, A. F., Hayles, A. B., Dockerty, M. B. and Love, J. G.: Encephalotrigeminal angiomatosis (Sturge-Weber disease) J.A.M.A. *167*:2169, 1958.

Petrozzi, J. W., Rahn, E. K., Mofensen, H. and Greensher, J.: Cutis marmorata telangiectatica congenita. Arch. Derm. *101*:73, 1970.

Raphan, W.: Multiple Hemangiomas of the skin, liver and intestinal tract. Helvet. Paediat. Acta *21*:56, 1966.

Riley, H. D., Jr. and Smith, W. R.: Macrocephaly, pseudopapilledema and multiple hemangiomata. Pediatrics *26*:293, 1960.

Rook, A., Wilkinson, D. S. and Ebling, F. J. G.: Textbook of Dermatology. Philadelphia, F. A. Davis Co., 1968.

Royle, H. E., Lapp, R. and Ferrara, E. D.: The Sturge-Weber syndrome. Oral Surg., Oral Med., Oral Path. *22*:490, 1966.

Schroder, E. and Helwig-Larsen, H. F.: Chronic hereditary lymphoedema (Nonne-Milroy-Meige s Disease). Acta Med. Scand. *137*:198, 1950.

Sharp, H. and Krivit, W.: Hereditary lymphedema and obstructive jaundice. J. Pediat. *78*:491, 1971.

Shim, W. K. T.: Hemangiomas of infancy complicated by thrombocytopenia. Amer. J. Surg. *116*:896, 1968.

Simpson, J. R.: Natural history of cavernous haemangiomata. Lancet *2*:1057, 1959.

Smith, D. W.: Recognizable Patterns of Human Malformation. Philadelphia, W. B. Saunders Co., 1970.

Touloukian, R. J.: Hepatic hemangioendothelioma during infancy: Pathology, diagnosis and treatment with prednisone. Pediatrics *45*:71, 1970.

Wacksman, S. J., Flessa, H. C., Glueck, H. I. and Will, J. J.: Coagulation defects and giant cavernous hemangioma. Amer. J. Dis. Child. *111*:71, 1966.

Wilmer, H. A.: Two cases of periarteritis nodosa occurring in the first month of life. Bull. Johns Hopkins Hosp. *77*:275, 1945.

Woerdeman, M. L.: Erythema gyratum perstans (Colcott Fox). Dermatologica *128*:392, 1964.

Wyburn-Mason, R.: Arteriovenous aneurism of midbrain and retina, facial nevi and mental changes. Brain *66*:163, 1943.

Zarem, H. A. and Edgerton, M. T.: Induced resolution of cavernous hemangiomas following prednisolone therapy. Plast. and Reconstr. Surg. *39*:76, 1967.

PLATE I

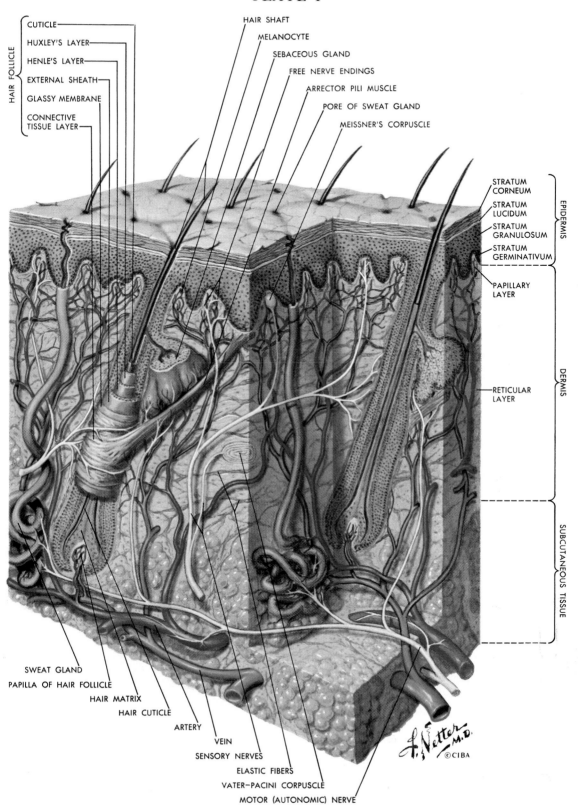

HAIR FOLLICLE
- CUTICLE
- HUXLEY'S LAYER
- HENLE'S LAYER
- EXTERNAL SHEATH
- GLASSY MEMBRANE
- CONNECTIVE TISSUE LAYER

HAIR SHAFT
MELANOCYTE
SEBACEOUS GLAND
FREE NERVE ENDINGS
ARRECTOR PILI MUSCLE
PORE OF SWEAT GLAND
MEISSNER'S CORPUSCLE

STRATUM CORNEUM
STRATUM LUCIDUM
STRATUM GRANULOSUM
STRATUM GERMINATIVUM
EPIDERMIS
PAPILLARY LAYER

RETICULAR LAYER
DERMIS

SUBCUTANEOUS TISSUE

SWEAT GLAND
PAPILLA OF HAIR FOLLICLE
HAIR MATRIX
HAIR CUTICLE
ARTERY
VEIN
SENSORY NERVES
ELASTIC FIBERS
VATER–PACINI CORPUSCLE
MOTOR (AUTONOMIC) NERVE

F. Netter, M.D.
©CIBA

Plate I. Cross section of skin. (From A. P. R. James: Common Dermatologic Disorders. CIBA Clinical Symposia. 19(2):38 [April–May–June], 1967.)

81

PLATE II

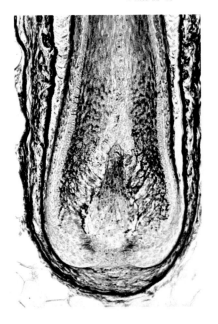

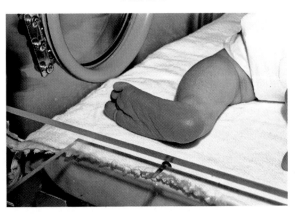

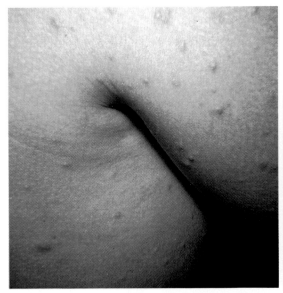

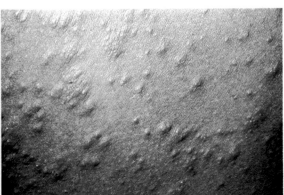

Plate II–A. Photomicrogaph of hair bulb. See also Figure 1–7, page 6. (Courtesy of Mr. A. C. Lonert.)
Plate II–B. Acrocyanosis. (Courtesy of Drs. David Fisher and John Paton.)
Plate II–C. Papules in a viral exanthem.
Plate II–D. Papules and vesicles (miliaria).

PLATE III

Plate III–A

Plate III–A

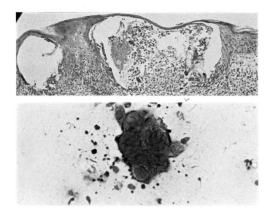

Plate III–B

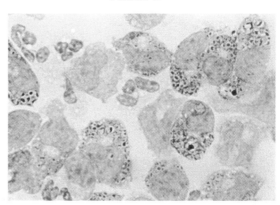

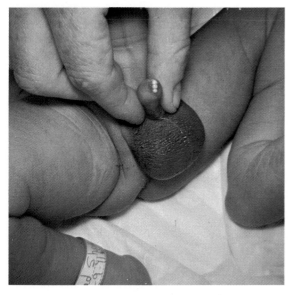

Plate III–C

Plate III–D

Plate III–A. Ballooning degeneration of the epidermal cells and the intraepidermal vesicle of Herpes simplex. (Courtesy of Merck Sharpe and Dohme.)

Plate III–B. Macrophages containing mucopolysaccharides. The cells were obtained using the skin window technique from a patient with Hurler's syndrome, (Giemsa Stain).

Plate III–C. Inclusion cysts of the penis.

Plate III–D. Sebaceous gland hyperplasia on the nose.

PLATE IV

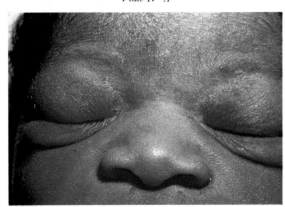
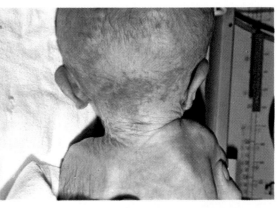
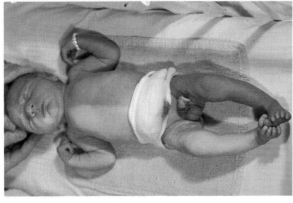
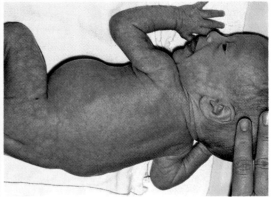
84

PLATE V

Plate V–B

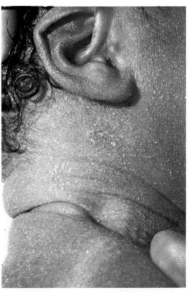

Plate V–A

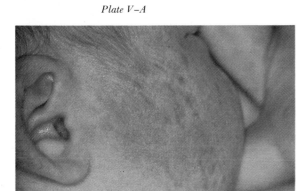

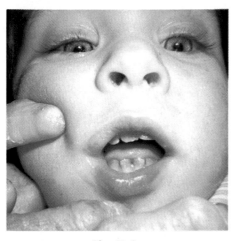

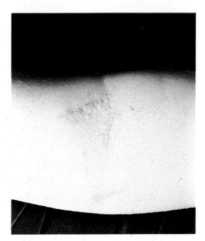

Plate V–C

Plate V–D

Plate V–A. Erythema toxicum.

Plate V–B. Miliaria crystallina.

Plate V–C. Pigmented teeth due to staining with porphyrins. This infant's teeth were stained by transplacental passage of porphyrins. He does not have porphyria.

Plate V–D. Epidermal nevus: small linear verrucous area.

PLATE VI

Plate VI–A

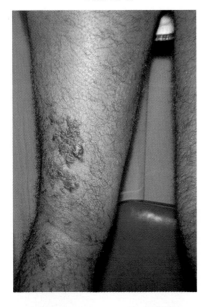

Plate VI–B

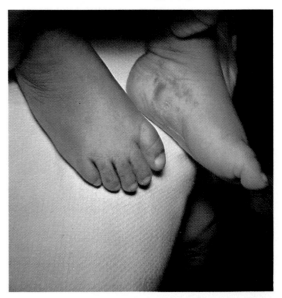

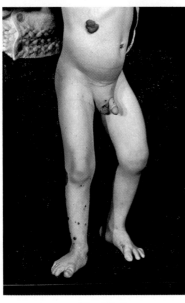

Plate VI–C

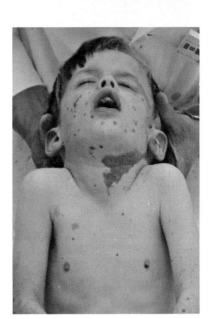

Plate VI–D

Plate VI–A. Epidermal nevus; verrucous hemangioma.

Plate VI–B. Epidermal nevus: benign congenital acanthosis nigricans.

Plate VI–C. The epidermal nevus syndrome. This patient has a verrucous nevus, pigmentary dysfunction, bony anomalies of the left hip, hypoplasia of the left side, and hemangiomas (right upper abdomen).

Plate VI–D. The epidermal nevus syndrome: verrucous linear nevi, multiple pigmentary anomalies including café-au-lait patches and vitiligo, left-sided hypoplasia and paresis, and hemangiomas.

PLATE VII

Plate VII–A

Plate VII–B

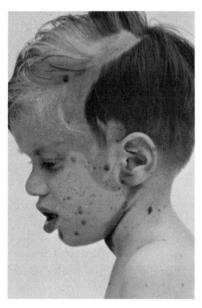

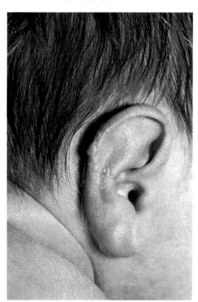

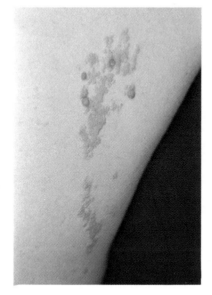

Plate VII–C

Plate VII–D

Plate VII–A. The epidermal nevus syndrome with large nevus sebaceous.
Plate VII–B. Small nevus sebaceous. (Courtesy of Drs. David Fisher and John Paton.)
Plate VII–C. Connective tissue nevus.
Plate VII–D. Nevus flammeus of the face.

PLATE VIII

Plate VIII–A

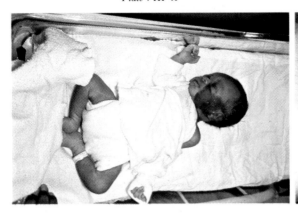

Plate VIII–B

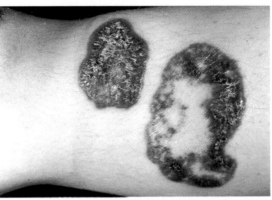

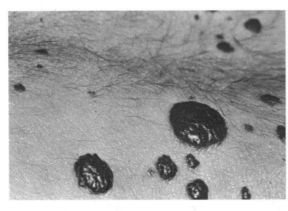

Plate VIII–C

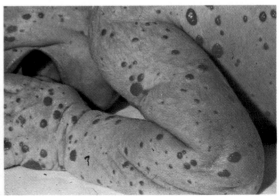

Plate VIII–D

Plate VIII–A. Nevus flammeus (port-wine stain). (Courtesy of Dr. Ruth Seeler.)
Plate VIII–B. Cavernous hemangioma undergoing involution.
Plate VIII–C. Disseminated hemangiomatosis. (Courtesy of Dr. James Ertle.)
Plate VIII–D. Disseminated hemangiomatosis. (Courtesy of Dr. James Ertle.)

PLATE IX

Plate IX–A

Plate IX–B

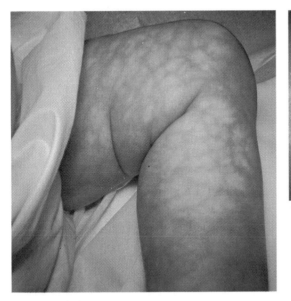

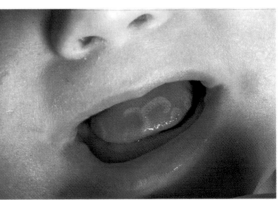

Plate IX–C

Plate IX–D

Plate IX–A.   Cutis marmorata telangiectata congenita.
Plate IX–B.   Familial annular erythema. (Courtesy of Dr. J. Martin Beare).
Plate IX–C.   Lymphangioma circumscriptum.
Plate IX–D.   Familial progressive hyperpigmentation. (Courtesy of Dr. Marvin Chernosky).

PLATE X

Plate X–A

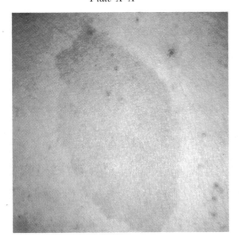

Plate X–B

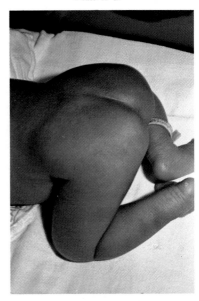

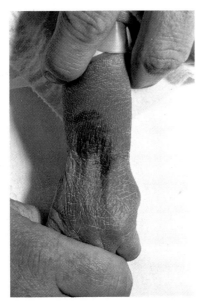

Plate X–C

Plate X–D

Plate X–A. Café-au-lait patch.
Plate X–B. Mongolian spot.
Plate X–C. Junction nevus.
Plate X–D. Incontinentia pigmenti (verrucous stage).

PLATE XI

Plate XI–A

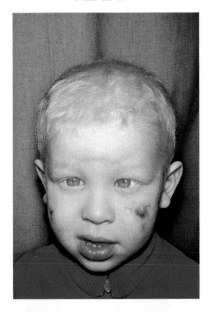

Plate XI–B

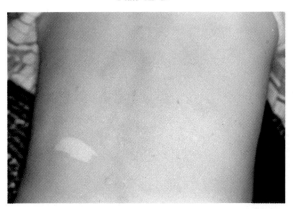

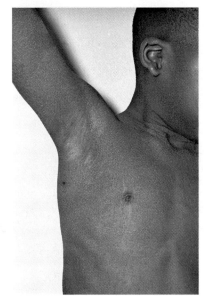

Plate XI–C

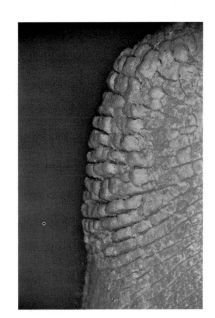

Plate XI–D

Plate XI–A. Albinism.
Plate XI–B. White macule and Shagreen patch (tuberous sclerosis).
Plate XI–C. X-linked ichthyosis. Axillae are spared.
Plate XI–D. Lamellar ichthyosis (non-bullous congenital ichthyosiform) of the knee.

PLATE XII

Plate XII–A

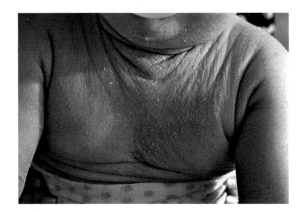

Plate XII–B

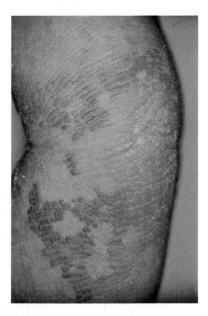

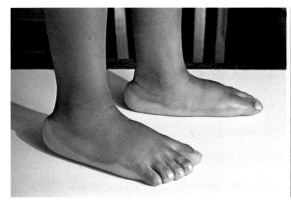

Plate XII–C

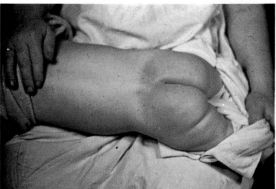

Plate XII–D

Plate XII–A.   Lamellar ichthyosis (non-bullous congenital ichthyosiform erythroderma).
Plate XII–B.   Bullous congenital ichthyosiform erythroderma.
Plate XII–C.   Hyperkeratosis of the soles (keratosis palmaris et plantaris).
Plate XII–D.   Early eczematous primary irritant diaper dermatitis.

PLATE XIII

Plate XIII–A

Plate XIII–B

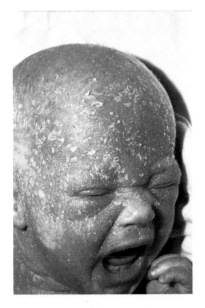

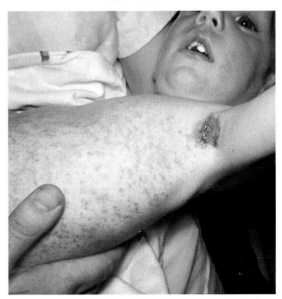

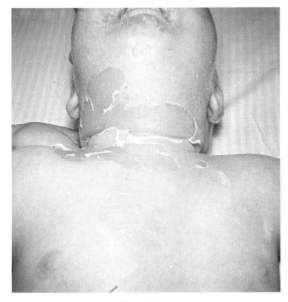

Plate XIII–C

Plate XIII–D

Plate XIII–A.   Leiner's disease.
Plate XIII–B.   Letterer-Siwe disease.
Plate XIII–C.   Toxic epidermal necrolysis (Lyell's syndrome, Ritter's disease).
Plate XIII–D.   Pseudomonas aeruginosa septicemia. (Courtesy of Dr. Ruth Seeler.)

PLATE XIV

Plate XIV–A

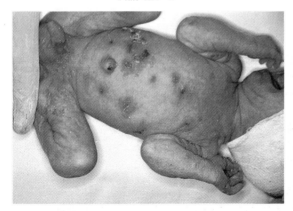

Plate XIV–B

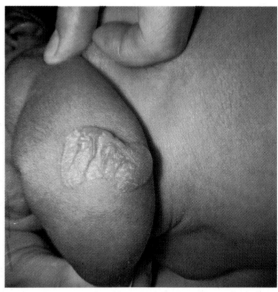

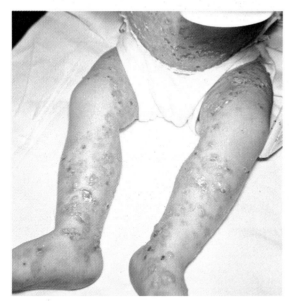

Plate XIV–C

Plate XIV–D

Plate XIV–A. Disseminated herpes simplex. (Courtesy of Dr. Robert J. Morgan.)
Plate XIV–B. Early blister of epidermolysis bullosa simplex (nonscarring, dominant).
Plate XIV–C. Dermatitis herpetiformis.
Plate XIV–D. Cytomegalic inclusion disease.

PLATE XV

Plate XV–A

Plate XV–B

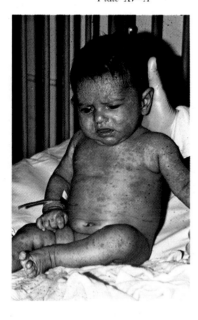

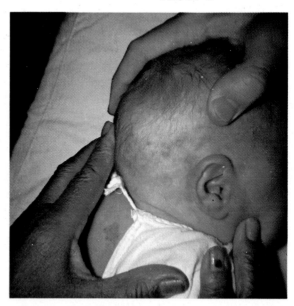

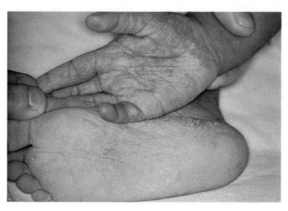

Plate XV–C

Plate XV–D

Plate XV–A. Congenital syphillis. Maculo-papular lesions. (Courtesy of Drs. David Fisher and John Paton.)
Plate XV–B. Lupus erythematosus. (Courtesy of Dr. David Fretzin.)
Plate XV–C. Letterer-Siwe disease.
Plate XV–D. Infantile acne. (Courtesy of Dr. David Fretzin.)

PLATE XVI

Plate XVI–A

Plate XVI–B

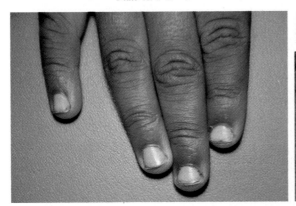

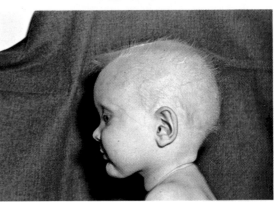

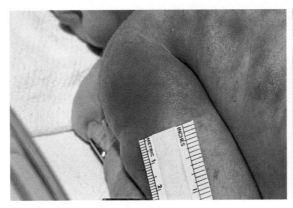

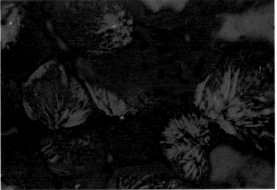

Plate XVI–C

Plate XVI–D

Plate XVI–A. Leukonychia. (Courtesy of Dr. David Fretzin.)
Plate XVI–B. Anhidrotic ectodermal dysplasia.
Plate XVI–C. Subcutaneous fat necrosis. (Courtesy of Dr. Ruth Seeler.)
Plate XVI–D. Anisotropic crystal formation in the affected area of subcutaneous fat necrosis. (Courtesy of Dr. David Fretzin.)

Chapter Ten

PIGMENTARY ABNORMALITIES

Melanin production normally is not at maximal function in the newborn skin. As a result, all babies, even Negro, Indian or Chinese, may look slightly tanned or red in color at birth. Within the first few weeks racial color becomes more evident because melanin production has been stimulated by exposure to light. For purposes of classification, it is useful to think of pathological pigmentary changes as diffuse or localized.

HYPERPIGMENTATION

Diffuse Hyperpigmentation

The intensity of cutaneous pigmentation must be considered in the light of the infant's genetic and racial background. What may be hyperpigmentation in one infant obviously may be normal for another. Diffuse hyperpigmentation in the newborn is a very unusual occurrence. It may be due to transplacental passage of therapeutic substances (e.g., androgens), a gene whose main effect is on the melanocyte, a hereditary disease with secondary pigmentary consequences, an endocrinopathy, a nutritional disorder or hepatic disease. In such cases, hyperpigmentation may be described as diffuse, but it may, in fact, be accentuated in certain areas such as the face, the genitalia, over the bony prominences or in the flexural creases (Fig. 10–1).

Melanism, an autosomal dominant disorder, is said to be "not uncommon" (Ebling, 1968). Melanism results in diffuse hyperpigmentation which is present at birth and increases until about five or six years of age. The face

and major body creases are affected and multiple melanocytic nevi may be found in association. *Familial progressive hyperpigmentation* (Plate IX–D, page 89) is a disorder very similar to melanism. Four members of a Negro

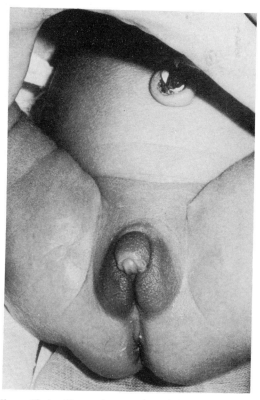

Figure 10–1. Hyperpigmentation of the perineum and clitoral hypertrophy resulting from androgen therapy during pregnancy.

family have recently been described with a spotty, progressive hyperpigmentation paralleled by an increase in the size and number of melanin granules in epidermal melanocytes (Chernosky, 1971).

Congenital Addison's disease may result from marked hypoplasia of the adrenal cortex, often secondary to pituitary aplasia (i.e., in anencephaly). The resulting lack of adrenal cortical hormones causes chronic weakness, anorexia, low blood pressure, wasting, salt loss and dehydration. The pigmentary changes in congenital Addison's disease consist of a diffuse increase in the normal coloring of the infant, although often less marked than in the adult, but seen in the same areas affected in the adult; that is, around nipples, genitalia, umbilicus, axillae, flexures, hands and buccal mucosa. The diagnosis is usually made by the discovery of associated findings. The hyperpigmentation of Addison's disease is due to an overproduction of β-melanocyte stimulating hormone (MSH) and ACTH so that primary pituitary failure mitigates the pigmentary changes (Fitzpatrick, 1971). It is interesting to note that vitiliginous spots may be found in association with Addison's disease. A similar progressive hyperpigmentation may also be seen in *hereditary adrenocortical unresponsiveness to ACTH* (Franks, 1970) and in *Fanconi's syndrome* (pancytopenia and multiple anomalies).

Both *pellagra* and *sprue* may give rise to a generalized or circumscribed intensification of pigmentation. These pellagrous changes may also occur in *Hartnup disease* (see Chap. 16) where a diffuse type of hyperpigmentation is most intense in light exposed areas. Rarely, the pigmentary changes in Hartnup disease may be seen in early infancy (Efron, 1971). Diagnosis of the specific deficiency is made from the patient's history and associated physical and laboratory findings.

Diffuse bronze discoloration of the skin may occur in a very early phase of *Niemann-Pick's disease* according to one author (Ebling, 1968), but another (Crocker, 1964) claims that the color changes are much overstated in the literature. Perhaps it should be noted here that the pigmentary changes seen in adult *Gaucher's disease* are not seen in the infantile form (Ebling, 1968). *Congenital biliary atresia, neonatal hepatitis* and other causes of intra- and extrahepatic cholestasis may give a bronze-green coloration to the skin due to bilirubin retention.

The authors have seen one child with a *monosomic G abnormality* whose cutaneous features included marked vascular lability as well as a diffuse bronze hyperpigmentation of the entire body.

Finally, *generalized hereditary lentiginosis,* inherited as an autosomal dominant trait, is characterized by numerous freckles which are present at birth and scattered over the entire body (or localized to one side). The disease is associated with nystagmus and mental retardation. Generalized lentiginosis has also been described as part of an hereditary syndrome which includes cardiac abnormalities, congenital deafness, oculomotor defects, granular cell myoblastomas and growth retardation (Moynahan, 1962; Caput, 1969; Gorlin, 1969; Clark, 1971; Selmanowitz, 1971). The freckles appear after the first year of life.

LOCALIZED HYPERPIGMENTATION: FLAT LESIONS

Café-au-Lait Spots. These may occasionally be seen in the newborn period. The lesions are flat, generally uniform in color, and vary from light brown in Caucasians to dark brown in Negroes (Plate X–A). Their significance varies with family history and associated systemic findings, as well as with size, shape and number of café-au-lait patches present. Single lesions under 3 cm in length and unassociated with a family history of neurofibromatosis are found in 19 per cent of normal children (Whitehouse, 1966). They have no special significance.

Neurofibromatosis (von Recklinghausen's multiple Neurofibromatosis). Neurofibromatosis (von Recklinghausen, 1886) has been known as an entity for almost a century, but the conspicuous aspects of the disorder had been known previous to that. In fact, Victor Hugo described its clinical features in Quasimodo, the hunchback of Notre Dame (Solomon, 1968). Hugo even imagined how the newborn babe with neurofibromatosis would appear (Hugo, 1831), but he simply described a miniature version of a fully developed adult case when, in fact, the only visible feature of the disease in the neonate may be single or multiple café-au-lait patches. These are usually 1.5 to 3 cm in length and greater than six in number. They occur bilaterally, and frequently are accompanied by symmetrical axillary, inguinal and nuchal freckling (Crowe, 1953). The pigmented lesions are occasionally present at birth, but more often appear later and increase in number with age, so that ultimately, 90 per cent of patients with neurofibromatosis have pigmented patches.

Neurofibromatosis occurs about once in every 3000 live births and is due to an autosomal dominant gene, although a positive family history is not always obtainable (possibly because of reduced penetrance and variable expressivity or because the patient represents a mutation). The clinical picture is that of early spotty hyperpigmentation, followed by the development of variable numbers of cutaneous and subcutaneous, soft, fleshy, unencapsulated tumors which appear in late childhood and adolescence. The tumors are usually asymptomatic and may also involve any internal organ, resulting in organomegaly. The expanding lesions may cause a wide array of symptoms, the most prominent of which are usually localized to the central or peripheral nervous system. Typically, the nervous system symptoms include eighth nerve syndromes (deafness, tinitus, dizziness and headache), trigeminal syndromes, deficits in the visual fields or spinal nerve root compression syndromes. A mild degree of mental retardation has been a frequent finding in those cases seeking help (Preston, 1952), but since minor variants of the disease may go unnoticed, this finding is probably not a prominent feature of the disease. Occasionally, huge, redundant, fleshy malformations may result from a massive neuroma deforming the face, a limb, the buttocks or thorax. These plexiform neuromas often also cause elephantiasis of the tissues in which they are found and may affect adjacent muscle and bone. Bony malformations in the form of cysts, scoliosis, hypertrophy, arciform bowing of the long bones, pseudarthroses and cranial defects are common (Holt, 1948). The oral cavity and teeth may also be involved. Five to 30 per cent of the cases of pheochromocytoma have been found in association with neurofibromatosis.

Histologically, the lesions demonstrate a marked accumulation of loose, unencapsulated whorled connective tissue, Schwann cells and some mast cells. There is a dearth of supporting collagen or elastic tissue in the lesions (Penfield, 1930). Recently, Fialkow et al. (1971) suggested that hereditary neurofibromas may result from the effect of a tumorigenic stimulus on cells at multiple foci. About 5 per cent of patients develop sarcomatous changes (Preston, 1952) in a peripheral tumor, and astrocytomas or glioblastomas in the central nervous system.

The management of an infant with café-au-lait pigmentation should include the following procedures: (1) the size, location and number of such lesions should be recorded; (2) a careful family and antecedent history should be obtained; (3) if there are less than three lesions and the family history is negative, no further action is required other than a bi-yearly examination for further lesions; (4) if the history is doubtful or positive, or if there are three or more lesions, then a biopsy of the skin is indicated for examination of the melanosomes by light and (where possible) by electron microscopy (see Albright's syndrome); (5) if the likelihood of neurofibromatosis exists, genetic counseling is indicated; (6) there is no reason to provide a dire prognosis for the affected infant since many patients have very minor forms of the disease; and, (7) yearly follow-up with complete physical examination is mandatory if neurofibromatosis exists.

Twenty-six per cent of those patients with *tuberous sclerosis* (see White Spots, page 106) also show café-au-lait spots (Hurwitz, 1970). The lesions of tuberous sclerosis are identical in appearance to those seen in neurofibromatosis, but very frequently are accompanied by leaf-shaped *white* macules.

Albright's Syndrome

In this syndrome the pigmented lesion is usually unilateral, elongated and large (more than 10 cm), with a ragged, irregular ("Coast of Maine") border (Fig. 10–2). Polyostatic fibrous dysplasia and endocrine dysfunction, resulting in sexual precocity in females, are associated with the pigmentary anomaly. The bony abnormalities may be unilateral or bilateral and result in "hockey stick" deformities of the femur and other long bones. Also affected are the pubis and skull (Gorlin, 1964). Endocrine changes, like bone changes, usually become apparent in the first decade, but vaginal bleeding may occur in the first month of life (Arlien-Soeborg, 1956). Pigmentary lesions have also been reported to occur (unusually) within the first few postnatal weeks. A possibly useful means of distinguishing the café-au-lait spot of neurofibromatosis from an insignificant lesion or the café-au-lait pigmentation of Albright's syndrome lies in the appearance of the melanosomes under the microscope (Johnson, 1970). When the epidermis of a melanotic plaque is incubated with DOPA, an increased number of melanocytes can be

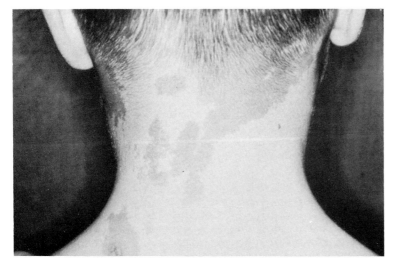

Figure 10–2. Albright's syndrome.

demonstrated (Johnson, 1971), but giant pigment granules are seen in melanocytes and keratinocytes from the affected areas in neurofibromatosis, and not in the café-au-lait spot of normal individuals or those of Albright's syndrome (Fitzpatrick, 1971).

Very large café-au-lait spots (hemithorax or more), associated with vitiliginous changes, vascular, bony and central nervous system abnormalities, as well as verrucous linear epidermal nevi (see Chap. 8), form part of the picture of the *epidermal nevus syndrome* (Solomon; 1968). Café-au-lait areas may also be seen on the skin of patients with *Silver's syndrome* (Vestermark, 1970).

Mongolian Spot, Nevus of Ota, Nevus of Ito. In Chapter six we discussed the common, ephemeral, dermal (spindle-shaped) melanocyte infiltrate which gives rise to Mongolian spot over the base of the spine and buttocks (Plate X–B). It has recently been shown in Japan (Hidano, 1971) that about 3 to 4 per cent of patients retain these spots in adult life. The natives of Samoa and Japan, as well as the American Indian and Negro, may exhibit a permanent, flat, slate blue hyperpigmentation, or *nevus of Ota* (Hidano, 1967), which has a unilateral orbital and zygomatic distribution. Very rarely, bilateral involvement has been reported (Gold, 1967). The eye may also have brown to black staining of the sclera, iris and fundus. The lesion is histologically identical to that of the Mongolian spot. A dense infiltrate of dendritic, spindle-shaped melanocytes is present in the dermis (Lever, 1967) and, rarely, in the underlying muscles or even the periosteum. A delto-trapezius localization of the same pathological process is called the *nevus of Ito* (Fig. 10–3). These conditions are usually quite charac-

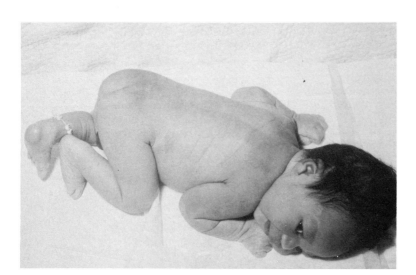

Figure 10–3. Nevus of Ito.

teristic clinically, and a diagnosis can almost always be made by inspection alone. A biopsy provides confirmatory evidence. Occlusive make-up is the most effective form of treatment. Excision is not advised and peeling techniques or dermabrasion do not remove the lesion completely, leaving a poor cosmetic result.

Flat Melanocytic Nevi (Junction nevi). Flat melanocytic nevi (Plate X–C) are found in about 3 per cent of newborn white infants (Pack, 1956) and in about 16 per cent of Negro infants (Lerner, 1958). Usually very few in number and brown or black in color (Fig. 10–4) these nevi vary in size from one to several centimeters. Occasionally they may involve the nail matrix (Fig. 10–5), resulting in a partially or completely pigmented nail. In the normal course of events, the number of junction nevi increases with age. In certain syndromes, such as neurofibromatosis, tuberous sclerosis, lentiginosis, xeroderma pigmentosum and bathing trunk nevi, there are increased numbers of flat melanocytic nevi present at birth. Histologic examination of the lesion is usually diagnostic, showing nests of cuboidal cells clustered at the junction of the dermis and epidermis and involving the

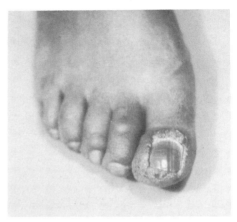

Figure 10–5. Compound nevus of the toe. The nail matrix produces a pigmented nail plate.

basal layer. (This is the reason why the term "junction" is used.) It is not necessary to routinely remove these lesions. A large speckled or very black lesion may be removed surgically and the defect grafted.

The Peutz-Jeghers Syndrome

The cutaneous features of the Peutz-Jeghers syndrome may be present at birth or develop soon thereafter (Dormandy, 1957). Characteristically, these lesions consist of oval pigmented macules, somewhat darker than freckles, which are distributed around the nose and mouth. The lips and oral mucosa are often involved, as are the hands, fingertips and nails. Macular hyperpigmentation is the only visible sign of this autosomal dominant disorder until adolescence, when the patient begins to suffer from attacks of intestinal intussusception—evidence of existing small bowel polyposis. The pigmentary change is due to an increase in the number of melanocytes in the basal layer and melanophages in the dermis. The intestinal polyps are adenomas, yet malignancy of the colon, rectum and stomach may coexist. With increasing age the pigmentary changes become less marked.

Xeroderma Pigmentosum. The speckled pigmentary changes in this disease are secondary to the induced inflammation of ultraviolet light and clinically resemble those seen in X-irradiation dermatitis (see Chap. 16).

Urticaria Pigmentosum (See Chap. 15).

Postinflammatory Hyperpigmentation. Hyperpigmentation may secondarily result from any banal inflammatory process in the skin and thus may have a multitude of causes, including primary irritant dermatitis, infec-

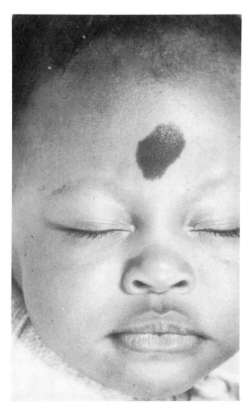

Figure 10–4. Junction nevus.

tious processes, panniculitis and hereditary diseases, such as epidermolysis bullosa. The hyperpigmentation may result from a greater number of melanosomes, increased melanin deposits in basal cells, increased numbers of keratinocytes, increase in the thickness of the stratum corneum or deposits of melanin in dermal melanophages.

LOCALIZED HYPERPIGMENTATION: RAISED LESIONS

Giant Hairy Nevus. The most important of the congenital melanocytic nevi is the *giant hairy (bathing trunk) nevus* (Fig. 10–6). Its importance lies not so much in the frequency of occurrence, which is quite low, but in its propensity for malignant degeneration. About 10 per cent of these patients develop malignant melanoma within the nevus (Reed, 1965; Greeley, 1965). These lesions, although present at birth, are probably not hereditarily transmitted. They constitute an overwhelming deformity. They may occupy 15 to 35 per cent of the body surface, involving a limb, or the entire trunk or buttocks. The lesion is usually unevenly pigmented, covering a spectrum from light brown to deep black. The affected skin may be leathery or of tortoise shell consistency and covered with dense long hair.

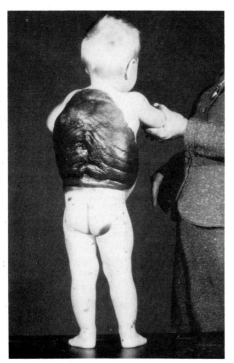

Figure 10–6. Bathing trunk nevus.

Almost invariably, numerous junction nevi, other dermal nevi and café-au-lait spots coexist elsewhere on the body. Leptomeningeal melanocytosis has been documented in many of these patients (Reed, 1965), and this latter complication may be manifested as seizures or other neurological abnormalities. Malignant melanoma of the meninges has also been reported (Hoffman, 1967).

Histologically, melanocytes of both cuboidal and spindle cell types, containing or lacking pigment, invade the entire dermis and junctional area. Indeed, the melanocytic invasion may extend to involve subcutaneous tissue, fascia or even underlying muscle (Solomon, 1968). Neural elements may also be found. Because of the significant incidence of malignant degeneration in these nevi, the hideous deformity and the intense pruritus which may accompany them, it is desirable to remove them as soon as possible. The infant should be old enough to withstand major surgery. The surgical approach is hampered when there is insufficient nevus-free donor skin to cover the defect, but segmental removal of the lesion and trimming the donor skin of small nevi may circumvent this difficulty (Solomon, 1968). Even using liberal criteria, not all lesions are operable. Removal of a giant nevus is a major undertaking which may lead to a rocky postoperative course complicated by infection, but when possible, the gain appears to warrant the risk involved.

Intradermal; Compound Nevi (Involvement of epidermal junction and dermis). Circumscribed, hairy and pigmented, these lesions may be present at birth. They occur everywhere but on the palms and soles, and are usually raised, warty and dome-shaped (Fig. 10–7). The melanocytic nevus cells are localized to the upper dermis around the appendages and contain variable amounts of pigment. The larger lesions (i.e., involving the dorsum of a hand) resemble the bathing trunk nevus in character, the smaller ones (2 to 4 cm in diameter) are simply benign moles. Usually the diagnosis presents no problem, nor does their surgical removal for cosmetic purposes. Occasionally, however, the lesions may occupy bizarre locations such as the eardrum or tip of the penis. The "kissing" nevus (Fig. 10–8) traverses the upper and lower eyelids and is separated by a normal eye. Localized nevi of this type usually are difficult to extirpate without consequent unacceptable deformity. It may be wise not to disturb the lesions in such cases.

Blue Nevus. Occasionally one may see a blue nevus (so called because of its Prussian blue color) at birth. Lund and Kraus (1962) have called these lesions dermal melanocytomas. They are usually 1 to 3 cm in size, oval, raised, dome-shaped tumors found on the upper half of the body and buttocks. They grow very slowly and have little or no known tendency to become malignant, but may be difficult to differentiate clinically from vascular tumors. Histologically, there are two types; one is identical to the Mongolian spot, while the other has clusters of round or cuboidal cells with a vacuolated pale cytoplasm. Excisional biopsy is at once diagnostic and curative.

Juvenile Melanoma (Spitz tumor). This is an uncommon benign tumor occurring in children between three and 10 years of age (Korting, 1969). The tumor is exceedingly rare in the newborn period, but occasionally this slow growing lesion may be seen in a one year old child in whom the history of the tumor goes back to birth. The lesion is a red-brown, fleshy nodule which, histologically, bears superficial resemblence to malignant melanoma. Juvenile melanoma is not a malignant tumor, and the presence of dermal telangiectasia, edema, giant cells and spindle cells helps to differentiate it from malignant melanoma (Lever, 1967). Excision is curative.

Epidermal Nevi (See also Chap. 8). Localized areas of hyperpigmentation are a constant feature of a variety of keratinocytic nevi of uncertain genetic nature, including

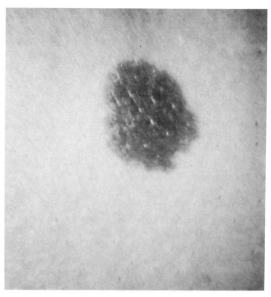

Figure 10–7. Compound melanocytic nevus.

nevus unius lateris, ichthyosis hystrix and *congenital acanthosis nigricans.* All of these entities may start within the first few weeks of life as a streaky, somewhat dirty looking patch with an ubiquitous distribution. The hyperpigmentation is the result of an increase in epidermal thickness or of a localized aggregation of melanin granules in the keratinocytes, but no increase in the number of melanocytes has been reported.

Incontinentia Pigmenti and Urticaria Pigmentosa (Mastocytosis). (See Chaps. 13 and

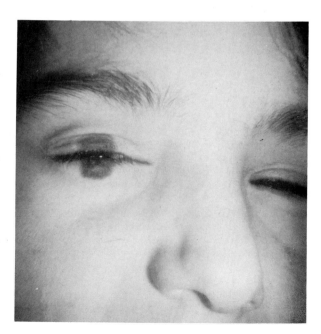

Figure 10–8. "Kissing" melanocytic nevus of the eyelids. (Courtesy of Dr. David Fretzin.)

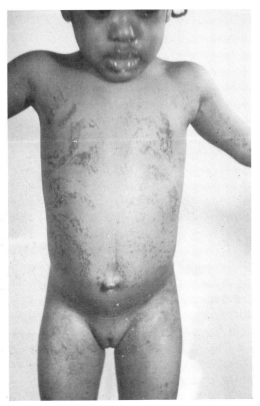

Figure 10–9. Incontinentia pigmenti.

15). Both of these conditions, which start as blistering diseases, may result in hyperpigmentation as a terminal feature of the process (Plate X–D). Very rarely do they result in pigmentary disturbance prior to three months of age. Incontinentia pigmenti (Fig. 10–9), after passing through its bullous and warty stage, ultimately leaves a whorled and feathered hyperpigmentation. Mastocytosis leaves a temporary, patchy hyperpigmentation after the tumor and urticarial stage have existed for some time.

HYPOPIGMENTATION

A diffuse or localized loss of cutaneous pigment in the neonatal infant may be due to heredity or a developmental disorder, or it may be acquired as a result of a nutritional disorder or postinflammatory change. Melanocytes may be absent, or they may be destroyed. Fitzpatrick (1971) has postulated four defects in biologic mechanisms that may cause hypopigmentation to occur: (1) formation of melanosomes; (2) formation of melanin; (3) transfer of melanosomes into keratinocytes; and (4) transport of melanosomes by keratinocytes.

These will be considered in discussing the following hypopigmentary diseases.

ALBINISM
(Complete albinism, oculocutaneous albinism)

This disease, which occurs in all races, has an incidence of between 1:5000 and 1:25,000, and the phenotypic picture is due to an autosomal recessive gene (Rook, 1968; Fitzpatrick, 1971). The affected infant usually has markedly reduced skin pigment, yellow or white hair, pink pupils, gray irides, photophobia and photosensitivity (Plate XI–A, page 91). There is a possibility that melanocytic nevi can develop and these may or may not be pigmented. In Negroes, the skin may be tan, and freckles can appear on exposure to light. The eyes often have nystagmus and a central scotoma with reduced visual acuity. Other associated abnormalities reported in albinism are small stature, mental retardation and coagulation disorders. Deafness may be found in association with complete oculocutaneous albinism as well as in partial albinism and other pigmentary anomalies (Konigsmark, 1972).

The biochemical defects responsible for this disease both result in a deficiency of tyrosinase function (Witkop, 1971). The first of these gives a negative hair-bulb tyrosine test, indicating a lack of the enzyme tryosinase. The second gives a positive hair-bulb tyrosine test and shows no deficiency of tyrosinase but is probably due to a defect in the enzymatic reaction which precedes the formation of DOPA from tyrosine. If tyrosinase is neither present nor able to function, tyrosine cannot be converted to DOPA. As a result the melanosomes do not pigment, and therefore never become melanin granules. Structurally, the melanosomes appear to be normal. Treatment consists of protection from ultraviolet light, since early actinic keratoses and squamous cell carcinomas are common occurrences in these patients.

PIEBALDISM
(Partial albinism)

Piebaldism is a rare inherited disease due to an autosomal dominant gene (Reed, 1967; Comings, 1966). It is present at birth but may not be evident in fair-skinned infants because of a lack of contrast in skin color. The differential diagnosis includes vitiligo (Fig. 10–10), achromic nevus, nevus anemicus, Waardenburg's syndrome, the amelanotic macules of tuberous sclerosis and Addison's disease. In piebaldism the hair and skin are affected. The amelanotic areas usually involve the widow's peak and anterior scalp, forehead (to the base of the nose), chin, thorax, trunk, back, mid-arm and mid-leg. There are normal islands of pigment within the hypomelanotic areas, and the distribution pattern is fairly constant. These two features, as well as the tendency of vitiligo to have its onset later than age six months, help to make the difficult differentiation of piebaldism from vitiligo. Examination of an amelanotic area by electron microscopy shows an absence of melanocytes or melanocytes with markedly deformed melanosomes. Comings and Odland (1966) believe the defect is due to an "incomplete ventral migration of melanoblasts from the neural crest or a defect in the differentiation of ventral melanoblasts to melanocytes." Repigmentation does not take place. An isolated white forelock may also occur as a minor variant of this phenomenon.

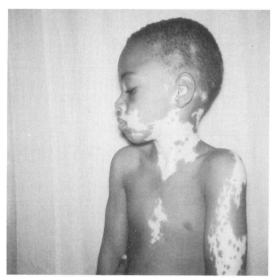

Figure 10–10. Vitiligo.

Phenylketonuria

A hereditary lack of L-phenylalanine hydroxylase is transmitted by an autosomal recessive gene (Jervis, 1937; Koch, 1967; Solomon, 1968). This biochemical defect results in a variety of neurological and cutaneous abnormalities, including mental retardation, seizures, diffuse hypopigmentation, eczema and photosensitivity. The inability to convert phenylalanine to tyrosine may lead to: (1) an accumulation of phenylalanine; (2) an accumulation of abnormal amounts of its metabolites, including phenylpyruvic, phenylacetic and O-hydroxy phenylacetic acids, as well as phenylacetyl glutamine; (3) a decrease in the formation of melanin; (4) a decrease or increase in other metabolites dependent on the tyrosine-to-melanin biochemical sequence; and (5) an inhibition of other metabolic processes because of the abnormal accumulation of phenylalanine and its catabolic residues.

The exact relation of these events to any of the clinical features of the disease remains a source of lively controversy. As far as the skin is concerned, it seems reasonably certain that the most likely cause of the hypopigmentation is the competitive inhibition of tyrosinase by excess phenylalanine, thus aggravating the lack of melanin substrate. It is not yet clear whether photosensitivity is indeed present as part of the syndrome or whether it simply reflects the decrease in melanin in the epidermis. The diagnosis of phenylketonuria is usually established soon after birth, since it is now routine pediatric practice to test the urine of the newborn for phenylketones. We need not enter into a discussion of dietary treatment here, but it is interesting to note that hair and skin darkening does occur with restriction of phenylanine intake and that the eczematous process may improve.

Chediak-Higashi Syndrome

The Chediak-Higashi syndrome is a rare disorder transmitted by an autosomal recessive gene. Its clinical features include diffuse, moderate reduction in cutaneous and ocular pigment, photophobia, hepatosplenomegaly and recalcitrant, recurrent infections. The leucocytes and other cells contain large granules, and this finding has its parallel in the melanocyte which produces giant melanosomes. It is not known why there is a clinical pigmentary deficit, but it appears to have little to do with true albinism. Windhorst et al. (1968) have speculated that the basic defect is due to a structural alteration in the lipoprotein matrix, giving rise to the abnormal melanosome (and granulocytic lysosomes). Thus, the melanin granules either are too easily destroyed or cannot be transferred to the keratinocyte (melanocytic impaction). Tyrosinase transfer may also be affected, or perhaps the abnormal melanosome does not serve as an adequate matrix for melanin deposition. The diagnosis may be made by family history, physical findings, laboratory demonstration of abnormal leucocytes and melanosomes and tracing the usual course of events which lead to death in childhood. Death results from a lymphoma-like process or infection. Hodgkin's disease has recently been reported as the fatal outcome in one case (Tan, 1971).

Klein-Waardenburg's Syndrome

The Klein-Waardenburg syndrome is inherited as an autosomal dominant condition. The most constant features of the disease are: Lateral displacement of the inner canthi of the eyes; a prominently broad nasal root; confluent eyebrows; loss of pigment in the iris (heretochromia iridum) and fundus; congenital deafness; a white forelock; and, cutaneous hypochromia (Waardenburg, 1951; Goldberg, 1966). The clinical picture is quite striking, and the diagnosis is usually not difficult. Although it is often limited to small areas, the hypopigmentation may be severe and extensive enough to resemble that of partial albinism. Since partial albinism may also have deafness associated with it (Reed, 1967), the distinction between these entities at times presents some difficulty. Also associated with Waardenburg's syndrome may be impaired speech, occurring with or without cleft palate.

Nevus Anemicus

Nevus anemicus is a pale, mottled, hand-sized area appearing on the trunk, and frequently is present in patients with neurofibromatosis. The lesions contain normal amounts of pigment but appear pale because of a vascular defect. Fleisher and Zeligman (1969) have shown that there is no decrease in the number of vessels in the affected area, but the vasculature within the nevus is apparently less responsive than the normal surrounding skin to endogenous vasodilatory mediators such as acetylcholine, histamine and serotonin. As a result, rubbing the area makes the pale, unresponsive lesion stand out in contrast to the vasodilated normal skin. Furthermore, it has also been suggested that the vessels within the lesion are undergoing sustained adrenergic vasoconstriction that may be overcome by sympathetic blockade (Greaves, 1970). This lesion should be contrasted with nevus achromicus (discussed in the next section). There is no effective treatment, however, the lesion is usually in a covered area, so there is little problem.

Nevus Achromicus

Present at birth, nevus achromicus is uni-lateral (in most cases), somewhat hypopigmented, irregularly shaped and of a bizarre streaky appearance (Coupe, 1967) It may be quite small or cover more than half the body. The hypopigmented area is quite uniform in color and the vessels within the lesion, in contrast to nevus anemicus, react normally to rubbing. The affected epidermis seems to have nonfunctioning or partially functioning melanocytes. This condition is probably not as rare as the paucity of literature would indicate. The authors have seen an affected infant with hemihypertrophy and profound mental retardation. In unusual cases, a similar hypopigmentary change may represent a terminal stage of incontinentia pigmenti.

WHITE SPOTS: TUBEROUS SCLEROSIS

Ninety per cent of infants with tuberous sclerosis have white macules that become apparent at birth or soon thereafter. They are about the size and shape of a European Mountain-Ash leaflet (Fitzpatrick, 1971). In fair-skinned infants the vitiliginous areas may be demonstrated by examining the skin with a Wood's lamp. The spots are variable in number and tend to affect the trunk and buttocks. The difference between these macules and the depigmented spots of vitiligo can be demonstrated by electron microscopy. The white macule of tuberous sclerosis has melanocytes with poorly pigmented melanosomes (Fig. 10–11), while in vitiligo, few or no melanocytes are found. The presence of white macules in a newborn infant strongly suggests that the infant has tuberous sclerosis; therein lies the importance of this unpretentious skin lesion (Hurwitz, 1970; Chao, 1959). It should be pointed out that not all white spots on the newborn infant seen with Wood's lamp are necessarily due to tuberous sclerosis. They may be nonspecific or indicate the presence of a developing hemangioma.

The syndrome accompanying tuberous sclerosis (epiloia, Bourneville's disease) consists of mental retardation, epilepsy, papular lesions on the face (adenoma sebaceum), peri and subungeal fibromas, shagreen patches, retinal glial tumors, calcification in the area of the basal ganglia and white spots. It is inherited as a dominant disease with frequent minor variants. The facial papules, long thought to be adenomas of the sebaceous glands, are in fact the fibrovascular tumors that characterize the disease. The lesions are

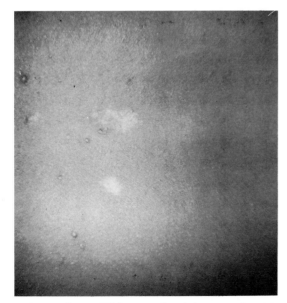

Figure 10–11. White macules (tuberous sclerosis). (Courtesy of Dr. David Fretzin.)

fleshy, red, and occupy the center of the face, particularly the region around the paranasal folds, but sparing the upper lip. These lesions usually become apparent after two years of age. The shagreen patches (Plate XI–B) are yellow or flesh-colored, pebbled, rough patches found on the back and around the sacral area. They contain excess collagen. Glial tumors are found in the retina and at the base of the brain. Hamartomas in the lung and kidney and rhabdomyomas of the heart are also frequently present. The latter lesions are said to lack potential for malignant transformation (Braverman, 1970).

White macules, many of which were present at birth, were found by Hurwitz and Braverman (1970) in 18 of 23 patients with tuberous sclerosis. One-hundred fifty-five children, including normal and mentally retarded children, as well as those with epilepsy not due to tuberous sclerosis, were studied as controls. In this control group one normal child was found to have a hypopigmented spot. In view of the high frequency of white macules present at birth in tuberous sclerosis, screening of all newborn infants with Wood's light is indicated. Detection of white spots should lead to careful consideration of family and antecedent history, histologic examination of the melanocytes in a lesion, frequent, careful follow-up with repeated physical examinations at appropriate intervals and, when the diagnosis has been established, parental genetic counseling.

MISCELLANEOUS CAUSES OF HYPOPIGMENTATION

A number of other conditions should be considered in the differential diagnosis of hypomelanosis. In *kwashiorkor* (McClaren, 1971) deficient protein intake may result in both an inadequate store of amino acid building blocks for construction of the protein matrix for the melanosome, as well as in a deficiency in phenylalanine and tyrosine for initiating melanin formation. The result is diffuse hypopigmentation of skin and hair. In black infants the clinical picture of marasmus, pale skin and reddish hair is diagnostic of kwashiorkor. The pigmentary changes are, of course, only part of the picture, since photosensitivity, purpura, excessive bruisability, scaling, erosions and complicating infection are frequently present as well.

The Cross-McKusick-Breen Syndrome (1967). This autosomal recessive hereditary disorder consists of mental retardation, spastic diplegia, diffuse hypopigmentation, microphthalmos and other severe ocular abnormalities.

Congenital Giant Halo Nevi (Berger,

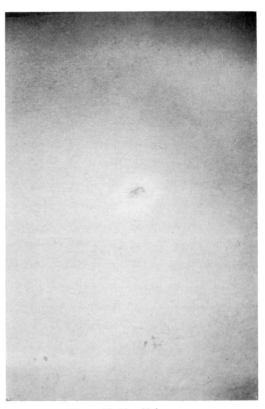

Figure 10–12. Halo nevus.

1971). A lesion has been reported in which giant junction nevi were found associated with a peripheral halo of depigmentation around each area of hyperpigmentation (Fig. 10–12). Ultrastructurally, in the white areas, there was a decrease in melanin, tyrosinase and melanosomes and an increase in Langerhans cells.

Finally, any *inflammatory reaction* in the skin may depress melanocyte function or even destroy melanocytes permanently, thus resulting in hypopigmentation.

REFERENCES

Albright, I., Butler, A. M., Hampton, A. O., and Smith, P.: Syndrome characterized by osteitis fibrosa disseminata, areas of pigmentation, and endocrine dysfunction, with precocious puberty in females. New Eng. J. Med. *216*:727, 1937.

Arlien-Soeborg, V. and Iverson, T.: Albright's syndrome. Acta Paediat. *45*:558, 1956.

Berger, R. S. and Voorhees, J. J.: Multiple congenital giant nevocellular nevi with halos. Arch. Derm. *104*:515, 1971.

Borberg, A.: Clinical and genetic investigations into tuberous sclerosis and von Recklinghausen's neurofibromatosis. Acta Psychiat. et Neurol. *71*(Suppl.): 11, 1951.

Braverman, I. M.: Skin signs of systemic diseases. Philadelphia, W. B. Saunders Co., 1970, p. 403.

Capute, A. J., Rimoin, D. L., Konigsmark, B. W., Esterly, N. B. and Richardson, F.: Congenital deafness and multiple lentigines. Arch. Derm. *100*:207, 1969.

Chao, D. H.-C.: Congenital neurocutaneous syndromes in childhood. J. Pediat. *55*:447, 1959.

Chernosky, M. E., Anderson, D. E., Chang, J. P., Shaw, M. W. and Romsdahl, M. M.: Familial progressive hyperpigmentation. Arch. Derm. *103*:581, 1971.

Clark, W. H., Jr. and Mihm, M. C.: Moles and malignant melanoma. *In* Fitzpatrick, T. B., Arndt, K. A., Clark, W. H., Jr., Eisen, A. Z., Van Scott, E. G. and Vaughan, J. H. (eds.): Dermatology in General Medicine. New York, McGraw-Hill, 1971.

Comings, D. E. and Odland, G. F.: Partial albinism. J.A.M.A. *195*:519, 1966.

Coupe, R. L.: Unilateral systematized achromic naevus. Dermatologica *134*:19, 1967.

Crocker, A. C.: The lipidoses. *In* Nelson, W. E. (ed.): Textbook of Pediatrics. 8th ed. Philadelphia, W. B. Saunders Co., 1964, p. 316.

Cross, H. E., McKusick, V. A. and Breen, W.: A new oculocerebral syndrome with hypopigmentation. J. Pediat. *70*:398, 1967.

Crowe, F. W. and Schull, W. J.: Diagnostic importance of café-au-lait spot in neurofibromatosis. Arch. Intern. Med. *91*:758, 1953.

Dormandy, T. L.: Gastrointestinal polyposis with mucocutaneous pigmentation. (Peutz-Jeghers syndrome). New Eng. J. Med. *256*:1093, 1141, 1186, 1957.

Ebling, F. S. and Rook, A.: Disorders of skin color. *In* Rook, A. J., Wilkinson, D. S. and Ebling, F. J. G. (eds.): Textbook of Dermatology. Philadelphia, F. A. Davis Co., 1968, p. 1111.

Efron, M. L. and Gallagher, W. F.: Cutaneous changes in errors of amino acid metabolism. *In* Fitzpatrick,

T. B., Arndt, K. A., Clark, W. H., Jr., Eisen, A. Z., Van Scott, E. G. and Vaughan, J. H. (eds.): Dermatology in General Medicine. New York, McGraw-Hill, 1971, p. 1115.

Fialkow, P. J., Sagebiel, R. W., Gartler, S. M. and Rimoin, D. L.: Multiple cell origin of hereditary neurofibromas. N. Eng. J. Med. *284*:298, 1971.

Fitzpatrick, T. B. and Mihm, M. C.: Abnormalities of the melanin pigmentary system. *In* Fitzpatrick, T. B., Arndt, K. A., Clark, W. H., Jr., Eisen, A. Z., Van Scott, E. J. and Vaughan, J. H. (eds.): Dermatology in General Medicine. New York, McGraw-Hill, 1971, p. 1591.

Fleisher, T. L. and Zeligman, I.: Nevus anemicus. Arch. Derm. *100*:750, 1969.

Franks, R. C. and Nance, W. E.: Hereditary adrenocortical unresponsiveness to ACTH. Pediatrics *45*:43, 1970.

Gold, D. H., Henkind, P., Sturner, W. Q. and Baden, M.: Oculodermal melanocytosis and retinitis pigmentosa. Amer. J. Ophthal. *63*:271, 1967.

Goldberg, M. F.: Waardenburg's syndrome with fundus and other anomalies. Arch. Ophthal. *76*:797, 1966.

Gorlin, R. J. and Pindborg, J. J.: Syndromes of the head and neck. New York, McGraw-Hill, 1964, p. 461.

Gorlin, R. J., Anderson, R. C. and Blaw, M.: Multiple lentigenes syndrome. Amer. J. Dis. Child. *117*:652, 1969.

Greaves, N. W., Birckett, D. and Johnson, C.: Nevus anemicus: A unique catecholamine-dependent nevus. Arch. Derm. *102*:172, 1970.

Greeley, P. W., Middleton, A. G. and Curtin, J. W.: Incidence of malignancy in giant pigmented nevi. Plast. and Reconstr. Surg. *36*:26, 1965.

Hidano, A.: Resistant mongolian spot in the adult. Letter to the Editor. Arch. Derm. *103*:680, 1971.

Hoffman, H. J. and Freeman, A.: Primary malignant leptomeningeal melanoma in association with giant hairy nevi. Report of two cases. J. Neurosurg. *26*:62, 1967.

Holt, J. F. and Wright, E. M.: Radiologic features of neurofibromatosis. Radiology *51*:647, 1948.

Hugo, V.: Notre-Dame de Paris. 3rd ed. Paris, Charles Gosselin Libraire, 1831.

Hurwitz, S. and Braverman, I. M.: White spots in tuberous sclerosis. J. Pediat. *77*:587, 1970.

Jervis, S. A.: Phenylpyruvic oligophrenia. Introductory study of 50 cases of mental deficiency associated with excretion of phenylpyruvic acid. Arch. Neur. and Psych. *38*:944, 1937.

Johnson, B. L. and Charneco, D. R.: Café-au-lait spot in neurofibromatosis and normal individuals. Arch. Derm. *102*:442, 1970.

Johnson, B. L. and Charneco, D. R.: The café-au-lait spot in "normal" persons in neurofibromatosis. Derm. Digest *10*:31, 1971.

Koch, R., Acosta, P., Fishler, K., Schaeffler, G. and Wohlers, A.: Clinical observations on phenylketonuria. Amer. J. Dis. Child. *11*:36, 1967.

Konigsmark, B. W.: Hereditary childhood hair loss and integumentary system disease. J. Pediat. *80*:909, 1972.

Korting, G. W.: Diseases of the Skin in Children and Adolescents. Philadelphia, W. B. Saunders Co., 1969, p. 184.

Lerner, A. B. and Lerner, M. B.: Congenital and hereditary disturbances of pigmentation. *In* Bibliotheca Paediatrica. Mod. Probl. Paediat. Basel, S. Karger, 1958.

Lever, W. F.: Nevocellular nevi and malignant melanoma. *In* Histopathology of the skin. 4th ed. Philadelphia, J. B. Lippincott Co., 1967, p. 725.

Lund, H. A. and Kraus, J. M.: Melanotic tumors of the skin. Fascicle 3, Atlas of Tumor Pathology. Armed Forces Institute of Pathology, Washington, D.C., 1962.

McLaren, D. S.: Cutaneous lesions in nutritional deficiencies. *In* Fitzpatrick, T. B., Arndt, K. A., Clark, W. H., Jr., Eisen, A. Z., Van Scott, E. J. and Vaughan, J. H. (eds.).: Dermatology in General Medicine. New York, McGraw-Hill, 1971, p. 1073.

Moynahan, E. J.: Multiple symmetrical moles with psychic and somatic infantilism and genital hypoplasia. Proc. Roy. Soc. Med. 55:959, 1962.

Pack, G. T. and Davis, J.: Moles, N.Y. J. Med. 56:3998, 1956.

Penfield, W. and Young, A. W.: The nature of Von Recklinghausen's disease and the tumors associated with it. Arch. Neur. and Psych. 23:320, 1930.

Preston, F. W., Walsh, W. S. and Clarke, T. W.: Cutaneous neurofibromatosis (von Recklinghausen's disease). Arch. Surg. 64:813, 1952.

Reed, W. B., Becker, S. W., Sr., Becker, S. W., Jr. and Nickel, W. R.: Giant pigmented nevi, melanoma and leptomeningeal melanocytosis. Arch. Derm. 91:100, 1965.

Reed, W. B., Stone, V. M., Boder, E. and Ziprkowski, L.: Pigmentary disorders in association with congenital deafness. Arch. Derm. 95:176, 1967.

Selmanowitz, V. J., Orentreich, N. and Felsenstein, J. M.: Lentiginosis profusa syndrome. Arch. Derm. 104:393, 1971.

Solomon, L. M.: Quasimodo's diagnosis. J.A.M.A. 204:190, 1968.

Solomon, L. M. and Desai, K.: Phenylketonuria. Cutis 4:1233, 1968.

Solomon, L. M., Altman, A. T. and Bader, K.: Management of giant nevus. Cutis 4:434, 1968.

Solomon, L. M., Fretzin, D. F. and Dewald, R. L.: The epidermal nevus syndrome. Arch. Derm. 97:273, 1968.

Tan, C., Etcubanas, E., Lieberman, P., Isenberg, H., King, O. and Murphy, M. L.: Chediak-Higashi syndrome in a child with Hodgkin's disease. Amer. J. Dis. Child. 121:135, 1971.

Vestermark, S.: Silver's syndrome. Acta Paediat. Scand. 59:435, 1970.

Von Recklinghausen, F.: Uber die Multiplen fibroma der Haut und inne Beziehung zu den Multiplen Neuromen. Berlin, A. Hirschwald, 1882.

Waardenburg, P. J.: A new syndrome combining developmental anomalies of the eyelids, eyebrows, and nose root, with pigmentary defects of the iris and head hair and with congenital deafness. Amer. J. Hum. Genet. 3:195, 1951.

Whitehouse, D.: Diagnostic value of the café-au-lait spot in children. Arch. Dis. Child. 41:316, 1966.

Windhorst, D. B., Zelickson, A. S. and Good, R. A.: A human pigmentary dilution based on a heritable subcellular structural defect—The Chediak-Higashi syndrome. J. Invest. Derm. 50:9, 1968.

Witkop, C. J., White, J. G., Nance, W. E., Jackson, C. E. and Desnick, S.: Classification of albinism in man. *In* Bergsma, D. (ed.): Birth Defects: Original Article Series. Part 12, Vol. 7. Skin, Hair and Nails. Baltimore, Williams and Wilkins Co., 1971.

Chapter Eleven

SCALING DISORDERS

The differential diagnosis of the scaly infant includes accentuation of physiologic desquamation, dysmaturity (placental insufficiency syndrome) and the various ichthyosiform dermatoses. In the first two entities, shedding of the skin is a transient phenomenon and the affected integument preserves its protective function. However, the infant with ichthyosis may have serious difficulty early in life and a diagnosis should be made, if possible, in the immediate neonatal period.

The normal infant with increased physiologic desquamation is most likely to have a gestational age between 40 and 42 weeks and to show peak shedding on approximately the eighth day of life. In a study of skin desquamation of the newborn, 75 per cent of 300 infants were found to have some scaling of the ankles on the first day of life (Griffiths, 1966). Moderate to severe desquamation occurred in only a small number of these infants but was of maximum intensity in all of the sites examined by the eighth day. No desquamation was observed in infants born prior to the 35th week of gestation, nor did those born between 35 to 40 weeks show more than a mild degree of shedding. An increase in frequency and degree of scaling occurred in infants of 40 to 42 weeks gestational age with desquamation decreasing after the 42nd week. An occasional normal infant may therefore show a marked degree of scaling, but such infants are usually readily distinguishable by their otherwise normal physical appearance and behavior.

In contrast to the normal infant with accentuated scaling, the dysmature infant exhibits

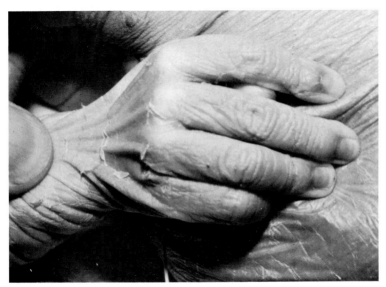

Figure 11–1. Dysmature infant. (Courtesy of Drs. David Fisher and John Paton.)

several identifying characteristics (Fig. 11–1). His gestational age may vary, but his weight will be low for his length. The body is lean with thin extremities and little subcutaneous fat. Vernix caseosa is absent. The skin is like parchment, dry and peeling, and shows meconium staining as do the nails and umbilical cord. The hair is long and abundant, and the nails are abnormally long. Other signs of chronic prenatal anoxia include elevation of the blood urea nitrogen, bilirubin, and hemoglobin, albuminuria and glycosuria (Sjöstedt, 1958).

Of the four major types of ichthyosis (Esterly, 1968), three may be symptomatic during the first month of life: *X-linked ichthyosis, nonbullous congenital ichthyosiform erythroderma* (CIE, lamellar ichthyosis) and *bullous congenital ichthyosiform erythroderma* (epidermolytic hyperkeratosis). *Ichthyosis vulgaris* (Wells, 1965), the most common and usually most benign form, is inherited as an autosomal dominant trait and rarely has its onset before the third month of life. It usually can be dismissed as a cause of scaling during the neonatal period. *"Harlequin fetus"* and *"collodion baby"* are descriptive terms for affected infants of a particular appearance but do not necessarily represent specific types of ichthyosis, although studies continue to differentiate these entities. Two other types of ichthyosis will be considered separately because their relationship to the previous four types remains unclear: ichthyosis linearis circumflexa and erythrokeratoderma variabilis (see Table 11–1). Epidermal nevi (including ichthyosis hystrix) and keratoderma of the palms and soles can be viewed as localized forms of abnormal keratinization.

In addition, there are a number of syndromes that include ichthyosis as a constant or variable feature. In some syndromes the clinical and histologic descriptions are insufficiently documented to permit classification of the ichthyosis. This group includes the Sjögren-Larsson syndrome, Rud's syndrome, Netherton's syndrome and Tay's syndrome. The signs and symptoms of Refsum's syndrome, in which an ichthyotic process may also be present, are not apparent until early childhood or later. The salient findings in these syndromes are summarized in Table 11–2.

Harlequin Fetus

The harlequin fetus, clinically the most severely affected ichthyotic infant, is so striking and grotesque that there is little chance of confusion with any other entity (Fig. 11–2). Virtually all of these infants succumb within the first hours or days of life and treatment is of little consequence to survival.

The skin of the harlequin fetus is hard, thick, gray or yellow in color with deep crevices running transversely and vertically and resembles tree bark or alligator hide. The fissures are reddish-brown or purple and have a moist and granular appearance. They are most prominent over areas of movement: the thorax; joints; groin; axillae; and neck. Rigidity of the skin about the eyes results in marked ectropion. Chemosis of the palpebral conjunctiva may completely obscure the globe, which is usually normal. The ears and nose are underdeveloped, flattened and distorted, and the lips are everted and gaping, producing a "'fish-mouth" deformity. The nails and hair may be hypoplastic or absent.

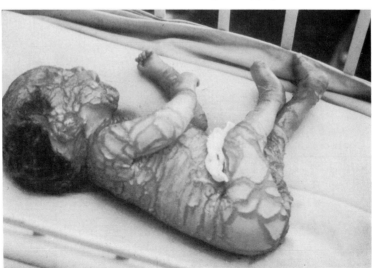

Figure 11–2. Harlequin fetus. (Courtesy of Dr. T. Briceño-Maaz.)

Table 11–1.

Condition	Inheritance	Age of Onset	Distribution
Ichthyosis vulgaris	Autosomal dominant	Usually after 3 months of life	1. Forehead and cheeks involved 2. Back more severely affected than abdomen 3. Limbs variably involved 4. Flexures spared 5. Increased palmar and plantar markings
Sex-linked ichthyosis	X-linked; female to male transmission	Birth to one year	1. Lateral face, neck and scalp most severely affected 2. Abdomen more severely involved than back 3. Limbs: total involvement common 4. Flexures variably affected; antecubital fossae and axilla more commonly in childhood, popliteal fossae in adulthood 5. Palms and soles normal
Nonbullous congenital ichthyosiform erythroderma (lamellar ichthyosis)	Autosomal recessive	Birth	1. Upper face more involved than lower face 2. Uniform generalized hyperkeratosis of trunk 3. Limbs also show generalized involvement 4. Flexures always affected (dry) 5. Palms and soles affected
Bullous congenital ichthyosiform erythroderma (epidermolytic hyperkeratosis)	Autosomal dominant	Birth to 6 months	1. Lower face more involved than upper face 2. Trunk variably affected 3. Limbs variably affected 4. Flexures always affected (moist) 5. Palms and soles usually affected
Ichthyosis linearis circumflexa	Autosomal recessive	Birth	1. Generalized migratory polycyclic lesions 2. Flexures hyperkeratotic
Erythrokeratoderma variabilis	Autosomal dominant	Birth	1. Face, buttocks, extensor surfaces and extremities for both hyperkeratotic plaques and erythematous areas

Extreme inelasticity of the skin is associated with flexion deformity of all joints of the limbs. The hands and feet are ischemic, hard and waxy in appearance and often have poorly developed distal digits, possibly due to pressure from hyperkeratotic bands. No consistent abnormalities have been found in other organ systems. The term "harlequin fetus" probably derives from the clown-like appearance of the face with the "O" shaped mouth, and from the triangular and diamond-shaped hyperkeratotic plaques on the body and limbs that resemble the traditional costume of the harlequin.

Microscopically, the skin shows an extremely thick stratum corneum which, in hairy areas, is perforated by fragmented and distorted hair shafts. The granular layer is normal, and the prickle layer (stratum malpighium) is hypertrophic without elongation of the rete ridges. Appendageal structures are well-developed, but the intraepidermal portion of the sweat ducts and follicles are plugged with hyperkeratotic debris. The dermis appears normal save for localized collections of inflammatory cells at the base of the fissures.

Several reports of affected siblings (Briceno-Maaz, 1963; Kessel, 1956) suggest that the disorder is inherited in an autosomal

Types of Ichthyosis

Associated Features	Scales	Histology
1. Localized shiny hyperkeratosis of knees and elbows 2. Atopic dermatitis common 3. Family history positive for atopic diseases in a high percentage of cases 4. Keratosis pilaris common	Fine, branny and white	1. Mild to moderate hyperkeratosis 2. Decreased to absent granular layer 3. Normal rete ridges
1. "Dirty" appearance due to character of scales 2. Only males affected 3. Occasionally have collodion membrane at birth 4. Deep corneal dystrophy on slit lamp examination 5. Normal cellular kinetics	Thick, dark brown and large	1. Moderate hyperkeratosis 2. Increased granular layer 3. Prominent rete ridges 4. Dermal perivascular infiltrate
1. Background erythroderma 2. Prematurity common 3. Occasionally have collodion membrane at birth 4. Harlequin fetus the most rare and severe 5. Ectropion present and often progressive 6. Increased epidermal mitotic rate	Flat, dark and large	1. Moderate hyperkeratosis with focal parakeratosis 2. Irregular increase in granular layer 3. Hypertrophic epidermis 4. Dermal perivascular infiltrate
1. Background erythroderma 2. Bullae during infancy and childhood 3. Increased epidermal mitotic rate	Small, yellow and shotty	1. Marked hyperkeratosis 2. Prominent granular layer 3. Papillomatous, hypertrophic epidermis 4. Vacuolization of epidermal cells with abnormal large keratohyaline granules
1. Background erythroderma 2. Hair shaft abnormalities (Netherton's syndrome) 3. Hyperhidrosis palms and soles (adults)	White, double edged scale bordering migratory lesions	1. Hyperkeratosis with focal parakeratosis 2. Acanthosis 3. Dilatation of dermal vessels 4. Mild perivascular infiltrate
1. Areas of discrete macular erythema, transient and migratory 2. May have thickened palms and soles	Thick, yellow-brown	1. Laminated stratum corneum 2. Focal parakeratosis 3. Prominent granular layer 4. Papillomatosis, irregular acanthosis 5. Elongated papillary capillaries

recessive fashion. Most authors believe that the harlequin fetus is a severe form of non-bullous CIE (Wells, 1965). Although the molecular defect is not known, on X-ray diffraction analysis of the horny layer from one harlequin fetus, a cross-β fibrous protein was identified as the major component (Craig, 1970). Since normal epidermal keratin contains mainly an α-fibrous protein but also has minor amounts of a cross-β protein (Baden, 1968), it is unclear whether the increased amount of cross-β protein represents an overproduction of the β-type substance or whether it is an abnormal protein derived from altered α-fibrous protein.

Frequent complications include difficulty in feeding owing to inelasticity of the lips, hypothermia, hypoventilation with secondary pneumonia and sepsis secondary to cutaneous infection. Although the disorder is rare and the prognosis is at present hopeless, knowledge of the genetic transmission of harlequin fetus is important in order to facilitate intelligent genetic counseling of parents of these infants.

Collodion Baby

The collodion baby (sometimes known as lamellar exfoliation of the newborn) is more

Table 11–2. Syndromes with Scaling Dermatosis

Condition	Age of Onset	Inheritance	Common Features	Inconstant Features
Netherton's syndrome	Birth	Autosomal recessive	1. Ichthyosis: usually ichthyosis linearis circumflexa or nonbullous congenital ichthyosiform erythroderma 2. Hair defects: trichorrhexis invaginata, pili torti, trichorrhexis nodosa, cup-like, braid-weave and rope-like deformities 3. Atopic diathesis: angioneurotic edema, rarely asthma, eczema	1. Aminoaciduria 2. Hypogamma-globulinemia
Sjögren-Larsson syndrome	Birth	Autosomal recessive	1. Mental retardation 2. Ichthyosis: nonbullous CIE 3. Spastic diplegia or quadriplegia	1. Degeneration of pigment epithelium of macula 2. Dysplasia of tooth enamel 3. Serrated teeth 4. Epilepsy 5. Hypertelorism 6. Dermatoglyphic abnormalities 7. Speech defects
Rud's syndrome	Infancy	Unknown	1. Ichthyosis: type unknown 2. Mental retardation 3. Epilepsy	1. Sexual infantilism 2. Gigantism 3. Dwarfism 4. Structural defects of hands and feet 5. Alopecia 6. Nerve deafness 7. Absent or hypoplastic teeth 8. Eye abnormalities
Conradi's syndrome	Birth	Autosomal recessive	1. Stippled epiphyses 2. Short femora or humeri with dysplasia of ends 3. Saddle nose 4. Cataract 5. Generalized erythema and scaling; follicular atrophoderma	1. Mental deficiency 2. Craniosynostosis 3. Various bony anomalies 4. Hypertelorism 5. Congenital heart defect 6. Hernia 7. Muscle fibrosis
Refsum's syndrome	First decade or later	Autosomal recessive	1. Atypical retinitis pigmentosa 2. Polyneuritis with progressive paresis and cerebellar signs 3. Elevated CSF protein 4. Ichthyosis: type unknown 5. Elevated serum phytanic acid	1. Anosmia 2. Deafness 3. Pupillary abnormalities 4. Skeletal anomalies 5. EKG changes
Tay's syndrome	Birth	Autosomal recessive	1. Ichthyosis 2. Hair defects; pili torti and trichorrhexis nodosa 3. Mental retardation 4. Growth retardation 5. Progeria-like appearance	1. Hypogamma-globulinemia (one patient)

common than the harlequin fetus and probably represents the phenotypic expression of
more than one genotype (Fig. 11–3). Affected infants usually develop nonbullous
CIE, but collodion membranes have also been
observed in patients with X-linked ichthyosis
and possibly may occur in a rare individual
with bullous CIE (Wells, 1966). In some
infants, the membrane is shed completely,
and the skin remains free of ichthyosis (Reed,
1972).

At birth the infant is encased in a cello-
phane-like membrane which may, by its
tautness, temporarily distort the facial features and distal portion of the extremities. A
partial membranous covering is less common.
The membrane is shiny and brownish-yellow,
resembling an envelope of collodion or oiled
parchment, and may be perforated by both
scalp and lanugo hair. Fissuring and peeling
of this covering begins shortly after birth, and
large sheets may desquamate, revealing
erythema of variable intensity. Complete
shedding of the collodion membrane may
take up to several months; in some infants,
the shedding takes place as an interrupted
process with reformation of a new membrane
over small areas of skin (Bloom, 1962).

Although these infants superficially resemble the harlequin fetus and a few transitional
cases have been reported, the collodion baby
is much less severely affected. Collodion
babies are frequently born prior to term
(Smeenk, 1966), but apart from the complications of prematurity, they usually do not have
a difficult neonatal course. No other organ
systems are affected and, after the membrane
has fissured over the thorax, restriction of
respiration is not a problem. Descriptions of
the histologic findings vary. Since the disorder is undoubtedly the result of genetic
heterogeneity rather than a specific entity,
one would expect the histologic pattern to
conform to that of an underlying disease. A
prolonged period of observation may be
required to predict the outcome and prognosis. Pedigree information and skin biopsy
are helpful in this regard. A diagnosis of
collodion baby alone is not adequate for genetic counseling, since the pattern of genetic
transmission will be determined by the specific type of ichthyosis present.

X-LINKED ICHTHYOSIS

The patient with X-linked ichthyosis may
present as a collodion baby or simply as a
scaly infant (Plate XI–C, page 000). In a large
English regional study (Wells, 1966) 17 per

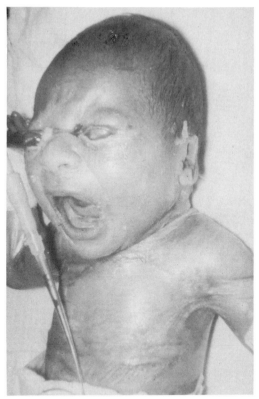

Figure 11–3. Collodion baby. (Courtesy of Dr. David
Fretzin.)

cent of such patients had a history of ichthyosis at birth, while 84 per cent were affected
by three months of age. In a later series
(Wells, 1967), 36 per cent were reputedly affected at birth and only 6 per cent were unaffected by three months of age.

Generally, the entire body surface is involved except for the palms and soles, the
central face and most of the flexural areas.
Involvement of one or two flexures occurs in
approximately 30 per cent of children.
Usually the axillae and antecubital fossae are
affected in childhood, but these areas are
spared in adulthood. In contrast, the popliteal fossae are affected more frequently in
later life. The scalp, neck, sides of the face,
anterior trunk and extensor surfaces of the
extremities tend to have the most prominent
scales in early childhood. The scales are large
and yellow to dark brown, giving the patient
an unwashed appearance, and may be shed
episodically in a profuse "moulting" (Fig. 11–
4). The internal organs are not affected in
this disorder.

Skin biopsy is helpful, although the histologic pattern resembles that of lamellar ichthyosis. There is moderate hyperkeratosis, a
well-developed granular layer, and acanthosis with prominent rete ridges. A well-

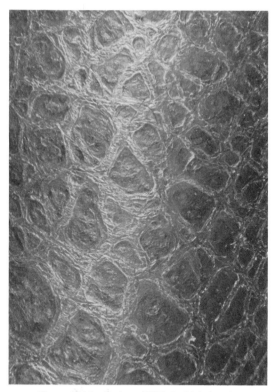

Figure 11–4. Scales of X-linked ichthyosis.

demarcated perivascular lymphocytic infiltrate is present in the dermis (Feinstein, 1970).

The disease is transmitted as an X-linked recessive trait; therefore, it is manifested only in males. Sisters of affected males may be heterozygous and may transmit the condition to their sons. Linkage with the Xg blood group provides additional eivdence for transmission on the X chromosome (Adam, 1969).

Deep corneal opacities have been described as a consistent finding in affected males (Sever, 1968). These are visible on slit lamp examination as discrete gray-white bodies resembling filaments, commas or dots which are diffusely distributed over the entire cornea. No decrease in visual acuity has been detected. The corneal changes appear at adolescence or in early adulthood (Jay, 1968). Since female carriers also have these lesions, corneal opacities may eventually prove to be a reliable marker for homozygous and heterozygous individuals.

NONBULLOUS CONGENITAL ICHTHYOSIFORM ERYTHRODERMA
(Lamellar ichthyosis)

Nonbullous CIE is a congenital disorder which is inherited as an autosomal recessive trait (Plate XI–D). Affected infants present with a brilliant and generalized erythema similar to that seen in Ritter's disease (see Chap. 13). Desquamation is universal, involving the flexures as well as other body surfaces (Fig. 11–5), but scaling is less prominent in infancy than it is later in childhood. Some of these infants are covered with a collodion membrane at birth (see preceding section). The palms and soles may show only increased markings or may be considerably thickened. Ectropion, often severe later in life, is not a problem during the neonatal period. Rapid growth of the hair and nails has been an inconstant finding.

These infants do relatively well in the neonatal period although macerated skin, particularly in the intertriginous areas, may serve as a portal of entry for bacterial organisms. As the infant grows older, the intense erythroderma fades somewhat and the scaling becomes more prominent with accentuation in the flexural areas. The scales vary in color from yellow to brown-black and, in some cases, form warty excrescences or thick, horny plates covering large areas (Plate XII–A, page 92).

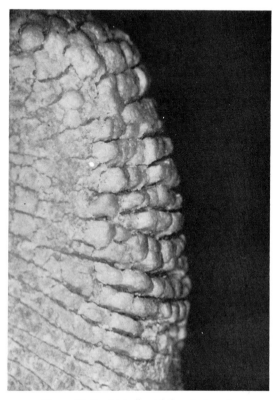

Figure 11–5. Lamellar ichthyosis (knee).

On histologic examination of sections from a skin biopsy, marked hyperkeratosis with patchy parakeratosis, an increased granular layer, acanthosis and papillomatosis are seen. A moderate, perivascular mononuclear inflammatory infiltrate is present in the upper dermis. Studies of epidermal cellular kinetics have shown that increased mitotic activity and a rapid epidermal cell transit time are characteristic of this disease (Frost, 1966). These findings suggest that the excessive proliferation of epidermal cells may account in part for the massive production of scale.

Family histories of infants with nonbullous CIE are consistent with an autosomal recessive mode of inheritance. Consanguinity is common in families with this disorder (Wells, 1965).

BULLOUS CONGENITAL ICHTHYOSIFORM ERYTHRODERMA
(Epidermolytic hyperkeratosis)

Infants affected with this condition have recurrent bullous lesions as well as erythema, dryness and peeling (Fig. 11–6). During the neonatal period the bullae may occur over widespread areas (Fig. 11–7), resulting in extensive denudation with secondary infection and sepsis (Fig. 11–8). In contrast to nonbullous CIE, an increased incidence of prematurity has not been noted. The disease is inherited as an autosomal dominant trait (Wells, 1965).

With increasing age the hyperkeratosis may remain generalized or may localize to the flexural regions. Scales are small, hard and shotty and are shed in large quantities (Plate XII–B). The palms and soles are usually normal but accentuated cutaneous markings and gross hyperkeratosis may occcasionally be seen. Ectropion is not a feature of this disease.

The blisters are the most characteristic manifestation of bullous CIE and differentiate this disorder from nonbullous CIE. Bullae occur in crops, vary from 0.5 cm to several centimeters in size and, in later childhood, are often localized to the lower portions of the legs. Secondary infection from β-hemolytic streptococci is a frequent occurrence and should be treated promptly with systemically administered antibiotics.

The histopathologic pattern is diagnostic in this disorder. The cells of the midepidermis and granular layer show extensive vacuolization and large clumped keratohyaline granules. Hyperkeratosis, papillomatosis and

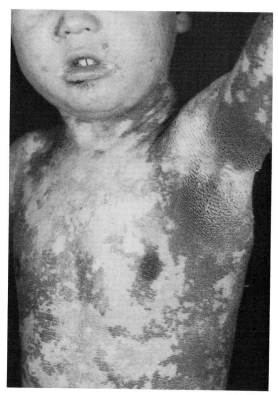

Figure 11–6. Bullous congenital ichthyosiform erythroderma.

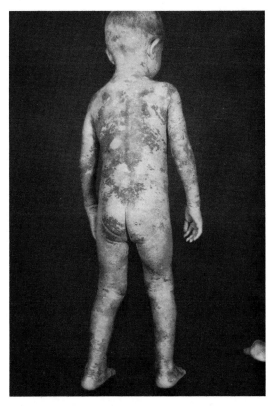

Figure 11–7. Bullous congenital ichthyosiform erythroderma.

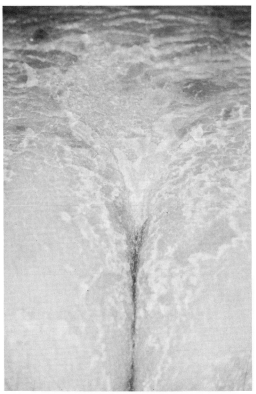

Figure 11–8. Bullous congenital ichthyosiform erythroderma in gluteal area.

acanthosis are all characteristic but may vary considerably in degree. The dermis is normal except for a small perivascular mononuclear cell infiltrate. Epidermal cellular kinetics are abnormal as in nonbullous CIE (Frost, 1966).

Ichthyosis Hystrix

This is a confusing term which has been applied to patients with lesions varying from mild to very severe whorled and linear hyperkeratoses (see also Chap. 10). The lesions may resemble porcupine quills or may form small segmental epidermal nevi. The histology in most cases is similar to that of bullous CIE (Zeligman, 1965). However, because of clinical and histological variability, the term should probably be used only in a descriptive sense to convey the clinical appearance of the hyperkeratotic lesions.

Differential Diagnosis and Treatment

The major types of ichthyosis are often a source of confusion for many physicians; exposure to large numbers of patients is necessary to become facile at recognition of the various forms of the disorder. In some instances the family history may be negative for

skin disease, and the clinical features, particularly in a newborn infant, may not be clearcut. A skin biopsy will often solve a diagnostic dilemma and should be included in the investigation of any infant with a scaling disorder. If X-linked ichthyosis is under consideration as a diagnostic possibility, an ophthalmological consultation, including slit lamp examination of the patient and family, may be helpful. Occasionally, a period of observation is necessary before a definitive diagnosis can be made, particularly for infants with collodion membranes. The diagnostic features of the four major types of ichthyosis are summarized in Table 11–1.

Apart from the dysmature infant and the rare normal infant with severe desquamation, erythrokeratoderma variabilis, ichthyosis linearis circumflexa and the ichthyotic syndromes must also be considered in the differential diagnosis of the scaling infant. Bullous CIE can be confused with epidermolysis bullosa or Ritter's disease: Neither scaling nor diffuse redness is usual in epidermolysis bullosa. In Ritter's disease erythroderma is characteristic, generalized scaling is absent and cultures of the blister fluid are positive for a Group II phage type *Staphylococcus aureus.* The bullae are flaccid, Nikolsky's sign is positive and the epidermis peels off in large sheets.

Therapy for ichthyosis is restricted almost entirely to topical preparations. The underlying principle is hydration of the skin and generous application of lubricants to retard evaporation or drying. A daily bath containing water dispersible bath oil should be followed immediately by application of ointments, creams or lotions to the entire body while it is still damp. Generally, ointments such as Aquaphor or petrolatum are more effective because they are relatively adherent. Frequent supplemental applications of lubricant throughout the day are also helpful, but prior hydration increases their effectiveness. In localized areas, a keratolytic agent such as salicylic acid incorporated into an ointment or oil may be utilized, particularly for very keratotic areas such as the scalp. A 10 per cent urea preparation in an ointment base is a moderately effective alternative in situations where lubricants alone are not beneficial. Topical vitamin A acid (0.1 per cent), currently undergoing investigational use, shows promise as a useful therapeutic modality for these disorders (Frost, 1969).

Detergents and soaps containing hexachlorophene should be avoided because they are irritating and drying, and toxic amounts of hexachlorophene might be absorbed. Soap substitutes or superfatted soaps may be used in place of conventional soaps. Exposure to harsh winter weather or extremely dry indoor heating should be avoided whenever possible. Secondary infections should be treated with appropriate antibiotic therapy. Areas which fissure or show a primary irritant dermatitis may be treated for brief periods with a topical corticosteroid preparation. Patients with widespread bullae (bullous CIE) may respond to a short course of systemically administered corticosteroids. Sedation with an oral antihistamine such as elixir of benadryl is often helpful in controlling the severe pruritus experienced by many of these infants.

ICHTHYOSIS LINEARIS CIRCUMFLEXA

This disorder is considered a variant of lamellar ichthyosis and is characterized by migratory, polycyclic scaly lesions, hyperkeratosis of the flexures and hyperhidrosis of the palms and soles. It is thought to be inherited in an autosomal recessive fashion (Hurwitz, 1971).

A diffusely red and scaly skin is noted at birth or during the first year of life. Numerous serpiginous lesions with raised erythematous, hyperkeratotic borders and a characteristic double-edged scale appear on the trunk and proximal extremities after a variable period of time. The flexural skin becomes hyperkeratotic and may have a brownish discoloration. Palms and soles are normal in appearance and hyperhidrosis has been reported, but only in adults. Since some of these patients may have defects of the hair shaft, a representative sample of hair should be examined microscopically (see Netherton's syndrome, page 120). The course is chronic with occasional brief spontaneous remissions. Treatment is the same as for other types of ichthyosis.

ERYTHROKERATODERMA VARIABILIS

Two morphologic components are present in this condition: sharply demarcated hyperkeratotic plaques with bizarre and irregular borders; and independent, discrete areas of macular erythema (also with geographic outlines) which change in size and location from day to day. Either type of lesion may predominate and both show considerable variability

(Cram, 1970). The disorder is inherited as an autosomal dominant trait.

Areas of predilection for the erythematous lesions are the face, buttocks and extensor surface of the extremities. Although the lesions are generally transient, some may become hyperkeratotic and fixed. The onset of erythematous macules is said to be associated with emotional upset or exposure to wind and cold. The hyperkeratotic plaques have a distribution similar to the erythematous lesions but usually tend to persist. The lesions are yellow-brown, thickened and covered with large greasy scales. The palms and soles may have a thickened stratum corneum. Hair, teeth and nails are normal as are other organ systems. Mild pain or pruritus in the lesions is occasionally noted.

Histopathologic findings include a laminated stratum corneum which frequently has a saw-toothed contour, occasional focal areas of parakeratosis, a prominent granular layer, papillomatosis and irregular acanthosis of the epidermis with suprapapillary thinning. Papillary capillaries are straight, elongated and surrounded by a mild mononuclear infiltrate. The epidermal proliferation rate is normal (Vandersteen, 1971).

ICHTHYOSIS SYNDROMES
Sjögren-Larsson Syndrome

The triad of ichthyosis, mental retardation and spastic diplegia constitutes the Sjögren-Larsson syndrome. Sjögren and Larsson (1957) first reported this syndrome in a group of 28 affected individuals, all of whom came from a coastal district in northern Sweden. Since that time individuals of diversified nationalities with this syndrome have been described. Many are siblings of unaffected parents, but consanguineous marriages occur frequently in these kindreds. The disease affects both sexes and appears to be inherited as an autosomal recessive trait.

Ichthyosis is present at birth and characterized by a fine, branny scaling with accentuation in the flexural areas. A variable degree of erythroderma is usually present. Palms and soles are hyperkeratotic but hair and nails are normal. Mental deficiency is severe and may necessitate institutional care. Spastic diplegia is marked in the legs and less severe or absent in the arms. Deep tendon reflexes are increased in the involved extremities and the Babinski sign is positive.

Ophthalmologic changes have been noted in 20 to 30 per cent of affected individuals.

Although the descriptions of the retinal lesions vary, all suggest a degenerative disturbance of the pigment epithelium. The exact age at which this feature has its onset is unknown, but fundus changes have been observed in patients as young as two years. Visual acuity is probably decreased in some instances. Fluorescein fundus angiograms demonstrate increased transmission of the choroidal vasculature in areas of hypopigmentation (Gilbert, 1968).

In addition to the usual features of this syndrome, occasional individuals have had dysplasia of tooth enamel, serrated teeth, epilepsy, dermatoglyphic abnormalities, hypertelorism, defective sweating and speech defects (Selmanowitz, 1967). No constant metabolic abnormalties have been found. The skin biopsy pattern is similar to that of nonbullous CIE.

Life expectancy is considerably shortened in these patients. Mental retardation is apparently static, but the spasticity may be progressive with deterioration of gait and other motor functions. Therapy is the same as for nonbullous CIE.

Rud's Syndrome

The clinical features of Rud's syndrome are oligophrenia, epilepsy and ichthyosis. Infantilism appears to be a less constant finding. The following associated anomalies have also been reported: dwarfism; partial gigantism; arachnodactyly; structural defects of the hands and feet; nerve deafness; hypoplastic or absent teeth; and alopecia. Eye defects include strabismus, retinitis pigmentosa, ptosis, nystagmus and blepharospasm.

Dermatologic descriptions of Rud's syndrome are scanty and there are no histologic studies documented; therefore, it is impossible to classify the ichthyosis. The cutaneous findings have varied from mild, generalized branny desquamation (MacGillivray, 1954) to severe ichthyosis resembling "snakeskin" (Ewing, 1955). The extensor surfaces of the extremities are most often involved and neither an erythrodermic component nor a predilection for the flexural areas has been noted.

Sexual infantilism may be manifested in the young child by the presence of hypoplastic genitalia and undescended or small, "soft" testicles. Mental retardation is moderate to severe. Both major and minor epilepsy occur, but in a few cases only an abnormal electroencephalogram has been found. Pertinent abnormal laboratory findings in a single affected male were low urinary gonadotropins, a reduced glucuronide fraction and an elevated sulfate fraction of the 17-ketosteroids (York-Moore, 1962).

Only a few cases of Rud's syndrome have been reported and none have occurred in documented pedigrees. More detailed genetic, clinical and metabolic data are needed to confirm the authenticity of this syndrome.

Netherton's Syndrome

Netherton's syndrome is characterized by ichthyosis, defects of the hair shaft and an atopic diathesis. In the initial descriptions, affected patients were thought to have nonbullous congenital ichthyosiform erythroderma (lamellar ichthyosis) and trichorrhexis invaginata (bamboo hair), an abnormality of hair in which the distal portion of the hair shaft is intersuscepted into the proximal portion, resulting in a ball-and-socket type deformity. More recent reports have clarified and broadened the scope of this syndrome.

The ichthyosis is usually present at birth. Flexural areas are always involved. A few patients have had an associated erythroderma that has been classified as nonbullous CIE, but the majority of cases appear to have typical ichthyosis linearis circumflexa (Hurwitz, 1970). Nails, teeth and mucous membranes are not affected.

The scalp hair is sparse, lusterless and short, and seems to fracture at defective sites along the hair shaft. Eyebrows, eyelashes and body hair may also be sparse. The most characteristic and unique microscopic hair abnormality is trichorrhexis invaginata. In some patients, a whole spectrum of defects has been observed including twisted hair (pili torti), nodal thickenings of the hair shaft (trichorrhexis nodosa), cup-like deformities, braid-weave, rope-like segments and variations in hair shaft diameter (Stevanovic, 1969). The hair shaft anomalies are readily detectable by examining plucked or cut hair with a dissecting microscope.

The most characteristic allergic manifestations are urticaria and angioneurotic edema, usually related to ingestion of nuts or other foods. Some patients have had asthma, anaphylactoid reactions, or, rarely, eczema (Altman, 1969). The first several patients reported to have Netherton's syndrome were all female, but since a few well-documented cases have been described in males, an autosomal recessive type of inheritance has been postulated. The histopathologic findings are similar to those seen in nonbullous

CIE and icthyosis linearis circumflexa. Examination of sections from the scalp usually shows an abnormality in the external and internal root sheath cells of follicles containing affected hairs (Stevanovic, 1969). No consistent metabolic defects have been noted. A few of the patients have been mentally deficient (Altman, 1969), but retardation is not considered to be a constant feature of the syndrome. The clinical diagnosis should be confirmed by skin biopsy and microscopic examination of representative hairs selected from various body sites.

Conradi's Disease

Infants with Conradi's disease (chondrodystrophia calcificans congenita) have an extensive array of anomalies affecting bone, joints, lens, skin, and occasionally, the cardiovascular and central nervous systems. The *sine qua non* of the disease is the finding of stippled epiphyses in the cartilaginous skeleton including, in some patients, the vertebral discs, joint capsules, larynx, trachea and hyoid bone. Epiphyseal changes are readily demonstrable on roentgenograms. Other common bony abnormalities include shortening of the femora and humeri, flexion contractures of the large joints and saddle nose secondary to dysplasia of the nasal bone. Less common bony anomalies are hip dysplasia, kyphosis, scoliosis, vertebral wedging, craniostenosis, polydactyly, syndactyly and asymmetrical hypoplasia of the bones of the hands and feet (Melnick, 1965). The most common eye anomaly is bilateral cataract with or without optic atrophy. Congenital heart defects,

high arched palate, hernias, mental and physical retardation, abnormal facies and hematologic disorders have also been described.

Skin changes (Fig. 11–9) have been noted in approximately 25 per cent of affected infants (Smith, 1970), and consist of universal or localized erythema in association with thick, white, adherent scales that may have a distinctive whorled pattern (Bodian, 1966). Some of these patients have been thought to have congenital ichthyosiform erythroderma. In Conradi's syndrome the nails and hair are normal but there is keratoderma of the palms and soles. The scaling and erythroderma decrease with age, but may be superseded by follicular atrophoderma, patchy alopecia and blotchy hyperpigmentation resembling the pattern seen in incontinentia pigmenti.

The frequency of consanguinity in families with affected children is high (12 to 33 per cent), and an autosomal recessive type of inheritance seems likely. Improvement in epiphyseal mineralization, skeletal growth and joint mobility occurs with age. The morbidity and mortality of Conradi's syndrome are related to the severity of the associated anomalies.

Tay's Syndrome

A new combination of abnormalities (ichthyosis, defective hair, progeria-like appearance, mental and growth retardation) has been described recently in three siblings of a Singapore family (Tay, 1971). Although the skin appears uniformly red and scaly at birth, by early childhood the erythroderma disappears and the hyperkeratosis is confined to

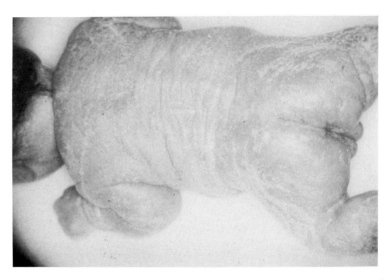

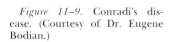

Figure 11–9. Conradi's disease. (Courtesy of Dr. Eugene Bodian.)

the face, trunk and extensor extremities, sparing the flexures. The palms and soles are thickened and fissured. This distribution of scaling, plus the diminished granular layer seen on skin biopsy, makes nonbullous congenital ichthyosiform erythroderma (the diagnosis suggested by the authors), seem unlikely.

In Tay's syndrome the scalp hair, eyebrows and eyelashes are sparse, short and brittle, fracturing easily with mild trauma. On microscopic examination, affected hairs show either twisting of the shaft (pili torti) or irregularly spaced transverse bands that are nonbirefringent with polarized light and, at the distal end of the shaft, become transected by a clear transverse fracture line.

Affected patients are dwarfed but the nature of the growth retardation has not been clarified. Intelligence quotients are low; however, patients are otherwise neurologically normal. The progeria-like appearance, characterized by lack of subcutaneous fat, beaked nose, sunken cheeks and bat-like ears, completes the syndrome. The presence of this entity in three of seven offspring of normal parents suggests an autosomal recessive mode of inheritance.

KERATODERMA OF THE PALMS AND SOLES

A number of hereditary disorders, many of them rare, are characterized by diffuse or localized hyperkeratosis of the palms (Fig. 11–10) and soles (Plate XII–C). Not all of these disorders are evident in infancy (Rook, 1968).

Tylosis, the most common of the palmoplantar keratodermas, is inherited in an autosomal dominant fashion and develops between birth and six months of age. The hyperkeratosis is diffuse, uniform and limited to the palms and soles, often with a sharply demarcated border surrounded by a band of erythema. Microscopically, there is increased thickness of the stratum corneum only. Because the horny layer may become markedly thickened, painful fissuring can result, particularly after trauma or dehydration. Extreme hyperkeratosis may be controlled to a degree by the use of a topical keratolytic agent, such as salicylic acid.

The less common palmoplantar keratodermas with onset in infancy are summarized in Table 11–3. Other inherited disorders in this group that are not present in infancy but become manifest later in childhood include keratoderma with carcinoma of the esophagus, punctate keratoderma, striate keratoderma, disseminate keratoderma with corneal dystrophy and circumscribed keratoderma (Rook, 1968). Hyperkeratosis of the palms and soles also occurs in hidrotic ectodermal dysplasia, pachyonychia congenita and pityriasis rubra pilaris.

FAMILIAL CONTINUAL SKIN PEELING

This rare disorder, also known as deciduous skin, is probably inherited as an autosomal recessive trait. Affected individuals are symptomatic in infancy with generalized and superficial desquamation similar to the peeling following a sunburn. There is no as-

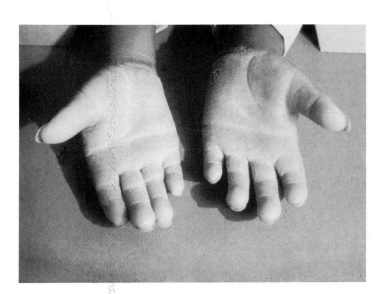

Figure 11–10. Hyperkeratosis of the palms (keratosis palmaris et plantaris).

Table 11–3. Keratoderma of Palms and Soles

Condition	Age of Onset	Inheritance	Clinical Features
Tylosis	Infancy	Autosomal dominant	1. Occasionally hyperhidrosis
Mutilating keratoderma	Infancy	Autosomal dominant	1. Fibrous bands on digits 2. Star-shaped keratoses dorsum of hands and feet 3. Knuckle-pads 4. Scarring alopecia variable 5. Occasionally high-frequency hearing loss
Progressive keratoderma	Infancy	Autosomal dominant	1. May involve dorsal hands and feet
Mal de Maleda	Infancy	Autosomal recessive	1. Redness of palms and soles 2. May involve dorsal hands and feet 3. Hyperhidrosis 4. Circumscribed hyperkeratosis on wrists, forearms, knees 5. Occasionally EEG abnormalities
Papillon-Lefevre syndrome	Infancy	Autosomal recessive	1. Erythema of palms and soles 2. Hyperhidrosis 3. Periodontosis with loss of teeth 4. Calcification of dura

sociated erythema. The entire body surface, except for the palms and soles, is involved and the peeling is accentuated by mild rubbing. Increased proliferation of epidermal cells has been demonstrated by *in vitro* autoradiographic studies (Kurban, 1969). The disorder is benign and symptoms may be relieved adequately with lubricants.

PSORIASIS

This disorder, common in adulthood and not uncommon in childhood, is exceedingly rare in infancy. Patients with infantile psoriasis may present with an erythroderma (Fig. 11–11), an infrequent variant of psoriasis (Scott, 1968), or with the more common localized or guttate forms (Watson, 1971). Oc-

casionally, psoriatic plaques may occur in the diaper region of the young infant and may not show the typical silvery scales because of the moist environment promoted by occlusive diapers and plastic pants. A strong family history of the disease, often in both paternal and maternal relatives, is usually obtained. Rarely, psoriasis will be congenital, not associated with family history, and have a poor prognosis (Lerner, 1972).

The histopathologic features characteristic of psoriasis are thickened parakeratotic horny layer, regular acanthosis of the epidermis, thinning of the epidermis overlying the dermal papillae, small epidermal microabscesses filled with polymorphonuclear leukocytes, dilatation of the dermal

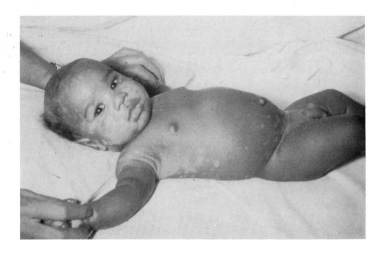

Figure 11–11. Psoriasis.

capillaries and a perivascular mixed inflammatory infiltrate. The epidermal cell turnover time is markedly accelerated.

In the absence of a positive family history and the classic histologic findings, psoriasis is an unlikely diagnosis in this age group. Differential diagnosis of the diffuse type includes Leiner's disease, nonbullous congenital ichthyosiform erythroderma and widespread atopic dermatitis (rare in the first month). Plaques and guttate lesions may be confused with seborrheic dermatitis, Letterer-Siwe disease and diaper dermatitis. Management of these patients is exceedingly difficult and may require an array of therapeutic agents. Topical corticosteroid therapy is the treatment of choice but antimitotic agents or systemically administered corticosteroids may be necessary to control the disease. Systemic medications should never be used for localized lesions of psoriasis in infancy or childhood.

REFERENCES

Adam, A., Ziprkowski, L. and Feinstein, A.: Linkage relations of X-borne ichthyosis to the Xg blood groups, and to other markers of the X in Israelis. Ann. Hum. Genet. *32*:323, 1969.

Altman, J. and Stroud, J.: Netherton's syndrome and ichthyosis linearis circumflexa. Arch. Derm. *100*:550, 1969.

Baden, H. P., Bonar, L. and Katz, E.: The fibrous proteins of epidermis. J. Invest. Derm. *50*:301, 1968.

Bloom, D. and Goodfried, M. S.: Lamellar ichthyosis of the newborn. Arch. Derm. *86*:336, 1962.

Bodian, E. L.: Skin manifestations of Conradi's disease. Arch. Derm. *94*:743, 1966.

Briceno-Maaz, T.: Two cases of congenital ichthyosis. Arch. Derm. *87*:230, 1963.

Craig, J. M., Goldsmith, L. A. and Baden, H. P.: An abnormality of keratin in the harlequin fetus. Pediatrics *46*:437, 1970.

Cram, D. L.: Erythrokeratoderma variabilis and variable circinate erythrokeratodermas. Arch. Derm. *101*:68, 1970.

Esterly, N. B.: The ichthyosiform dermatoses. Pediatrics *42*:990, 1968.

Ewing, J. A.: The association of oligophrenia and dyskeratoses. Part III. The syndrome of Rud. Amer. J. Ment. Defic. *10*:575, 1955.

Feinstein, A., Ackerman, A. B. and Ziprkowski, L.: Histology of autosomal dominant ichthyosis vulgaris and X-linked ichthyosis. Arch. Derm. *101*:524, 1970.

Frost, P. and Weinstein, G. D.: Topical administration of vitamin A acid for ichthyosiform dermatoses and psoriasis. JAMA *207*:1863, 1969.

Frost, P., Weinstein, G. D. and Van Scott, E. J. The ichthyosiform dermatoses. II. J. Invest. Derm. *47*:561, 1966.

Gilbert, W. R., Smith, J. L. and Nyhan, W. L.: The Sjögren-Larsson syndrome. Arch. Ophthal. *80*:308, 1968.

Griffiths, A. D.: Skin desquamation in the newborn. Biol. Neonat. *10*:127, 1966.

Hurwitz, S., Kirsch, N. and McGuire, J.: Reevaluation of ichthyosis and hair shaft abnormalties. *103*:266, 1971.

Jay, B., Black, R. K. and Wells, R. S.: Ocular manifestations of ichthyosis. Brit. J. Ophthal. *52*:217, 1968.

Kessel, J. and Friedlander, F. C.: Harlequin foetus. Arch. Dis. Child. *31*:53, 1956.

Kurban, A. K. and Azar, H. A.: Familial continual skin peeling. Brit. J. Derm. *81*:191, 1969.

Lerner, M. R. and Lerner, A. B.: Congenital psoriasis. Arch. Derm. *105*:578, 1972.

MacGillivray, R. C.: The syndrome of Rud. Amer. J. Ment. Defic. *59*:67, 1954.

Melnick, J. C.: Chrondrodystrophia calcificans congenita. Amer. J. Dis. Child. *110*:218, 1965.

Reed, W. B., Herwick, R. P., Harville, D., Porter, P. S. and Conant, M.: Lamellar ichthyosis of the newborn. Arch. Derm. *105*:394, 1972.

Rook, A., Wilkinson, D. S. and Ebling, F. J. G.: Textbook of Dermatology. Philadelphia, F. A. Davis Co., 1968.

Scott, R. B. and Surana, R.: Erythrodermic psoriasis in childhood. Amer. J. Dis. Child. *116*:218, 1968.

Selmanowitz, V. J. and Porter, M. J.: The Sjögren-Larsson syndrome. Amer. J. Med. *42*:412, 1967.

Sever, R. J., Frost, P. and Weinstein, G.: Eye changes in ichthyosis. JAMA *206*:2283, 1968.

Sjögren, T. and Larsson, T.: A clinical and genetic study, oligophrenia in combination with congenital ichthyosis and spastic disorders. Acta Psychiat. et Neurol. Scand. *32* (suppl. 113):1, 1957.

Sjostedt, S., Engelson, C. and Rooth, G.: Dysmaturity. Arch. Dis. Child. *33*:123, 1958.

Smeenk, G.: Two families with collodion babies. Brit. J. Derm. *78*:81, 1966.

Smith, D. W.: Recognizable Patterns of Human Malformation. Philadelphia, W. B. Saunders Co., 1970, p. 210.

Stevanovic, D. V.: Multiple defects of the hair shaft in Netherton's disease. Brit. J. Derm. *81*:851, 1969.

Tay, C. H.: Ichthyosiform erythroderma, hair shaft abnormalities, and mental and growth retardation. Arch. Derm. *104*:4, 1971.

Vandersteen, P. R. and Muller, S. A.: Erythrokeratodermia variabilis. Arch. Derm. *103*:362, 1971.

Watson, W. and Farber, E. M.: Psoriasis in childhood. Pediat. Clin. N. Amer. *18*:875, 1971.

Wells, R. S.: Genetic classification of ichthyosis. Arch. Derm. *92*:1, 1965.

Wells, R. S. and Jennings, M. C.: X-linked ichthyosis and ichthyosis vulgaris. JAMA *202*:485, 1967.

Wells, R. S. and Kerr, C. B.: Clinical features of autosomal dominant and sex-linked ichthyosis in an English population. Brit. Med. J. *1*:947, 1966.

York-Moore, M. E. and Rundle, A. T.: Rud's syndrome. J. Ment. Defic. Res. *6*:108, 1962.

Zeligman, I. and Pomeranz, J.: Variations of congenital ichthyosiform erythroderma. Arch. Derm. *91*:120, 1965.

Chapter Twelve

ECZEMA

The term "eczema" is a source of bewilderment to those who are not acquainted with the vagaries of the word's usage. It may have different meanings in American and European literature. Some consider the term "eczema" to be synonomous with "dermatitis." For the purposes of this discussion, it may be useful to think of *eczema* as a "genus" of skin disorder, and less specific than one of its "species," for example, *atopic eczema*. *Dermatitis*, without a qualifying adjective, is a less definitive term since it simply refers to an inflammation of the skin which may result in a spectrum of lesions varying from acute necrosis and ulceration to simple erythema. A comparison of some "species" of eczema is shown in Table 12–1. The eczematous process plays its tune with a more limited scale of patho-

Table 12–1. Features of Atopic Dermatitis, Primary Irritant Dermatitis, and Infectious Dermatitis in the Newborn

	Atopic Dermatitis	*Primary Irritant*	*Infectious Dermatitis*
Age of onset	Usually not before 3 months, rarely at end of first month, not at birth	Any time during first month	Any time
Family history	High incidence of respiratory allergy, hay fever, atopic dermatitis	None	May have bacterial carrier in family
Skin lesions	Weeping, vesicular, scaling; little lichenification before 4 months. Extensor surfaces, cheeks, ears and scalp. Symmetrical. Rarely diaper area alone	Bright red, weeping. Less scaling. Any site may be involved but mostly diaper area, perianal area. May not be symmetrical	Weeping, much crusting. Perioral, nasal, umbilical and diaper areas. Punched out ulcers frequent on buttocks, perineum
Pruritus	Marked, precedes lesion	May be variable—follows lesions	Little
Culture	Often negative	Often negative	Positive—*Staphylococcus aureus* Streptococci Enterococci *Candida albicans* Pseudomonas
Other skin lesions	Associated "seborrheic" lesions, ichthyosis vulgaris frequent. Not seen until after 3 months of age.	Usually none	Usually none. May be a complication of congenital defects. Bullous lesions frequent
Consequence of delay in treatment	May improve spontaneously	Usually gets worse locally	Usually gets worse locally; satellite lesions develop nearby and at a distance
Incidence	Very rare	Very common	Common

Table 12–2. Causes of Eczema in the Newborn

Exogenous		Endogenous	
		With the cutaneous process predominant	*Cutaneous process secondary to a systemic process
Primary irritant	Contact dermatitis		
Allergic		Infantile eczema, atopic seborrhea, "cradle cap"	Wiskott-Aldrich syndrome
			Congenital sex-linked agammaglobulinemia
			Leiner's disease with C₅ dysfunction
Bacteria	Infection	Desquamative erythroderma	Ataxia-telangiectasia
			Chronic granulomatous disease
Fungi			Phenylketonuria
		Ritter's disease	Ahistidinemia
Light	Physical agents		Mucopolysaccharidoses
		Congenital ichthyosiform erythroderma	Hartnup disease
Cold			Acrodermatitis enteropathica
			Gluten-sensitive enteropathy
Heat		"Diaper dermatitis"	Anhidrotic ectodermal dysplasia
			Histiocytosis X
Allergic component	Insect bites		Long arm 18 deletion syndrome
			Hereditary acrokeratotic poikiloderma

Leiner's disease with C_5 dysfunction

*This list is not all-inclusive. Many additional reports exist wherein an eczematous process forms part of a syndrome.

logic notes. Lesions of eczema may have a temporal or spatial relationship to each other; that is, a lesion may evolve from one stage to another, or, several stages may be present simultaneously on different parts of the body.

There are four phases of eczema, any one of which may persist as the dominant feature depending on the age of the patient, the local physiologic characteristics of the skin involved and the persistence of the underlying cause. All phases are characterized by pruritus. The initial stage (1) is *erythema*, which proceeds to (2) formation of microvesicles and *weeping* or oozing. The epidermal response to the injurious process then causes a burst of rapid epidermal mitotic activity which leads to (3) *scaling*. (4) Finally, *lichenification* (thickening of the skin with increased visibility of normal skin markings) and *pigmentary disturbances* (usually, an initial increase followed by decrease in pigmentation) supervene. In the young infant, the first three stages predominate and lichenification is not seen.

Histologically, these four stages are represented by (1) vasodilation (accompanied locally by the release of vasoactive substances including histamine, acetylcholine, kinins, serotonin, norepinephrine, prostaglandins and others not yet chemically defined), and (2) infiltration of acute and chronic inflammatory cells into the epidermis. Next follows edema of the Malpighian layer which in turn causes rupture of intercellular bridges, mi-

crovesicle formation (spongiosis) and loss of epidermal integrity. (3) Epidermal proliferation and imperfect formation of a new stratum corneum, some cells of which may retain their nuclei (parakeratosis), can then be seen. This results in (4) thickening of the dermis and epidermis because of downward proliferation of the rete ridges (acanthosis). The histologic features are comparable for all of the eczemas except when the infiltrate causing it is of a specific type (e.g., histiocytosis X).

It can be perceived from the preceding discussion that recognition of eczema is not difficult. But since its course and clinical picture may be quite variable, it is often difficult to distinguish different types of eczema from one another, and the histologic picture may not be helpful.

Although the causes of eczema in the adult comprise a formidable list, the causes of this disorder in the newborn are less numerous. Furthermore, the most common types of eczema in the adult are among the least common in the newborn. Indeed, *eczema is a much less common disorder in the neonatal period than in an infant older than two months of age.*

During the first month of life, the causes of eczema (see Table 12–2) may be considered under two broad categories: *exogenous* and *endogenous*. The *exogenous* causes include primary irritant contact dermatitis, physical agents (light, cold or heat), allergic eczematous contact dermatitis and infection. The *endogenous* group may, for the purposes of discussion, be divided into those disorders in which the skin is predominantly involved and those in which the cutaneous eruption reflects serious systemic disease.

EXOGENOUS CAUSES OF ECZEMA

Irritating chemical substances, excessive washing, chafing, prolonged exposure to solar light, cold and wind and infection with bacteria and fungi, more frequently cause an eczematous eruption during the neonatal period than allergy to food or topically applied agents.

PRIMARY IRRITANT ECZEMATOUS CONTACT DERMATITIS

In this common type of eczema the site of eruption varies somewhat with the etiologic agent. Saliva may be irritating to the face and chin, and fecal secretions irritating to the buttocks. Detergent bubble bath may cause a scaly, itchy eruption with a widespread distribution, but it most often affects the cheeks, buttocks, throat and extensor surfaces of the limbs. Preparations commonly applied to the diaper area, such as proprietary antiseptic agents and harsh soaps containing mercury, phenol, tars, salicylic acid or sulphur, may cause an acute, erosive diaper dermatitis (Fig. 12–1) which can become eczematous (Plate XII–D, page 92) and spread from the original site of involvement to cover the entire body. For this reason, it is imperative to have very specific information from the mother about substances that have been applied to the infant's skin. We have found that this

aspect of the history is frequently neglected, resulting in confusion for both physician and parent as to the cause of a refractory eczema. Infant skin, for example, may not tolerate phenolated petrolatum, while the medication usually does no harm to adolescent skin. When an agent is discovered to which an infant, but not his older brother, is susceptible, an error frequently is made in assuming that the sensitivity must have an allergic basis. A primary irritant will cause a skin eruption in all infants if used in adequate concentrations, but it will not necessarily affect older children at that concentration. The skin of the infant is more permeable and susceptible to damage, and some areas, such as the eyelids or scrotum, are even more vulnerable than others.

ALLERGIC ECZEMATOUS CONTACT DERMATITIS

In the first month of life allergic reactions to topically applied agents are extremely rare. If such an event does occur, one should expect to see a well-circumscribed weeping lesion in the area of application. A diffuse eczematous cutaneous reaction to a systemically administered drug may also occur in the newborn as a result of transplacental passage of certain drugs (i.e., bromides) (Hodgeman, 1971), but like allergic contact dermatitis, drug eruptions are exceedingly rare during this period.

PHYSICAL AGENTS

Excessive exposure to summer sunlight, chafing wind or a warm, humid atmosphere

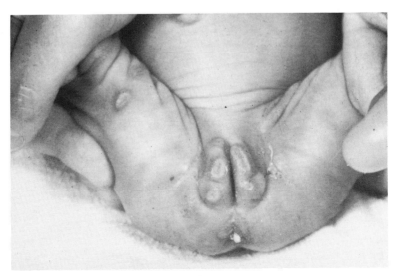

Figure 12–1. Erosive and eczematous diaper dermatitis resulting from primary irritation.

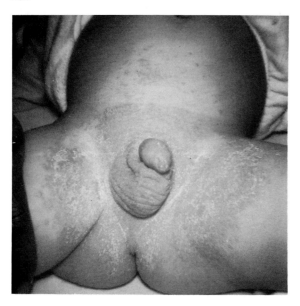

Figure 12–2. Candidal diaper dermatitis.

can produce a dermatitis which, in the very young infant, may mimic the early phases of the eczematous response. A blistering sunburn reaction may be a cutaneous expression of excessive exposure to ultraviolet light; however, in the child with inherited light-sensitivity (see xeroderma pigmentosum, porphyria and Hartnup disease), exposure to minimal amounts of sunlight may result in eczema. During the winter months a mild, self-limiting eczematous eruption may occur on cheeks and hands as a result of exposure to the elements. During the summer months miliaria (see Chap. 6) may become widespread and eczematized.

INFECTIOUS ECZEMA

The diaper area is frequently the site of an erosive and eczematous reaction caused by primary irritation and infection. When infections exist, the organisms found are usually *Staphylococcus aureus* and gram-negative enterococci, especially *Escherichia coli*. In one study, *Candida albicans* (Fig. 12–2) was cultured from the diaper area in 77 per cent of infants with diaper dermatitis (Montes, 1971). These authors also frequently found a mixed infection that lead them to suggest that synergistic action between the bacterial and fungal organisms might contribute to the pathogenesis of the dermatitis. In contrast, other investigators have not noted appreciable differences in skin flora on the buttocks of infants with diaper dermatitis in comparison to normal controls, nor have they demon-

strated a high incidence of candidal infection in the diaper dermatitis group (Brookes, 1971). The buttocks only or the entire diaper area may be involved. The lesions start as erythematous patches which may coalesce, become erosive, weep and result in punched-out ulcers. If *Candida albicans* is the causative agent, the intertriginous areas are most often affected and the central area of dermatitis is surrounded at the periphery by satellite pustules.

ENDOGENOUS ECZEMA AS A PREDOMINANTLY CUTANEOUS PROCESS

The infant who develops a localized or diffuse eczematous process during the first month of life but who otherwise appears to be in good health constitutes a diagnostic problem with several possible solutions.

ATOPIC DERMATITIS

There are several synonyms for this disorder, including atopic eczema, infantile eczema, constitutional eczema, and so on.

Although atopic dermatitis (Fig. 12–3) is probably the most common cause of an eczematous eruption after the second or third month of life, *it is very uncommon during the first month* (Rostenberg, 1968; Rostenberg, 1971; Solomon, 1966; Norins, 1971; Solomon, in press). This diagnosis should not be made lightly during this period and prac-

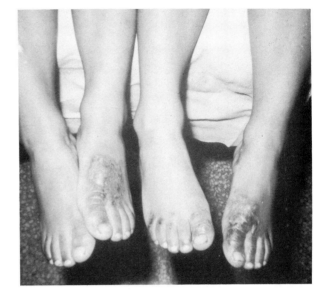

Figure 12–3. Atopic dermatitis in uniovular twins. There is remarkably identical involvement.

tically never should be considered during the first week of life. Contrary to opinion, there is little evidence to incriminate allergy as a cause of atopic dermatitis, and diet probably has little to do with its provocation. On examining the data one would have to conclude that atopic dermatitis is probably a hereditarily determined metabolic defect resulting in increased vulnerability to a wide variety of itch stimuli.

The diagnosis of atopic dermatitis may be considered under the following set of circumstances: (1) if there is onset of a highly pruritic, erythematous, scaly and oozing eruption involving the cheeks, scalp, extensor surfaces of arms, legs and diaper area, and associated at times with similar patchy lesions on thorax and abdomen; (2) if a child is otherwise healthy and a systemic cause for the eczematous eruption has been ruled out (see following section); (3) if an eruption tends to be persistent if untreated but responds quickly to topical therapy and environmental control (see following section); (4) where a strong family history of asthma, hay fever and eczema exists; (5) where an exogenous cause, such as infection or contact dermatitis, has been excluded as a primary cause of the eruption; and (6) in the absence of histologic evidence of congenital ichthyosiform erythroderma.

If the above criteria have been met, it is likely (but by no means certain) that the three to four week old infant has atopic dermatitis. A positive cutaneous reaction to intradermally injected egg albumen, the presence of peripheral eosinophilia or an abnormal blanching reaction to intradermally administered acetylcholine (the delayed blanch test, [Hinrichs, 1966]) may be misleading factors and are not adequate criteria for the diagnosis.

Seborrheic Dermatitis and Leiner's Disease

The term "seborrhea" or "seborrheic dermatitis" refers to a condition characterized by greasy scaling associated with patchy redness, fissuring and occasional weeping. It may be seen from this description that, morphologically, there is enormous similarity between the scaly phase of eczema and that of seborrheic dermatitis. The confusion increases by the use of the term "seborrheic eczema." Furthermore, seborrheic lesions involving the scalp, ears and perineal folds (Fig. 12–4) are often seen as part of atopic dermatitis. Many cases of seborrheic dermatitis that are diagnosed with assurance when first seen may, on prolonged observation, evolve into typical atopic dermatitis. It is almost impossible on strictly morphological grounds to determine that seborrheic dermatitis will not become atopic dermatitis. Perhaps it would be more accurate to consider eczema as the basic process and greasy scaling as one of its morphologic components, just as weeping is a second component and lichenification, a third.

In the first week or two after birth a scaly dermatitis of the scalp (*cradle cap* or *milk crust*) is a common occurrence (Beare, 1968). It is without major significance, although

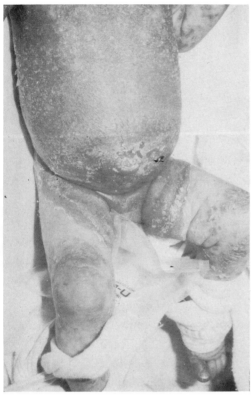

Figure 12–4. Seborrheic type of eczema and candidiasis of the diaper area.

frequently a source of worry for parents. Its cause is not known but some believe it to be a minor variant of seborrhea.

In the third or fourth week a more widespread process may involve the scalp, ears, forehead and flexural areas. The lesions are scaly, well-circumscribed and apparently not pruritic. The child seems well. The eruption may last three to six weeks or longer, heal and never reappear, or it may evolve into more typical symptoms of atopic dermatitis with pruritus and weeping. It is this transformation which is a source of controversy. It is possible that seborrheic dermatitis of the neonate is: (1) a single disease entity; (2) a disorder with multiple causes; and (3) a very early stage of atopic dermatitis. At this time, however, not enough is known to draw any conclusions. We believe it is sufficient to recognize the seborrheic picture and to treat it as such without giving the parents a prognosis concerning the development of atopic dermatitis.

Leiner's Disease (Fig. 12–5). In some infants between two and four months of age, the seborrhea may become generalized, resulting in a full-blown exfoliative erythroderma, or Leiner's disease (Plate XIII–A). It has been pointed out by Jacobs and Miller (1972) that certain familial cases of Leiner's disease have an ominous prognosis. These authors refer specifically to those infants with generalized exfoliative dermatitis starting within a week or two of birth and associated with severe diarrhea, recurrent gram-negative infections, wasting and death. These infants were found to suffer from a defect in function of the fifth component of complement (C_5). The C_5 dysfunction resulted in decreased opsonic activity of the patient's serum with poor enhancement of phagocytosis. Infants with Leiner's disease and severe diarrhea should have a functional assay of C_5, not merely an immunochemical quantitative

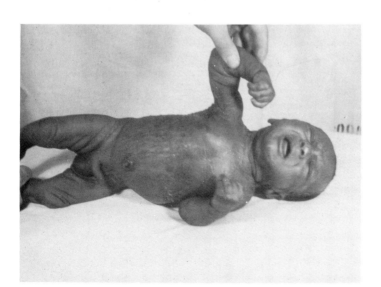

Figure 12–5. Leiner's disease (seborrheic dermatitis).

assay. The administration of fresh plasma was a lifesaving procedure for the patients reported.

Ritter's Disease (Toxic epidermal necrolysis; scalded skin syndrome)

In its very early stages Ritter's disease (see chapters on infection and bullous diseases) can resemble the erythematous phase of eczema so closely that discrimination between the two may at first be difficult (Fig. 12–6). In general, Ritter's disease is rapidly progressive, the infant is more toxic and the lesions are less pruritic. The lesions of Ritter's disease quickly develop a characteristic bullous or scalded skin appearance, whereas large bullae or areas of epidermal necrosis do not occur in uncomplicated eczema. The finding of *Staphylococcus aureus* phage type 71 or 55/71 in Ritter's disease should resolve the dilemma.

Congenital Ichthyosiform Erythroderma

Infants with congenital ichthyosiform erythroderma may develop a transient ec-

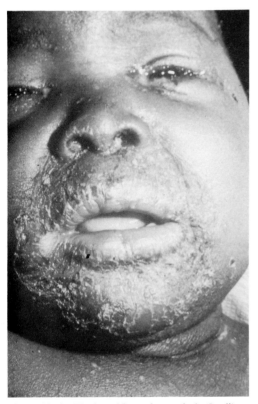

Figure 12–6. Toxic epidermal necrolysis (Lyell's syndrome, Ritter's disease).

zematous phase. The presence of an eruption *from the time of birth*, the overriding ichthyotic character of the disease, familial occurrence and the characteristic histologic and electron microscopic picture of congenital ichthyosiform erythroderma help to establish the diagnosis (see Chap. 11).

Diaper Dermatitis (Napkin dermatitis)

From the preceding discussion it becomes evident that the causes of an eczematous eruption in the diaper area are multiple. Probably the most common causes are infection and primary irritant contact dermatitis. At the end of the first month, uncommon causes include seborrheic dermatitis and allergic dermatitis. In order to exclude other etiologic agents, bacterial and fungal cultures from the affected area are mandatory.

All ointments that possibly contain primary irritants should be discontinued, but skin testing is not advised. Urine and feces may be quite irritating if prolonged contact with skin is permitted, either because of their biologic catabolites or because they foster bacterial contamination of the area. It is for this reason that frequent diaper changes are desirable. Most important, evaporation of water must not be impeded. Plastic panties are impermeable, resulting not only in bacterial and fungal overgrowth, but also in maceration of the skin and a localized increase in temperature which in turn fosters continued inflammation. The authors of this volume have differing opinions concerning the use of plastic panties. Both of us agree that their use on infants without skin disease may not be desirable but that it is inevitable considering the advantages and freedom they offer to mother. We further agree that the use of plastic panties in the acute weeping stage of diaper dermatitis is so deleterious to the healing process that they must be avoided. The most troublesome decision, however, concerns their use in the subacute stages of dermatitis. One of us (NBE), the mother of four children, feels that the impracticality of frequent diaper and crib sheet changes is not outweighed by the benefit of a possibly more rapid healing period. The other (LMS), a male with behindsight, feels that plastic panties are always deleterious to the healing process and should be avoided in all infants with diaper dermatitis.

Some texts refer to an entity labeled "intertrigo." This term describes a symmetrical, moist eruption in the skin folds or creases. The same elements discussed in diaper dermatitis are valid for any consideration of intertrigo.

ECZEMA AS A CUTANEOUS EXPRESSION OF A SYSTEMIC DISEASE

An eruption very much like that of atopic dermatitis may occur as a major or minor expression of systemic disease (Rostenberg, 1968). In all of these diseases (see Table 12–2), the eruption is of secondary importance since the systemic process is a source of more serious concern. In some diseases, the eruption often has a characteristic feature, in addition to eczema, which may provide clues to the underlying processes. Diagnosis of these disorders is usually not difficult for the alert physician.

IMMUNE DEFICIENCY DISEASES

Wiskott-Aldrich Syndrome

A severe recalcitrant eczematous eruption (Fig. 12–7) is part of the disorder first described by Aldrich and colleagues in 1954. Eczematous dermatitis, together with recurrent infection and thrombocytopenia, constitute this syndrome. It is transmitted by an X-linked recessive gene and characterized by defects in cell-mediated and humoral immunity. The latter factors include lack of delayed hypersensitivity reactions and low levels of IgM. Blaese (1968) has postulated that these patients have a broad defect in the processing or recognition of antigens even though lymphocytes may be present in normal numbers. Oppenheim (1970) has shown that lymphocytes from affected individuals are defective in their ability to undergo transformation in the presence of an appropriate antigenic stimulus. The immune deficiency in these patients may be related to the epinephrine-adenyl cyclase-protein kinase system, since Kuramoto (1970) has shown that the platelets from three patients with Wiskott-Aldrich syndrome did not aggregate normally in the presence of epinephrine. In an interesting study, Berman (1971) has demonstrated that partial correction of the immune deficiency by administration of transfer factor did not improve the eczematous condition.

Clinically, the patient has a short life expectancy, usually with death supervening within two to three years. The dermatitis may appear soon after birth and involves the scalp,

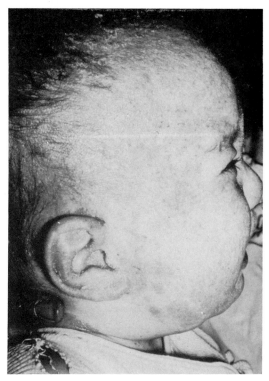

Figure 12–7. Wiskott-Aldrich syndrome.

face and flexural areas, as well as the buttocks. Multiple infections are common, with the ears being particularly vulnerable. The dermatitis does not respond to treatment and a purpuric component is often in evidence, mixed with the eczema. The purpuric element is particularly helpful in resolving the diagnostic difficulty. Generalized exfoliative dermatitis frequently precedes the terminal event, which may be precipitated by acute pulmonary bacterial or viral infection.

Ataxia Telangiectasia

Ataxia telangiectasia is transmitted by an autosomal recessive gene and is manifested by cerebellar ataxia, ocular and cutaneous telangiectasia (appearing in the fifth year or later), repeated respiratory infections, diminished serum and secretory IgA, diminished immediate and delayed hypersensitivity, hypoplasia or absence of the thymus and growth failure (Louis-Bar, 1941; Rosen, 1971).

Reed and associates (1966) noted an eczematous dermatitis in three of 22 patients with ataxia telangiectasia that was not accompanied by hay fever or asthma. The finding of eczema in immunologically deficient patients is of particular interest since it contrasts sharply with the currently held view that atopic dermatitis is a disease of allergic hypersensitivity.

Sex-Linked Agammaglobulinemia

Peterson (1965) observed atopic dermatitis in four of 23 infants and children with sex-linked agammaglobulinemia. The dermatitis was identical in appearance to mundane eczema. The association of these two findings is of interest for the same reasons mentioned in the previous section. If atopic dermatitis is caused by the presence of IgE, it is difficult to understand how these patients may demonstrate the dermatitis yet presumably have no IgE.

METABOLIC DISEASES

An eruption resembling eczema may be associated with several metabolic disorders. Patients with *phenylketonuria* (see Chap. 10) have an incidence of atopic dermatitis between five and 10 times greater than that of the normal population. The eruption is identical to that of atopic dermatitis in the normal infant. The presence of hypopigmentation, mental growth arrest and the finding of phenylketones in the urine identify the underlying disorder.

Ahistidinemia (Snyderman, 1963). A histidine deficient diet resulted in the development of an eczematous eruption in five of six infants under three months of age. Administration of histidine reversed the process within 24 hours.

Mucopolysaccharidoses (see Chap. 15). Three of 22 patients with one of the mucopolysaccharidoses were found to have typical atopic dermatitis (Peterson, 1965). Apart from this, these patients may also have a dry, scaly, thickened and immobile skin which is the clinical expression of mucinous deposits in the epidermis and dermis. A biopsy and mucin stains will help confirm the diagnosis.

Hartnup disease (see Chap. 16). An eczematous, pellagra-like dermatitis aggravated by sunlight is one of the symptoms of Hartnup (or H) disease. The distribution of the eruption with a sharp limitation to exposed areas, its characteristic flare after exposure to sunlight and the associated finding of excessive urinary excretion of indole derivatives of tryptophan and other biochemical abnormal-

ities, will separate the eruption of Hartnup disease from other eczematous processes.

HEREDITARY DEFECTS

A less known, but extremely common feature of *hereditary anhidrotic ectodermal dysplasia* (see Chap. 17) is atopic dermatitis. Reed and associates (1970) studied three such patients and found that they had an eczematous eruption in the flexural areas associated with hay fever and asthma. In three cases of anhidrotic ectodermal dysplasia seen by one of us (LMS) during the past four years, a dermatitis indistinguishable from atopic dermatitis was present.

Weary et al. (1971) have described a dominantly inherited disorder, *hereditary acrokeratotic poikiloderma*, in 10 members of a family group. The disease started at about one month of age as a vesico-pustular eruption on hands and feet. At age three months or so, atopic dermatitis developed and was gradually accompanied by diffuse cutaneous atrophy (poikiloderma). Keratotic plaques ultimately appeared on the hands.

In *Long Arm 18 Deletion Syndrome* (Insley, 1967), a high incidence of atopic dermatitis has also been found. The syndrome consists of small stature, mental retardation, microcephaly and mid-facial hypoplasia in combination with anomalies of the skeleton, ears, heart and genitalia. Six of 24 such patients have had atopic dermatitis (Smith, 1970).

OTHER CONDITIONS

Several other systemic diseases may cause an eczematous eruption that could give rise to confusion in diagnosis.

Histiocytosis X. The cutaneous features of Letterer-Siwe's disease (see Chap. 15) may be extremely varied, but one frequent finding is an eczematous dermatitis (Fig. 12–8), often accompanied by petechiae or frank ecchymoses (Plate XIII–B). The areas most often involved are the scalp and neck, the axillae, groin and diaper area. The affected child may appear ill. On examination one may find fever, anemia, hepatosplenomegaly, lymphadenopathy, bone tumors and mucocutaneous involvement. A biopsy of skin shows masses of histiocytes, eosinophils and the other features characteristic of histiocytosis X.

Gluten-Sensitive Enteropathy. Eczema may be associated with gastro-intestinal mal-

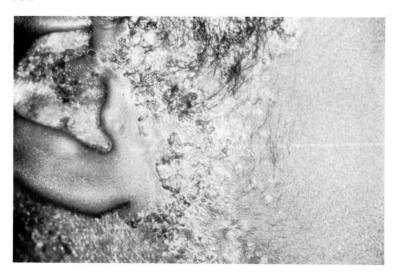

Figure 12-8. Letterer-Siwe disease.

absorption (Editorial, 1965). Cooke et al. (1953) found that 20 of 100 patients with gluten-sensitive enteropathy had a desquamating eczematous eruption of the hands, legs, forearms and face. The eruption seemed to vary in intensity with the underlying enteropathy. Friedman and Hare (1954) also described eczema in four cases of gluten-sensitive enteropathy and steatorrhea. The eczematous eruption fluctuated in intensity, becoming worse each time the patients were exposed to gluten and improving on a gluten-free diet. Fry (1965) found that 59 of 70 patients with eczema given d-xylose showed no evidence of impaired intestinal absorption. In contrast, Shuster and Marks (1965) found steatorrhea in 9 of 10 patients with eczema which these authors believed was related to the dermatitis.

Acrodermatitis Enteropathica. One of the presenting features of acrodermatitis enteropathica (see Chap. 13) may be a weeping eczematous eruption with a highly characteristic distribution involving the perioral areas, limbs and diaper area. The nails are often dystrophic and severe hair loss develops. Lesions in the characteristic distribution, accompanied by diarrhea and failure to thrive, should point to the diagnosis.

TREATMENT

A general discussion relative to the symptomatic treatment of a variety of skin disorders is included in Chapter 5, but perhaps a special section on the treatment of the eczematous process is in order here. The man-

agement of dermatitis associated with systemic disease is essentially one of treating the underlying problem. Treatment of the eczematous dermatitis which results from one of the exogenous or uncomplicated endogenous types is as follows:

Clothes. Impermeable diapers sustain an environment conducive to aggravating the dermatitis, and woolens and silks may be irritating. Cotton and washed linen provide an acceptable covering and frequent diaper changes are helpful.

Topical Therapy. When bacterial or fungal infections exist, appropriate antibacterial or antifungal ointments based on the results of culture and sensitivity studies are indicated. Weeping lesions should be treated with compresses or by bathing in tepid water, protective ointments (simple zinc oxide paste) and nonmedicated powders (talcs) should be applied after each diaper change, and soiled ointments and pastes should be removed with mineral oil. A more extensive eczematous eruption should be treated for short periods with 1 per cent hydrocortisone cream. A scaly eruption on the scalp may be treated by frequent shampooing with an antiseborrheic agent, such as Sebulex shampoo or Fostex cream followed by 1 per cent salicylic acid or 3 per cent sulfur in cold cream. The bathing routine is described in Chapter 5. It should be stressed, however, that infants with diffuse dermatitis lose heat readily and are intolerant of even mild temperature or humidity changes. For these reasons, humidification in winter and air conditioning in summer are desirable.

Systemic Therapy. Systemic corticosteroids should be avoided in the treatment of eczema. Where itching is severe, chloral hydrate may be used as a sedative. Elixirs of antihistamines such as benadryl or chlortrimeton are also acceptable. Systemic antibiotics are usually unnecessary unless a cutaneous infection has been demonstrated.

REFERENCES

Aldrich, R. A., Steinberg, A. G. and Campbell, D. D.: Pedigree demonstrating a sex-linked recessive condition characterized by draining ears, eczematoid dermatitis and bloody diarrhea. Pediatrics *13*:133, 1954.

Beare, J. M. and Rook, A.: The newborn. *In* Rook, A., Wilkinson, D. S. and Ebling, F. J. G. (eds.): Textbook of Dermatology. Philadelphia, F. A. Davis Co., 1968, p. 112.

Berman, S. C.: Transfer factor and Wiskott-Aldrich syndrome. Chicago, Proc. Inst. Med. *28*:441, 1971.

Blaese, R. M., Strober, W., Brown, R. S. and Waldmann, T. A.: The Wiskott-Aldrich syndrome. Lancet *1*:1056, 1968.

Brookes, D. B., Hubbert, R. M. and Sarkany, J.: Skin flora of infants with napkin rash. Brit. J. Derm. *85*:250, 1971.

Cooke, T. W., Peeney, A. L. P., and Hawkins, C. F.: Symptoms signs and diagnostic features of idiopathic steatorrhea. Quart. J. Med. *46*:59, 1953.

Editorial: Eczema and gastrointestinal malabsorption. Brit. Med. J. *1*:941, 1965.

Friedman, M. and Hare, P. S.: Gluten sensitive enteropathy and eczema. Lancet *1*:521, 1965.

Fry, L.: d-Xylose absorption in patients with eczema. Brit. Med. J. *1*:967, 1965.

Hinrichs, W. L., Logan, G. B. and Winkelmann, R. K.: Delayed blanch phenomenon as an indication of atopy in newborn infants. J. Invest. Derm. *46*:189, 1966.

Insley, J.: Syndrome associated with a deficiency of part of the long arms of chromosome No. 18. Arch. Dis. Child. *42*:140, 1967.

Jacobs, J. C. and Miller, M. E.: Fatal familial Leiner's disease: A deficiency of the opsonic activity of serum complement. Pediatrics *49*:225, 1972.

Kuramoto, A., Steiner, M. and Baldini, M. G.: Lack of platelet response to stimulation in the Wiskott-Aldrich syndrome. New Eng. J. Med. *282*:475, 1970.

Louis-Bar, M.: Sur un syndrome progressif conprenant des telangiectasies capillaires, cutanées et conjonctivales symétriques, a disposition naevoide et des troubles cérébelleaux. Confin. Neurol. *4*:32, 1941.

Montes, L F., Pitullos, R. F., Hunt, D., Narkates, A. J. and Dillon, H. C.: Microbial flora of infants skin. Arch. Derm. *103*:400, 1971.

Norins, A.: Atopic Dermatitis. Ped. Clin. N. Amer. *18*: 801, 1971.

Oppenheim, J. J., Blaese, R. M. and Waldmann, T. A.: Defective lymphocyte transformation and delayed hypersensitivity in Wiskott-Aldrich syndrome. J. Immunol. *104*:835, 1970.

Peterson, R. D. A.: Immunologic responses in infantile eczema. J. Paediat. *66*:224, 1965.

Reed, W. B., Lopez, D. A. and Landing, B.: Clinical spectrum of anhidrotic ectodermal dysplasia. Arch. Derm. *102*:134, 1970.

Reed, W. B., Epstein, W. L., Boder, E. and Sedgewick, R.: Cutaneous manifestations of ataxia-telangiectasia. J.A.M.A., *195*:746, 1966.

Rosen, F. S.: The thymus gland and the immune deficiency diseases. *In* Samter, M. (ed.): Immunological Diseases. 2nd ed. Boston, Little Brown and Co., 1971, p. 497.

Rostenberg, A., Jr. and Solomon, L. M.: Atopic Dermatitis and Infantile Eczema, *In* Samter, M. (ed.): Immunologic Diseases. 2nd ed. Vol. II. Boston, Little Brown and Co., 1971, p. 920.

Shuster, S. and Marks, J.: Dermatogenic enteropathy: a new cause of steatorrhea. Lancet *1*:1367, 1965.

Smith, D. W.: Recognizable Patterns of Human Malformation. Philadelphia, W. B. Saunders Co., 1970, p. 50.

Snyderman, S. E., Boyer, A., Roctman, E., Holt, L. E., Jr. and Prose, P. H.: The histidine requirement of the infant. Pediatrics *31*:786, 1963.

Solomon, L. M.: Atopic Dermatitis. *In* Moschella, S., Hurley, H. and Pillsbury, D. (eds.): Dermatology, 2nd ed. W. B. Saunders Co., Philadelphia. In Press.

Solomon, L M. and Beerman, H.: Atopic dermatitis. Am. J. Med. Sci. *252*:478, 1966.

Weary, P. E., Manley, W. F. and Graham, G. F.: Hereditary acrokeratotic poikiloderma. Arch. Derm. *103*:409, 1971.

Chapter Thirteen

VESICO-BULLOUS ERUPTIONS

Blistering diseases in the neonatal period may be caused by infection, congenital disease, an infiltrative process or by disease of unknown origin. The proper management of the problem depends on the etiology of the disease or, when this is not known, on an understanding of the pathogenesis of the particular type of blister encountered. Basic to this understanding is knowledge of the level of blister formation within the skin.

Blister sites may be either epidermal or subepidermal. In the epidermis, the blister may be very high (subcorneal), midepidermal or basal. The midepidermal blister may be formed by primary separation of intercellular contacts (acantholysis), by secondary edematous disruption of intercellular contacts (spongiosis) or by intracellular injury, such as one sees in viral infections (Braun-Falco, 1969). This simplistic scheme will be referred to in discussing the various disease entities. The diagnosis of a blistering disease usually requires some genetic information, laboratory studies relative to finding an infectious agent, knowledge of the general state of the infant's health, an immediate past history of the infant and mother, description of the morphological characteristics of the eruption and biopsy of the involved skin. The biopsy should be taken from a typical fresh, small young lesion, and preferably should include some normal surrounding skin.

Treatment of erosive lesions with steroids and antibiotics should be tempered by the fact that infants may not handle these substances in the same manner as adults and that increased permeability of the skin may result

in excessive absorption (McCracken, 1969; Feiwal, 1969).

BACTERIA

BULLOUS IMPETIGO OF THE NEWBORN

(The synonym "pemphigus neonatorum" should no longer be used, since the disease has no relation to adult pemphigus.)

The lesions of impetigo usually appear after the first few days of life, in contrast to the congenital blistering diseases that may be present at birth. The blisters range in size from small vesicles to large, flaccid bullae filled with a straw-colored fluid. These soon rupture, leaving a red, moist, denuded area. The distribution of the lesions over the body surface is variable. There may be only a few lesions or the greater part of the body may be involved. The blisters are most likely to rupture at the site of pressure or trauma (back and skin folds) but will probably maintain their structure at the sites where the stratum corneum is thickest (palms and soles). When the epidermis is shed in large sheets, Ritter's disease should be suspected (see following section). The organism most frequently involved is a coagulase positive, phage Group II *Staphylococcus aureus*. Since certain phage types (i.e., type 71) are so frequently incriminated (Howells, 1961), it is believed by some (Arbuthnot, 1969) that certain strains are particularly prone to cause blister formation;

136

however, the host environment may also play a role.

The diagnosis is made by smear (for Gram's stain) and culture of the blister fluid. If the peripheral white blood count is elevated, the differential may show a leukocytosis with shift to the left. In atypical cases skin biopsy may be helpful, showing an intraepidermal (subcorneal or midepidermal) bulla filled with polymorphonuclear leukocytes. Blood cultures are mandatory, as is investigation and culture of those having contact with the infant, including nursery personnel, in order to find the source of the organism. The infant should be placed in strict isolation and observed carefully for signs of sepsis. A high degree of suspicion during examination of other infants in the nursery is the most effective means of preventing epidemic spread of the infection. Nursery personnel caring for the premature should use an aseptic technique in handling infants to prevent infection.

Adequate treatment should be instituted without delay. Topical therapy consists of compresses of sterile water or normal saline, to which 0.1 per cent silver nitrate may be added. Systemic antibiotics are indicated and should adequately cover the etiologic probabilities until culture results are available.

With extensive disease, fluid and electrolyte replacement therapy may be required. Recovery in a majority of cases is complete within several days, and usually there is little scarring. Perhaps a cautionary note about hexachlorophene would be appropriate. This substance is widely used in a variety of vehicles in the treatment of impetigo. It should be noted that hexachlorophene may be readily absorbed through damaged skin and cause systemic toxicity, resulting in seizures and other manifestations. Impetigo in the very young infant is best treated with systemic antibiotics.

RITTER'S DISEASE
(Toxic epidermal necrolysis;
Lyell's disease; scalded skin syndrome)

This disease is an extremely severe bullous eruption seen primarily in young children and in the elderly, but which has been reported at all ages (Koblenzer, 1967; Lyell, 1967; Melish, 1971). The infant develops a rapidly spreading bullous eruption in which the bullae become confluent and the skin is shed in sheets on minimal trauma (Plate XIII–C, page 93). Frequently, the entire epidermis may be shed from a limb in a glove-like fashion. The skin is brightly erythematous with pale areas of necrotic epidermis interspersed with intact blisters, giving the appearance of "scalded" skin (Fig. 13–1). The oral mucosa and particularly the conjunctivae are often involved; the infants generally appear toxic and may suffer severe fluid loss. The cause of Ritter's disease in infants is most frequently *Staphylococcus aureus*, phage type 71, but other Group II phage types have been incriminated. In older children and adults the same syndrome may be caused by drugs.

The differential diagnosis in the first few weeks of life may include Leiner's disease, bullous congenital ichthyosiform erythroderma, epidermolysis bullosa and bullous erythema multiforme. These diagnostic possibilities may be excluded by a lack of seborrheic scaling on the scalp and elsewhere (Leiner's), a negative family history (congenital ichthyosiform erythroderma, epidermolysis bullosa) and the presence of the appropriate histopathologic findings. It is more difficult to exclude erythema multiforme bullosum. Lyell believes that both disorders may, in fact, be concurrent in some cases. When this does occur, the toxic epidermal necrolysis is more likely to be related to drug ingestion and to be present in an older individual. A positive diagnosis of Ritter's disease is established by its clinical evolution, biopsy findings and bacteriologic examination and culture of blister fluid. Staphylococci recovered from such lesions should be phage typed whenever possible. As with bullous impetigo, blood cultures are mandatory, and the infant should be maintained in strict isolation. Histopathologically, the blister is found most often in the midepidermis, and is characterized by acute cellular death and acantholysis with minimal inflammation. Subepidermal bullae may also be seen.

Treatment includes prompt administration of systemic antibiotics with coverage for a penicillin-resistant organism, fluid and electrolyte replacement and measures to assure maintenance of body temperature. In cases of clear-cut staphylococcal disease, corticosteroids may be contraindicated (Melish, 1971), although there is disagreement about the usefulness of this therapy in the severely ill infant. Intravenous use of corticosteroids should be dictated more by the state of the infant's general health than by the presence of a blistering disease per se. Topical therapy

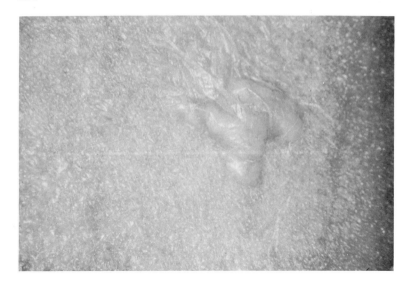

Figure 13–1. (See also Plate XIII-C). Early blister of toxic epidermal necrolysis.

should include cool sterile water or isotonic saline compresses during the exudative phase and emollients during the healing phase. As the infant improves, rapid resolution of the process, without scarring, is the usual outcome.

PSEUDOMONAS AERUGINOSA
(Hall, 1967)

The skin lesions of *Pseudomonas aeruginosa* infection in the newborn have a characteristic appearance and herald an accompanying septicemia (Fig. 13–2). The umbilicus can serve as a portal of entry for the organism, and omphalitis may be the earliest lesion. Such infections are most commonly seen in the premature infant and occur when the organism finds a favorable medium for growth on macerated skin in the high moisture con-

tent of the incubator environment (Plate XIII–D).

The lesions appear as grouped opalescent vesicles with a surrounding band of erythema that rapidly becomes green, pustular and hemorrhagic. These rupture to form indolent punched-out ulcers with a necrotic base surrounded by areas of violaceous cellulitis (Geppert, 1952). Once the diagnosis is suspected and the appropriate cultures obtained, parenteral antibiotic therapy should be initiated immediately. With widespread lesions, the prognosis is exceedingly grave.

LISTERIOSIS

On rare occasions infection with *Listeria monocytogenes*, a gram-positive bacteria, may cause a fulminating disease in the neonatal period (Weinberg, 1971). The infant is often

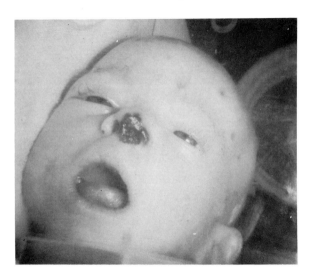

Figure 13–2. Nasal ulcer due to *Pseudomonas aeruginosa.*

moribund and the usual cutaneous features include petechiae, papules, pustules and rarely, vesicles. The associated systemic manifestations are hepatosplenomegaly, central nervous system depression and meconium staining of the skin; identification of the organism from smear of the meconium spinal fluid or skin lesion helps to establish the diagnosis. (See also Chap. 14.)

CONGENITAL SYPHILIS

The majority of neonates with congenital syphilis have typical maculopapular lesions; however, a small number may acquire a bullous eruption. Bullae are occasionally present at birth but more often develop during the first few days of life on the palms and soles. The blisters appear on an area of dusky redness, are of irregular size and contain a cloudy or hemorrhagic liquid teeming with spirochaetes. As the blisters rupture they leave a denuded area which readily macerates or dries and crusts. The diagnosis is made by demonstrating *T. pallidum* on darkfield examination of the blister fluid. (See Chap. 14.)

EPIDERMAL VIRAL LESIONS

The vesicles of variola, vaccinia, varicella, herpes zoster and herpes simplex have similar histologic patterns (Lever, 1967). The causative virus may be found in early lesions; thus, aspirated fluid may be a source of virus to be identified by culture on the appropriate medium. The vesicle is situated in midepidermis. There is marked destruction of individual cells, and acantholysis is an important feature. The result of this cellular demise is ballooning degeneration. Eosinophilic mononuclear and multinucleated "balloon" cells may be seen on a smear carefully prepared from scraping the base of a fresh vesicle, then staining with Giemsa's stain (the Tzanck test). These "balloon" cells are most frequently seen in the herpes group (varicella-zoster; simplex), but are occasionally found in the pox group (variola; vaccinia). A young viral blister may also be roughly identified according to the type of viral inclusion body found in the degenerated cells.

VARICELLA-ZOSTER

Since the incubation period of varicella is about 10 to 23 days, it is believed by most observers (Newman, 1965; Brunell, 1967) that varicella occurring within the first 10 days of life has been acquired in utero. The eruption is vesicular and morphologically indistinguishable from varicella occurring at a later age. Neonatal varicella may progress to a fatal outcome, but widespread dissemination occurs much less frequently than in neonatal herpes simplex. Rinvick (1969) reported a case in which the mother had varicella near the end of the first trimester. The infant, born at 41 weeks gestation, had multiple anomalies, as well as round scars and a linear zosteriform scar on the leg. The author believed that the infant's modified response (the zoster pattern) was the result of varicella-zoster (V-Z) antibodies acquired transplacentally from the mother.

The diagnosis of varicella in the newborn is confirmed by a rise in the V-Z antibody titer and by changes in the cutaneous biopsy,

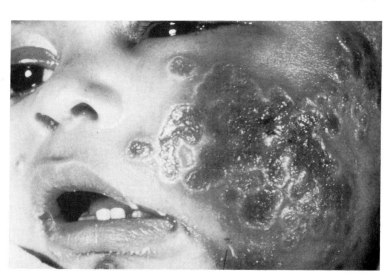

Figure 13–3. Vaccinia in an older infant.

which shows a midepidermal bulla with the characteristic ballooning degeneration. Treatment is supportive and should include the administration of gamma globulin.

Variola and Vaccinia

The vaccinia virus may cross the placental barrier, a phenomenon recognized by Jenner. Fetal vaccinia (Fig. 13–3) may result from vaccination of the mother and often ends in abortion or stillbirth. Similarly, maternal variola usually results in a spontaneous termination of the pregnancy. Lynch's review (1932) of the cutaneous aspects of neonatal variola and vaccinia remains an excellent source of information on the subject. The more recent literature was reviewed by Harley and Gillespie (1972), who also reported an infant who survived congenital vaccinia but was born with severe ocular damage, hypoplastic bone changes and cutaneous scars.

HERPES SIMPLEX

Herpesvirus hominis infection is frequently a fatal disease in the newborn and must be distinguished from other causes of vesico-bullous eruptions (Plate XIV–A, page 94). Although *Herpesvirus hominis* is ubiquitous and is thought of as a common benign infectious agent in childhood (Catalano, 1970), its role in neonatal mortality is gaining recognition. The clinical spectrum and outcome of this disease in the neonatal period has been extensively reviewed by Nahmias (1970). In newborn infants, the genital strain of the virus (type 2) has been the responsible agent in more than 80 per cent of reported cases (Nahmias, 1970). Widespread dissemination of the virus is related to the virulence of the strain, the age of the patient and, possibly, an absence of maternal antibodies. It would be of interest to determine whether the known susceptibility of adult patients with atopic dermatitis to the spread of certain viral infections can be transmitted to their offspring, and thus be another predisposing factor in herpes neonatorum. The disease may be acquired in utero (Nahmias et al., 1967) or post partum. Systemic involvement almost always results in cardiorespiratory manifestations, hepatocellular necrosis, varying degrees of ocular disease (Hagler, 1969), coagulopathy (Miller, 1970), and, less commonly, disease of the central nervous system. Death is frequently the outcome (Torphy, 1970).

Clinical cutaneous features vary from a few vesicles to a generalized vesico-bullous eruption (Torphy, 1970). Linear zosteriform lesions have also been noted (Nahmias, 1970). The diagnosis may be made by cutaneous biopsy and by isolation and identification of the virus and typing of the strain. Systemically administered 5-iodo-2'-deoxyuridine may prove to be a useful treatment for this severe form of infection, but the data are too scarce as yet to determine its efficacy and safety. Topical treatment is usually not very effective in speeding recovery, but cleanliness may reduce secondary bacterial contamination of the lesions. Cesarean section should be considered in instances of known maternal genital herpes infection, particularly if rupture of the membranes has not yet occurred (Kozinn, 1957; Dobias, 1957; Dvorak, 1966; Chilgren, 1969).

CANDIDA

Cutaneous candidiasis (Fig. 13–4) in infancy may be a mild episodic disease, a chronic affliction or may result in disseminated infection and death. The latter two forms may be associated with multiple en-

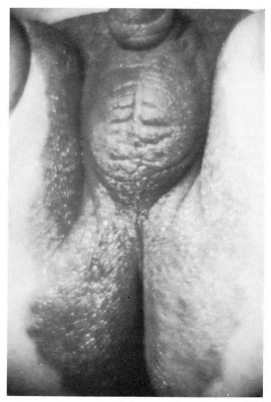

Figure 13–4. Vesico-bullous and erosive candidal diaper dermatitis.

docrinopathies (Blizzard, 1968) or with a defect in a chemical mediator necessary for immunological potency and defense against Candida (Kirkpatrick, 1970).

Candidiasis may occur at any age, but it is often seen in the neonatal period. Oral infection (thrush) is acquired at birth during passage through the vaginal canal; therefore, the incidence is highest in infants of mothers with untreated vulvovaginitis (Shrand, 1961). Clinical lesions are often not apparent until eight or nine days of life and are characterized by adherent, white, friable, pseudomembranous patches on an inflammatory base and distributed over the buccal mucosa, tongue, gums and occasionally in the posterior pharynx. The organism may be identified by Gram's stain or potassium hydroxide preparation (see Chap. 4) of material removed from a plaque as well as by routine cultures. Treatment with oral nystatin suspension for a week to 10 days is usually effective.

Occasionally *intrauterine infection* occurs and infants affected in this way may present with severe systemic involvement (Dvorak, 1966), diffuse cutaneous and paronychial lesions (Sonnenschein, 1964) or with infection of the fetal adnexae and umbilical cord (Aterman, 1968). The lesions on the umbilical cord are circumscribed, whitish yellow, flat and a few millimeters in diameter. Intrauterine infection is thought to occur either by a transplacental route or via ruptured or intact placental membranes from the infected vagina. The diagnosis can be made in infants with a widespread skin eruption or umbilical cord lesions, by culture and examination of infected epithelial tissue. Response to conservative therapy has been prompt in some cases, but infants with disseminated infection usually do not survive.

Cutaneous lesions may be vesicular with an areola of erythema. The vesicles become confluent, forming a moist erosion surrounded by satellite pustules (Fig. 13–5). This vesicopustular form of the disease most often begins in the genital and periumbilical areas.

Chronic mucocutaneous candidiasis is a special form of infection, often associated with endocrinopathy or immunologic deficiency disease (Valdimarsson, 1970). The mouth, nose, vagina, eyelids, scalp, hands, feet and nails may show weeping erythematous lesions covered with macerated crusts, as well as superficial, dry scaly patches.

Candidal granuloma is characterized by deep granulomatous lesions with heaped-up verrucous surfaces and horn-like projections. The diagnosis is made by identifying the yeast on Sabouraud's agar. Treatment depends on the extent of involvement; however, this form of disease is often refractory to therapy.

Specific candidicidal agents include nystatin and amphotericin B. The latter can be used both systemically and topically. The most frequent candidal eruption, mild involvement of the diaper area, is simply treated by applying nystatin powder, cream or ointment or amphotericin B lotion at each diaper change. Other topical antibiotics generally do little to help the situation. Impermeable plastic panties are to be avoided and frequent diaper changes are desirable. Although oral nystatin is usually not necessary, a significant percentage of infants are gastrointestinal carriers of the organism and simultaneous administration of the oral preparation may, on occasion, be helpful in a recalcitrant candidal diaper eruption.

ARTHROPOD INDUCED BLISTERS

A variety of arthropods may cause blisters that are preceded by erythema and wheals, followed by a superficial or, occasionally, a deep slough (Derbes, 1971). Bites and stings are not common causes of blister formation

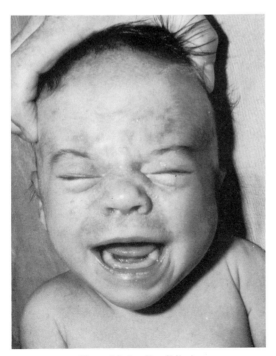

Figure 13–5. Candidiasis.

in the neonatal period, but when they occur they are often a source of mystery because the victim cannot recount the history of the bite, and the attacker is only occasionally caught in the act of aggression.

A single or a few localized, acute lesions, often in a linear arrangement, are suggestive of arthropod bites. *Millipedes* (Diplopoda) exude an irritant poison and *centipedes* (Chilopoda) inject an irritant by biting. In both cases, stinging erythema, purpura and occasionally blister formation are produced. Of the arachnids, *scorpions* and the *brown recluse spider* (Loxocelles reclusa) are particularly troublesome. Scorpion bites occur in tropical or subtropical regions and may be fatal to an infant. The usual cutaneous reaction to the scorpion's bite progresses from intense inflammation through evanescent blister to gangrenous slough. Associated systemic reactions may include mounting restlessness, autonomic dysfunction and convulsions. The gangrenous slough, which may be preceded by a hemorrhagic bulla, is also characteristic of the brown recluse spider bite. This spider appears to be extending its territory; in recent years specimens have been found as far north as suburban Chicago.

The genitalia of the *blister beetle* (family Meloidae) contain cantharidin, a vesicant. When this material comes in contact with the skin, a subepidermal blister is formed. This will heal without scarring if treated promptly to avoid infection.

Bees, wasps, fleas, moths, butterflies, flies, mosquitoes and *bed bugs* all usually cause wheals and papules associated with pain of varying degrees and pruritus leading to excoriation. Rarely, in the very young, they may produce blisters and diagnosis is dependent on the observer's high degree of suspicion.

The treatment of arthropod bites includes cleansing of the affected area, local anti-inflammatory therapy (cool compresses), management of frequent secondary infection, and, when systemic symptoms indicate, antivenom or corticosteroids. *Mite* infestations (scabies) may cause a variety of symptoms, as well as secondary bacterial infections (see chapter on infections).

HEREDITARY CAUSES OF BLISTERING DISEASES

EPIDERMOLYSIS BULLOSA

The term "epidermolysis bullosa" refers to a group of hereditary defects characterized by intraepidermal or subepidermal blisters produced as a result of minor degrees of trauma (Pearson, 1962; Cross et al., 1968;

Table 13–1.   Types of Nonscarring Epidermolysis Bullosa

Disorder	Inheritance	Age of Onset	Clinical Features	Localization of Blister
Epidermolysis bullosa simplex	Autosomal dominant	Birth or early infancy	1. Bulla heal without scarring 2. Bulla on entire body surface but most common on legs and feet 3. Lesions induced by mild trauma 4. Nails may be affected but regrow 5. May have erosions mistaken for cutaneous aplasia at birth	1. Basal layer of epidermis
Epidermolysis bullosa letalis (Herlitz)	Autosomal recessive	Birth	1. Nonscarring bullae, if uncomplicated 2. Generalized distribution except for palms and soles 3. Perioral involvement and scalp lesions characteristic 4. Vegetating granulomas at sites of old blisters 5. Loss of nails but no digital fusion 6. Oral lesions common 7. Moderate to severe anemia 8. Failure to thrive 9. Defective dentition	1. Dermal-epidermal separation between plasma membrane of basal cell and basement membrane
Bullous eruption of hands and feet (Cockayne-Weber)	Autosomal dominant	First year of life or later	1. Bulla on palmar, plantar and dorsal surfaces, rarely occurring elsewhere 2. Bullae heal without scarring 3. Difficult to produce blisters with trauma	1. Cytolysis of suprabasal cells with marked dyskeratosis

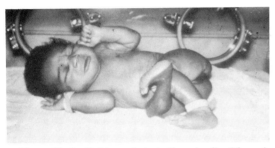

Figure 13–6. Epidermolysis bullosa letalis. There is a large erosion over the right tibia, and dorsiflexion of the foot.

Pearson, 1971). For this reason, Pearson (1971) prefers to call this group of diseases the "mechanobullous diseases." Multiple names have been applied to these entities, resulting in confusion compounded by eponymic profusion. At this time, it is not possible to simplify the classification without prolonged explanation and extensive historical review—a task beyond the scope of this book. We will, however, indicate the major classes of epidermolysis bullosa, their clinical-pathologic picture and mode of inheritance.

Nonscarring Epidermolysis Bullosa

Epidermolysis bullosa may be grouped into two major types: those that may result in complete healing without scarring and those that inevitably produce scars. *Nonscarring epidermolysis bullosa* (Table 13–1) has two modes of transmission: (1) autosomal recessive (epidermolysis bullosa letalis); and (2) autosomal dominant (epidermolysis bullosa simplex). The term "nonscarring" refers to the manner in which an *uncomplicated* blister may heal. In the recessive form, unfortunately, few blisters heal without complication.

Epidermolysis Bullosa Letalis. This disorder is usually present at birth. Sheets of epidermis loosen after minimal trauma, leaving moist erosions of varying size on the legs, scalp, thorax, diaper area, around the mouth and on the oral mucosa. The nail beds are frequently involved and the nails are soon lost, but digital fusion does not occur. Not infrequently there is a large denuded lesion on the pretibial area and, in two cases seen by one of the authors (LMS), there were congenital fixed anteflexion deformities of the foot (Fig. 13–6). Anal and esophageal lesions also occur but are usually not as troublesome clinically as in the recessive dystrophic type. Many lesions heal spontaneously and completely, but large lesions may become infected, ulcerate and remain the sites of vegetating granulomas (Fig. 13–7). Septicemia and anemia complicate the picture. The life span in the majority of patients is usually short, but occasional children have survived, although they exhibit severe growth retardation and recalcitrant anemia. Interpretations of the histopathologic picture in this disease are not in complete agreement, but electron microscopic investigation has shown that blisters form *between* the basement membrane of the epidermis and the plasma membrane of the basal cells. The blisters, therefore, lie at the junction of dermis and epidermis. The cause of the separation is unknown. Treatment is usually protective, palliative and dictated by the complicating features. Systemic corticosteroids, blood transfusions and iron therapy used in times of crisis may prolong life. High doses of an oral iron preparation should be given from birth.

Epidermolysis Bullosa Simplex. In the *autosomal dominant form* of nonscarring epidermolysis bullosa, lesions may be present at birth or appear shortly thereafter in areas of trauma related to delivery. The legs, feet and scalp show erosions (occasionally mistaken

Figure 13–7. Epidermolysis bullosa letalis.

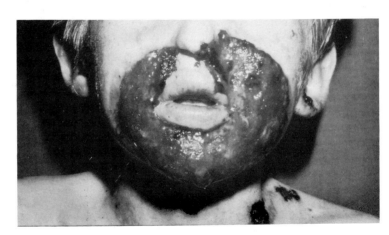

for cutaneous "aplasia") that heal slowly but, if uncomplicated, without scars. In this, as in most forms of epidermolysis bullosa, blisters may readily be elicited by gentle rubbing. Mild trauma will result in blister formation within a few hours (Plate XIV–B, page 94) and these "fresh" lesions may be used for histopathologic examination. The bullae may contain blood and can be surrounded by some erythema. Secondary infection with staphylococci, streptococci, gram-negative organisms or candida is common (Fig. 13–8). The nails may be involved (in unusual cases) but will regrow in time. A warm humid environment enhances the pathologic process. In contrast to the recessive form of nonscarring epidermolysis bullosa, the infants are usually in good general health.

Histopathologically, the diagnostic blister of the dominant form is found in the basal layer of the epidermis, and results from disintegration of the basal cells. This cytolysis, as seen by electron microscope, is initiated in the perinuclear region and spreads centrifugally to involve the entire basal cell. The cause is unknown, but intracellular enzymatic activation of a proteolytic process has been suggested. Topical treatment is similar to that used for epidermolysis bullosa letalis. Systemic steroids are rarely needed, and the prognosis for life is good.

Scarring Epidermolysis Bullosa

Scarring epidermolysis bullosa (also called polydysplastic and dystrophic epidermolysis bullosa) similarly has two modes of hereditary transmission: autosomal recessive (Figs.

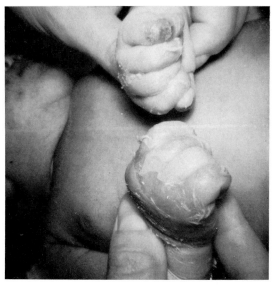

Figure 13–8. Epidermolysis bullosa, dominant nonscarring type.

13–9 and 10): and autosomal dominant. This classification is shown in Table 13–2. An "acquired" type of epidermolysis bullosa has also been described but does not occur in infants.

Recessive Scarring Epidermolysis Bullosa. This disease is often seen in consanguineous families. Erosions, frequently hemorrhagic, and blisters may be present at birth, especially about the feet, and, in contrast to the nonscarring group, milia may mark the site of healed blisters. Usually trauma precedes the blister formation. The toe and finger lesions heal with pseudofusion of the digits and loss of the nails (Fig. 13–11). As the fingers become immobile (usually over

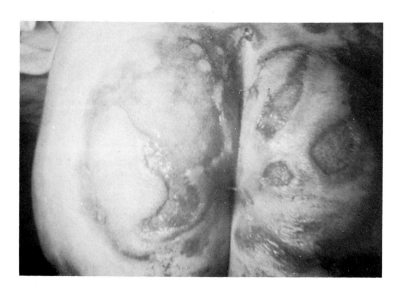

Figure 13–9. Erosive diaper dermatitis: epidermolysis bullosa, recessive scarring type. (Courtesy of Dr. Alan Lasser.)

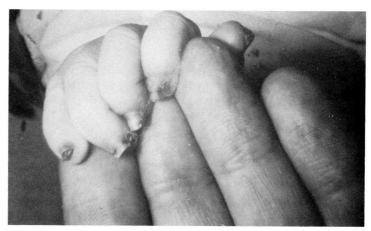

Figure 13–10. Nail changes in epidermolysis bullosa, recessive scarring type. (Courtesy of Dr. Alan Lasser.)

several years' time), the hands and arms become fixed in a flexed position and contractures ensue. Mitten-like envelopment of the hands is characteristic (Fig. 13–11). Repeated episodes of blistering, infection and scar formation result in severe deformities, loss of hair, buccal mucosal scarring, dysphagia due to esophageal involvement and retarded physical and sexual development. Visceral amyloidosis, hyperglobulinemic purpura, clotting abnormalities and refractory anemia are associated with this severe, life-limiting disease.

The electron microscopic changes in the scarring forms (recessive, dominant and acquired) are identical and said to be diagnostic of this group. There is a sharp separation just *beneath* the basement membrane (subepidermal bullae). The normal basal layer anchoring fibrils are absent. The defect probably lies in the connective tissue of the dermis immediately adjacent to the basement membrane of the epidermis. Eisen (1969) has demonstrated elevated levels of collagenase in the epidermis and subepidermal connective tissue of these patients and Hollman (1971) has found a very low level of dermatan sulfate in the skin of one patient.

Treatment for scarring epidermolysis bullosa is essentially the same as for the nonscarring forms. Steroids may be palliative if used intermittently, particularly for esophageal lesions (Katz, 1969), and surgery for flexion deformities and release of the digits may be useful in selected cases. Iron therapy for anemia and control of supervening infection is necessary. High concentration topical steroid ointments have been found to be helpful in some cases of the scarring types.

Table 13–2. Types of Scarring Epidermolysis Bullosa

Disorder	Inheritance	Age of Onset	Clinical Features	Localization of Blister
Dominant dystrophic	Autosomal dominant	Early infancy and later	1. Milia and soft wrinkled scars at sites of bullae 2. Mucous membrane lesions mild 3. Tremendous variability in extent of involvement 4. Nails often involved; deforming scarring of hands and feet, rarely severe	Dermal-epidermal separation beneath basement membrane
Recessive (polydysplastic) dystrophic	Autosomal recessive	Birth	1. Bullae heal with scarring and milia formation 2. Fusion of digits characteristic 3. Severe oral and esophageal involvement 4. Teeth dysplastic 5. Retardation of growth and development 6. Moderate to severe anemia	Dermal-epidermal separation beneath basement membrane

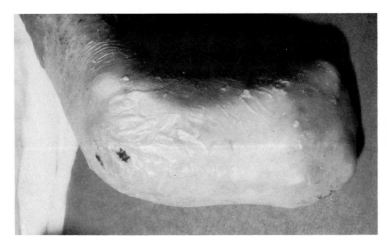

Figure 13–11. Epidermolysis bullosa, recessive scarring type. The hand has acquired a cutaneous envelope.

Dominant Scarring Epidermolysis Bullosa. This form is less severe than the recessive type. Lesions may be present at birth, but often appear later, and are usually limited to the hands, feet and sacrum. Nails may be lost, but deforming scars and contractures are not frequent. The lesions heal with soft, wrinkled scars. Keloids may occur in predisposed individuals. Hypo- and hyperpigmentation are often found at sites of old lesions, as are milia. Instead of a blister, red plaques may result from injury. Mucous membrane lesions do occur but tend to be mild. General health is usually unimpaired.

GENERAL CARE OF INFANTS WITH EPIDERMOLYSIS BULLOSA

The routine care of an infant with epidermolysis bullosa is often exceedingly difficult. Even minimal trauma is likely to result in extensive denudation and several precautionary measures must be taken. Devices available for feeding infants with cleft palates, such as rubber bulb syringes, should be used in place of conventional bottles since the latter may aggravate oral lesions and stimulate the formation of perioral bullae as a result of vigorous sucking and perioral contact. Soft, nonabrasive materials should be used for crib coverings and clothing, and metal closures on clothing and diaper pins should be avoided. Paper tape is a convenient and atraumatic means of holding diapers together. Occasionally, the use of a sheepskin pad may be helpful. All equipment such as cribs, infant seats and strollers should be well-padded. Toys should be made of soft material or foam rubber.

Bathing the young infant may result in loss of large areas of epidermis due to handling. Sponge baths with water containing dispersible bath oil will often suffice until the infant is able to sit without support in a tub. If superficial infection is present, a diluted hexachlorophene preparation may be used to wash limited areas but should be thoroughly rinsed off. Denuded areas may be treated with an antibiotic ointment such as Polysporin and covered with nonadherent dressing. Adhesive tape should never be applied to the skin since large areas of epidermis will be torn off on its removal. Large bullous lesions may be punctured and the collapsed blister left in place as a protective covering. Damaged nails should not be avulsed since this practice may lead to hemorrhage from the paronychial tissue. Adherent nasal crusts may be loosened with saline nose drops and vaseline but these should not be forcibly removed.

Oral and esophageal lesions often create severe nutritional problems since the infant may refuse his feedings. Topical benadryl or viscous xylocaine applied to the mouth just before feeding will help to alleviate pain. Feedings of cereal may have to be thinned considerably with milk, and solid foods should be puréed to facilitate swallowing. High protein and iron-containing foods should be offered early in infancy to keep up with protein and blood loss of the skin lesions. Dysphagia secondary to esophageal lesions may require brief, intensive courses of orally administered corticosteroids in high doses (Katz, 1967). Dilatation by bouginage may be necessary in older patients if there is no response to steroid therapy.

High doses of supplemental iron are required from early infancy. Iron deficiency, chronic infection and hemorrhage all play a role in the characteristic chronic anemia. Radioisotope studies of protein turnover, erythrocyte survival and ferrokinetics in two brothers with epidermolysis bullosa letalis (Hruby and Esterly, unpublished data) have confirmed an iron deficiency state but demonstrate that the anemia is complicated by chronic inflammation and protein loss via the skin. Absorption of oral iron preparations has been shown to be adequate. Routine immunizations, except vaccination, can be administered to most infants.

CONGENITAL PORPHYRIA
(Erythropoietic porphyria)

The porphyrias may be defined as a group of hereditarily determined defects (quantitative and qualitative) in heme synthesis, resulting in a variety of systemic and cutaneous manifestations. We will not discuss all the porphyrias in this chapter since only the autosomal recessive form of the disease, congenital erythropoietic porphyria (not to be confused with erythropoietic protoporphyria), may result in mutilating skin lesions during the neonatal period. In addition to developing skin lesions, patients with erythropoietic porphyria excrete large amounts of uroporphyrin I and varying amounts of coproporphyrin and may suffer from hemolytic anemia.

Clinically, the first sign may be a pink-stained diaper due to the presence of uroporphyrin I in the urine. The infant then exhibits marked photosensitivity in the 3200 to 4500 Å range, resulting in erythema and a vesico-bullous eruption on the exposed sites (particularly on the ears), as well as signs of systemic toxicity. The eruption often becomes ulcerated and secondarily infected. This causes scarring and loss of nails, digits and cartilaginous protuberances (ears and nose). Cartilage may acquire a red pigment. When the teeth erupt they are stained pink-brown. Keratoconjunctivitis, synblepharon, pigmentary disturbances, marked cutaneous fragility and a diminished life expectancy complete the terrible picture of suffering these patients endure.

Histologically, the subepidermal blister may be difficult to distinguish from that of scarring epidermolysis bullosa. The diagnosis is established by a positive family history, identification of the excess urinary porphyrins and the characteristic photosensitivity. Genetic counseling of the parents is mandatory and management of the infant should include protection from light exposure, application of a sunscreen preparation to exposed areas, treatment of anemia and infection and, in some cases, splenectomy.

Bullous Congenital Ichthyosiform Erythroderma

The bullous form of congenital ichthyosiform erythroderma is mentioned as a possible source of confusion in the differential diagnosis of bullous diseases in the neonate. The most frequent finding in congenital ichthyosiform erythroderma is a widespread scaly integument (see Chap. 11), but the eruption has a bullous phase, the clinical correspondent of the characteristic epidermolytic histologic changes. For this reason Pearson (1971) classifies this disease with the mechanobullous eruptions. A biopsy from a small lesion examined by light or with electron microscopy (Wilgram, 1966) will provide a diagnosis. Treatment, until now, has been relatively ineffective, even in a palliative sense.

INCONTINENTIA PIGMENTI

Incontinentia pigmenti is a hereditary disorder affecting the skin, skeletal system, heart, eye and central nervous system (Carney, 1951; Reed, 1967; Pallisgaard, 1969). Its mode of inheritance is probably that of an X-linked trait, and it is lethal in the majority of affected males (Carney, 1970). As a result, the disease is extremely uncommon among living newborn males, and a high frequency of abortion has been noted among female carriers (Gordon, 1970).

The cutaneous lesions are usually present at birth and undergo three distinct morphological stages. The initial lesions are inflammatory bullae that erupt in crops, usually in a linear distribution (Fig. 13–12). These are succeeded by pigmented, warty excrescences which gradually resolve and form flat pigmented patterns of whorls and brushstroke lines. These bizarre pigmented lesions represent an end stage, although pigmentation may occasionally accompany some of the early lesions. The blistering lesions occur on the trunk or limbs and vary in density from few to many. Nails and hair may also be affected and eosinophilia may be present during the bullous phase of the disease.

The diagnosis should be suspected if inflammatory bullae arranged in lines are found in a female infant; in addition, ocular and skeletal abnormalities may be present. Faulty dentition, microcephaly and abnormalities of the central nervous system may also occur, but may not be evident during

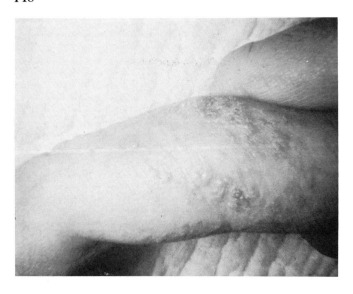

Figure 13–12. Incontinentia pigmenti, bullous phase. (Courtesy of Dr. Alan Lasser.)

the neonatal period. Biopsy of a small blister shows an inflammatory dermatitis in which there are subcorneal vesicles filled with numerous eosinophils. The differential diagnosis includes erythema toxicum neonatorum and other bullous diseases. The evolution of the cutaneous process results in a histologic pattern of pigment-laden macrophages in the upper dermis during the third or end stage, and helps to identify the disease.

No specific therapy is required for the skin lesions; if inflammation becomes excessive during the bullous phase, treatment with compresses and topical corticosteroids may be helpful. Genetic counseling is advisable for the parents.

INFILTRATIVE DISEASES CAUSING BLISTERS

MAST CELL DISEASES
(Mastocytosis, urticaria pigmentosa)

Blisters are a common manifestation of cutaneous mast cell disease up to three years of age (Robinson, 1962; Miller, 1965; Carney, 1970). The clinical findings are those of single or multiple bullous lesions that occur primarily on the trunk, limbs or scalp. These are associated with an urticarial wheal and leave an area of hyperpigmentation (see also Chap. 15). The bullous lesions of urticaria pigmentosa in the infant are replaced by wheals during childhood, if the disease persists. This transition from blister to wheal demonstrates the difference in the strength of epidermal attachment in the infant in contrast to the child and adult (see Chapter 1).

Rarely, a generalized bullous eruption may be the presenting picture in mastocytosis. The diagnosis can be established by cutaneous biopsy, and the demonstration of a subepidermal bulla and its associated mast cell infiltrate, which is characterized by intracellular metachromatically staining granules. Localized mast cell tumors which blister may be treated by simple excision if only one or two lesions are present. If the lesions are multiple, a conservative approach is indicated, consisting of topical steroids and orally administered antihistamines.

HISTIOCYTOSIS X

Histiocytosis X is the name given to a group of clinically dissimilar disorders with common histological features, including proliferation of histiocytic macrophages in organs containing elements of the reticuloendothelial system (see also Chap. 15). Letterer-Siwe disease is its most malignant form, occurring during the first few years of life. It may appear as a congenital disease and has been so reported in 17 cases in the literature (Reid, 1969; Hertz, 1968). In the context of the present discussion, it is interesting to note that although hemorrhagic, bullous and vesicular lesions may occur as part of this grave disease, this type of skin lesion is most unusual. The most common cutaneous findings of Letterer-Siwe disease are purpuric lesions intermingled with and underlying a torpid, eczematous scaly dermatitis. Examination of a section from a biopsy of the skin should demonstrate the diagnostic histologic picture of Letterer-Siwe disease.

OTHER BULLOUS DISEASES

Acrodermatitis Enteropathica

A rare disorder, acrodermatitis enteropathica is considered to be inherited as an
autosomal recessive trait, and is characterized
by an acute vesico-bullous eruption occurring
around the mouth, genitalia and on the distal
parts of the extremities (Cairns, 1968; Cash,
1969). Onset may be as early as the third
week of life, but more frequently occurs
later in infancy. Failure to thrive, glossitis,
stomatitis, hair loss, verrucous lesions on the
hands and nail dystrophy are additional features of the disease. Chronic, severe diarrhea
is the most serious manifestation and may be
life threatening. Secondary infection with
Candida albicans is a common complication.
The disease has been attributed to a defect in
tryptophan metabolism but more likely is due
to an abnormality in the physiological disposition of unsaturated fatty acids and the synthesis of essential fatty acids (possibly arachidonic acid), but the pathogenesis has not yet
been firmly established (Cash, 1969). An immunological defect may also coexist in some
patients with this disease (Rennart, 1971).
Diodoquin is effective in controlling the disease and may be required for protracted
periods. In some infants the diarrhea has
failed to remit on diodoquin therapy alone
but has responded rapidly to the replacement
of cow's milk with human breast milk in the
diet. The reasons for the success of this therapy are unknown.

Juvenile Dermatitis Herpetiformis

This disease, rarely found in the first
month of life, has been shown to be different
from juvenile bullous pemphigoid (Ganpule,
1967; Sneddon, 1968). The small, clear, tense
blisters appear in crops (Plate XIV–C, page
94) in an otherwise healthy infant (occurring more often in boys than in girls), usually
on the genitalia, buttocks, face and around
the joints (Fig. 13–13). The lesions may be
highly pruritic and resemble impetigo. In
contrast to impetigo, the lesions are usually
sterile and the blisters are located *below* the
epidermis. The disease generally recurs in
bouts until its spontaneous resolution months
or years later. During the acute phases, sul-
fapyridine or dapsone may prevent blister
formation. In juvenile bullous pemphigoid,
as in the adult form, there are fixed and
circulating antibasement membrane antibodies and these may be demonstrated by
an in vitro immunofluorescent test (Jordon,

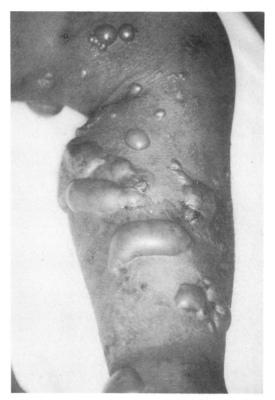

Figure 13–13. Dermatitis herpetiformis.

1970; Bean, 1970). Bullous pemphigoid in
the young child may be clinically indistinguishable from juvenile dermatitis herpetiformis.

REFERENCES

Arbuthnott, J. P., Gemmell, C. G., Kent, J. and Lyell, A.:
Haemolysin and enzyme patterns of coagulase-posi-
tive staphylococci isolated from toxic epidermal necrolysis, Ritter's disease and impetigo contagiosa. J.
Med. Microbiol. 2:479, 1969.

Aterman, R.: Pathology of Candida infection of the umbilical cord. Amer. J. Clin. Path. 49:798, 1968.

Bean, S. F., Good, R. A., and Windhorst, D. B.: Bullous
pemphigoid in an 11 year old boy. Arch. Derm.
102:205, 1970.

Blizzard, R. M. and Gibbs, J. H.: Candidiasis: Studies
pertaining to its association with endocrinopathies
and pernicious anemia. Pediatrics 42:231, 1968.

Braun-Falco, O.: The pathology of blister formation. *In*
Kopf, A. and Andrade, R. (eds.): Year Book of Der-
matology. Chicago, Year Book Medical Publishers,
Inc., 1969.

Brunell, P. A.: Varicella-zoster infections in pregnancy.
JAMA 199:315, 1967.

Cairns, R. J.: Metabolic and nutritional disorders. *In*
Rook, A., Wilkinson, D. S. and Ebling, F. J. G. (eds.):
Textbook of Dermatology. Philadelphia, F. A. Davis
Co., 1968, p. 1599.

Carney, R. G.: Incontinentia pigmenti. Arch. Derm.
64:126, 1951.

Carney, R. G. and Carney, R. G., Jr.: Incontinentia pigmenti. Arch Derm. 102:157, 1970.

Cash, R., and Berger, C. W.: Acrodermatitis enteropathica: Defective metabolism of unsaturated fatty acids. J. Pediat. *74*:717, 1969.

Catalano, P. M.: Broadening spectrum of herpes virus hominis (herpes simplex). Arch. Derm. *101*:364, 1970.

Chilgren, R. A. and Hong, R.: The cellular immune defect in chronic mucocutaneous candidiasis. Lancet *1*:1286, 1969.

Cross, H. E., Wells, R. S. and Esterly, J. R.: Inheritance in epidermolysis bullosa letalis. J. Med. Genet. *5*:189, 1968.

Derbes, V. J.: Arthropod bites and stings. *In* Fitzpatrick, T. B., Arndt, K. A., Clark, W. H., Jr., Eisen, A. Z., Van Scott, E. J. and Vaughan, J. H. (eds.): Dermatology in General Medicine. New York, McGraw-Hill, 1971, p. 1940.

Dobias, B.: Moniliasis in children. Amer. J. Dis. Child. *99*:234, 1957.

Dvorak, A. M. and Gavaller, B.: Congenital systemic candidiasis. N. Eng. J. Med. *274*:540, 1966.

Eisen, A. Z.: Human skin collagenase: Relationship to the pathogenesis of epidermolysis bullosa dystrophica. J. Invest. Derm. *52*:449, 1969.

Feiwel, M.: Percutaneous absorption of topical steroids in children. Brit. J. Derm. *81*:113, 1969.

Ganpule, M.: Juvenile dermatitis herpetiformis. Brit. J. Derm. *79*:221, 1967.

Geppert, L. J., Baker, H. J., Copple, B. I. and Pulaski, E. J.: Pseudomonas infections in infants and children. J. Pediat. *41*:555, 1952.

Gordon, H. and Gordon, W.: Incontinentia pigmenti: Clinical and genetical studies of two familial cases. Dermatologica (Basel) *140*:150, 1970.

Hagler, W. S., Walters, P. V. and Nahmias, A. J.: Ocular involvement in herpes simplex virus infection. Arch. Ophthal. *82*:169, 1969.

Hall, J. H., Callaway, J. L., Tindall, J. P. and Smith, J. G., Jr.: Pseudomonas aeruginosa in dermatology. Arch. Derm. *97*:312, 1967.

Harley, J. D., and Gillespie, A. M.: A complicated case of congenital vaccinia. Pediatrics. *50*:150, 1972.

Hertz, C. G. and Hambrick, G. W.: Congenital Letterer-Siwe disease. Amer. J. Dis. Child. *116*:553, 1968.

Hollman, E. P. M. J., Mier, P. D., Van de Staak, W. J. B. M., Urselmann, E. and Warndorff, J. A.: Cutaneous acid mucopolysaccharides in some dermatoses. Brit. J. Derm. *85*:421, 1971.

Howells, C. H. L. and Jones, H. E.: Two outbreaks of neonatal skin sepis caused by *Staphylococcus aureus*, phage type 71. Arch. Dis. Child. *36*:214, 1961.

Jordon, R. E., Bean, S. F., Triftshamser, C. T. and Winkelmann, R. K.: Childhood bullous dermatitis herpetiformis. Arch. Derm. *101*:629, 1970.

Katz, J., Gryboski, J. P., Rosenbaum, H. M. and Spiro, H. M.: Dysphagia in children with epidermolysis bullosa. Gastroenterol. *52*:259, 1967.

Kirkpatrick, C. H., Chandler, J. W. and Schimke, R. N.: Chronic mucocutaneous moniliasis with impaired delayed hypersensitivity. Clin. Exp. Immunol. *6*:375, 1970.

Koblenzer, P. J.: Acute epidermal necrolysis. Arch. Derm. *95*:608, 1967.

Kozinn, P. J., Taschdjian, C. L., Dragutsky, K. and Minsky, A.: Cutaneous candidiasis in early infancy and childhood. Pediatrics *20*:827, 1957.

Lever, W. F.: Histopathology of the skin. 4th ed. Philadelphia, J. B. Lippincott Co., 1967, p. 365.

Lyell, A.: A review of toxic epidermal necrolysis in Britain. Brit. J. Derm. *79*:662, 1967.

Lynch, F. W.: Dermatologic conditions in the fetus with particular reference to variola and vaccinia. Arch. Derm. *26*:997, 1932.

McCracken, G. H., Jr., Eichenwald, H. F. and Nelson, J. D.: Antimicrobial therapy in theory and practice. II. Clinical approach to antimicrobial therapy. J. Pediat. *75*:923, 1969.

Melish, M. E. and Glasgow, L. A.: Staphylococcal scalded skin syndrome: The expanded syndrome. J. Pediat. *78*:958, 1971.

Melish, M. E., and Glasgow, L.: The staphylococcal scalded-skin syndrome: Experimental model. New Eng. J. Med. *282*:1114, 1970.

Miller, D. R., Hanshaw, G. B., O'Leary, D. S. and Hnilicka, J. V.: Fatal disseminated herpes simplex virus infection and hemorrhage in the neonate. J. Pediat. *76*:409, 1970.

Miller, R. C. and Shapiro, L.: Bullous urticaria pigmentosa in infancy. Arch. Derm. *91*:595, 1965.

Nahmias, A., Alford, C. A. and Korones, S.: Infection of the newborn with *Herpesvirus hominis*. Advances in Pediatrics. Vol. 17, p. 185, 1970.

Nahmias, A. J., Josey, W. E. and Naib, Z. M.: Neonatal herpes simplex infection. JAMA *199*:164, 1967.

Newman, C. G. H.: Perinatal varicella. Lancet *2*:1159, 1965.

Pallisgaard, G.: Incontinentia pigmenti in a newborn boy. Acta Dermatovener. *49*:197, 1969.

Pearson, R. W.: The mechanobullous diseases. *In* Fitzpatrick, T. B., Arndt, K. A., Clark, W. H., Jr., Eisen, A. Z., Van Scott, E. J. and Vaughan, H. J. (eds.): Dermatology in General Medicine. New York, McGraw-Hill, 1971, p. 621.

Pearson, R. W.: Studies on the pathogenesis of epidermolysis bullosa. J. Invest. Derm. *39*:551, 1962.

Reed, W. B., Carter, C. and Cohen, T. M.: Incontinentia pigmenti. Dermatologica (Basel) *134*:243, 1967.

Reid, M. J. and Gottlieb, B.: Congenital histiocytosis X. Calif. Med. *111*:275, 1969.

Rennert, O., Julius, R., Schulkind, M. and Sprinkle, T.: Acrodermatitis enteropathica with dysgammaglobulinemia. Soc. Ped. Res. (April) 1971 (abstract).

Rinvik, R.: Congenital varicella encephalomyelitis in surviving newborn. Amer. J. Dis. Child. *117*:231, 1969.

Robinson, H. M., Kile, R. L., Hitch, J. M. and Robinson, R. C. V.: Bullous urticaria pigmentosa. Arch. Derm. *85*:346, 1962.

Shrand, H.: Thrush in the newborn. Brit. Med. J. *2*:1530, 1961.

Sneddon, I. B.: Juvenile pemphigoid. *In* Rook, A., Wilkinson, D. S. and Ebling, F. J. G. (eds.): Textbook of Dermatology. Philadelphia, F. A. Davis Co., 1968, p. 1187.

Sonnenschein, H., Taschdjian, C. L. and Clark, D. M.: Congenital cutaneous candidiasis. Amer. J. Dis. Child. *107*:260, 1964.

Torphy, D. E., Ray, G. C., McAlister, R. and Du, J. N. H.: Herpes simplex virus infection in infants: A spectrum of disease. J. Pediat. *76*:405, 1970.

Valdimarsson, H., Holt, L., Riches, H. R. C. and Hobbs, J. R.: Lymphocyte abnormality in chronic mucocutaneous candidiasis. Lancet *1*:1259, 1970.

Weinberg, A. N. and Swartz, M. N.: *Listeria monocytogenes* infections. *In* Fitzpatrick, T. B., Arndt, K. A., Clark, W. H., Jr., Eisen, A. Z., Van Scott, E. J. and Vaughan, J. H. (eds.): Dermatology in General Medicine. New York, McGraw-Hill, 1971, p. 1739.

Chapter Fourteen

INFECTIONS

Infections in the fetus and newborn may have a profound and adverse effect on normal growth and development. Although many infectious diseases, such as herpes simplex and cytomegalic inclusion disease, are relatively innocuous in the child or adult, they may cause widespread systemic involvement with serious, permanent sequelae in the neonate. We have tried in this chapter to include diseases that are primarily skin infections or have cutaneous manifestations and briefly to delineate the scope of their systemic effects; however, no attempt has been made here to discuss thoroughly all infections affecting the newborn infant. (Infections that are predominantly manifested by blisters have been discussed in the chapter on vesicobullous eruptions.) We have used this approach because we feel it might be more helpful to the clinician, when presented with a specific skin lesion, to think in terms of a differential diagnosis of the lesion, rather than of a category of disease.

BACTERIAL INFECTIONS

STREPTOCOCCAL INFECTIONS

Group A Streptococci are known to colonize in the newborn infant and have been responsible for a number of nursery epidemics (Geil, 1970; Dillon, 1966). The organism is usually introduced into the nursery by one of two major sources. The first is the nursery personnel who may harbor streptococci in the respiratory tract or in skin lesions. Alternatively, maternal carriers with organisms in the respiratory or vaginal tract may provide another possible reservoir. The umbilical stump appears to be a primary site of colonization. Frank streptococcal omphalitis may not be apparent until several days after discharge from the nursery. Umbilical infections due to this organism are usually indolent and result in a moist, granulating umbilical stump, often with seropurulent discharge and surrounding erythema; occasionally pustular lesions are present on the adjacent abdominal wall. Paronychia, conjunctivitis (Geil, 1970) and vaginitis (Dillon, 1966) have also resulted from infection with group A streptococci. Dillon (1966) reported an infant with fever, seizures, keratitis and skin lesions resembling erysipelas. Group A streptococci were isolated from the patient's blood and cerebrospinal fluid.

Since streptococci are a not infrequent cause of neonatal meningitis and sepsis, recovery of streptococci from the skin or umbilicus of newborn infants should alert physicians immediately to institute surveillance measures in the nursery. Personnel should be investigated for active streptococcal infection and for presence of the organism in the respiratory tract. Anal carriage has also been reported in certain individuals (Schaffner, 1969), and should not be overlooked as a potential source of the organism. Possible maternal reservoirs include the respiratory tract, vagina, anus and infected episiotomy wounds.

Controlling nursery outbreaks due to group A streptococci has at times been difficult. Isolation or treatment of carriers is mandatory. Penicillin should be administered systemically to infected infants for a 10-day period. Additional measures such as careful handwashing, fomite control and isolation of infected infants should also be instituted. One outbreak, which could not be controlled by the administration of penicillin as prophylaxis, finally disappeared when bacitracin ointment was routinely applied to the umbilical stumps of all nursery infants (Geil, 1970).

The group B streptococcus can also be a serious pathogen and has been implicated in neonatal septicemia (Eickhoff, 1964). The maternal vagina is considered to be the major source of the organism and, in one study (Hood, 1961), a 5 to 6 per cent vaginal carrier rate was demonstrated among pregnant women. The organisms colonize both the nasopharynx and the umbilicus of the infant and can be the cause of indolent inflammatory umbilical lesions or skin abscesses (Ribble, 1967). Penicillin is the treatment of choice.

STAPHYLOCOCCAL INFECTIONS

(See Chapter 13.)

LISTERIOSIS

Listeria monocytogenes (Fig. 14–1), although an infrequent cause of infection in humans, occasionally produces purulent meningitis or disseminated miliary granulomatosis in the newborn infant (see also Chap. 13). Both the septicemic form and meningitis, which is often combined with the generalized granulomatous form, can be acquired transplacentally and result in death in utero. Infection evident in the early neonatal period was probably transmitted during delivery from the maternal genital tract. Although some in-

vestigators feel that the preterm infant is most susceptible to this organism, other studies do not confirm this hypothesis (Nichols, 1962; Hood, 1961).

Infants with both forms of the disease may present with irritability, poor feeding, diarrhea, vomiting, fever, a full or bulging fontanelle and respiratory distress. The omphalitis evident in some infants with meningitis suggests that the umbilical area may be a portal of entry (Nichols, 1962). A characteristic skin eruption, which occurs in a small percentage of these infants, consists of small grayish-white papules or papulopustules that may resemble miliary abscesses and often contain the disease organism. These lesions are concentrated on the back and lumbar area, but may be widespread and involve both the oropharynx and the conjunctiva where they appear as small, white foci. At autopsy similar miliary granulomas have been seen throughout the viscera, particularly in the lungs, spleen, liver, pharynx, intestines, adrenals and brain (Erdmann, 1962). Less specific skin manifestations have been described in listeriosis but it is unclear from the descriptions whether or not the eruptions are directly related to the infection. Generalized or localized erythemas, petechiae and purpura, morbilliform and roseola-like eruptions have all been noted (Dincsoy, 1965).

Spinal fluid is a good source of organisms for culture, but they may also be isolated from the skin, blood, or in some instances, the meconium. The organism grows readily on standard culture media and is usually found to be sensitive to a wide variety of antibiotics. Systemic antibiotic therapy should be insti-

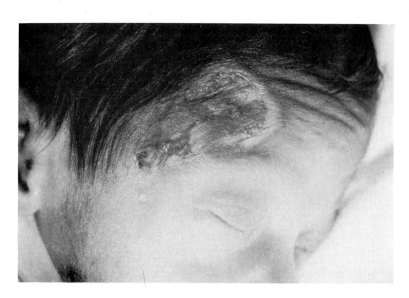

Figure 14–1. Staphylococcal infection of a traumatic scalp wound. (Courtesy of Drs. David Fisher and John Paton.)

tuted promptly if listeriosis is suspected, as many infants recover completely if they are treated early.

PSEUDOMONAS

(See Chapter 13.)

HEMOPHILUS VAGINALIS INFECTION

Hemophilus vaginalis, in reality a Corynebacterium, is known to reside in the vagina and may be the cause of overt vaginitis in the adult. Infection in the pregnant woman has, on rare occasion, been associated with ascending endometritis, amnionitis, congenital sepsis or abortion. One instance of neonatal skin infection presenting as occipital scalp nodules has also been reported (Platt, 1971).

The *Hemophilus vaginalis* is a nonmotile, nonencapsulated, pleomorphic, gram-variable rod which will grow on a variety of media but requires a CO_2 enriched environment. It is usually found to be sensitive to penicillin, tetracycline, chloromycetin, erythromycin, kanamycin and bacitracin *in vitro*. Skin abscesses due to this agent should be vigorously treated with aqueous soaks and with systemically administered antibiotics, depending on the sensitivities of the strain cultured.

MIMA AND HERELLEA

Mima polymorpha and *Herellea vaginicola* are benign residents of the skin, vagina and conjunctiva in a small proportion of normal individuals. Nevertheless, they occasionally have been implicated as the causative agents in septicemia, genitourinary tract infections, meningitis, synovitis, endo-carditis and skin infections. A number of victims have been newborns; therefore, Mima and Herellea should be regarded as pathogens when isolated in pure culture from a sick infant (de Torregosa, 1961). Primary skin lesions due to these organisms have a characteristic appearance. They are sharply demarcated with an elevated erythematous base surmounted by a cluster of 1 to 3 mm pustules (Dexter, 1958). The lesions tend to be indolent if untreated.

Mima and Herellea are gram-negative pleomorphic rods that grow well on standard culture media but are occasionally confused with Neisseria. Since sensitivity patterns differ for the various strains, antibiotic therapy should be based on *in vitro* tests of the patient's organism.

See also Chapter 13 for further discussion of these topics.

VIRAL INFECTIONS

(Herpes simplex, variola, vaccinia and herpes zoster are discussed in Chapter 13.)

CUTANEOUS

Molluscum contagiosum (Fig. 14–2) is a benign viral disease of the skin which is seen frequently in older infants and children. The infecting agent is a member of the pox virus group. Characteristic lesions are discrete, waxy papules of an ivory, yellow or pink hue, and may vary in size from 1 mm to 1 cm, often with a central umbilication. When opened, a firm plug of cheesy material can be expressed. Although the lesions are self-limited, they will slowly enlarge and are autoinoculable; therefore, it is usually appropriate to remove them by curettage, with light application of liquid nitrogen or by pricking with a small needle and expressing the plug.

If the diagnosis is uncertain, the plug obtained from a lesion may be examined under the microscope after clearing debris with 10 per cent potassium hydroxide (see Chap. 4). Frequently, typical molluscum bodies can be visualized in this manner without resorting to biopsy. A biopsy is pathognomonic, showing downward growth of the epidermis in multiple lobules and homogeneous eosinophilic inclusions in the basal epidermal cells which become more basophilic as they move toward the surface of the epidermis.

An infant has been reported with molluscum lesions noted within one week of birth (Mandel, 1970). The youngest patient previously reported was six weeks of age (Young, 1926). The occurrence of molluscum contagiosum in infants is of interest since it has been shown that the disorder may be transmitted by sexual contact (Lynch, 1968). Mothers of affected infants should be examined for lesions, particularly in the vaginal area.

Warts on both the skin and mucous membranes are rare in the neonatal period but presumably can occur. The authors have seen older infants with mucous membrane warts (condylomata acuminata): moist, papillomatous growths that arise on the mucosa of the anus, genitalia and mouth, or on the adjacent skin. These lesions will increase in size and spread to contiguous areas if not treated promptly. The treatment of choice is 15 per cent podophyllin in compound tincture of benzoin applied to the lesions for three hours and then washed off. Applications should be repeated weekly until the lesions have disap-

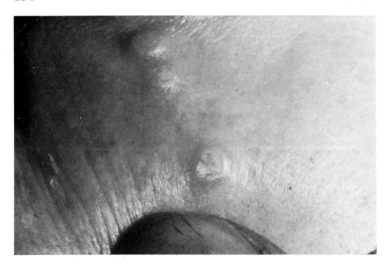

Figure 14–2. Molluscum conta-giosum.

peared. Because of possible confusion with the condylomata of syphilis (condylomata lata), serologic tests for syphilis should always be obtained.

Flat warts (verruca plana) and common warts (verruca vulgaris), should they occur in this age group, may be treated by the more conservative measures advised in any standard dermatology textbook. All types of human warts are caused by a virus included in the papova group.

SYSTEMIC DISEASES

Cytomegalic Inclusion Disease

Cytomegalovirus infection in the newborn infant is a congenitally acquired disease which results in involvement of many organs and tissues (Plate XIV–D). Affected infants are often born prematurely or are below average birth weight for their gestational age. Typical clinical manifestations include hepatosplenomegaly, jaundice, anemia, thrombocytopenia, lethargy, respiratory distress, microcephaly, convulsions and chorioretinitis. Petechiae and purpura are common cutaneous findings but generalized papular eruptions have also been described (Hanshaw, 1966). Brough and his colleagues (1967) reported three infants with a generalized papulonodular eruption similar to that seen in the rubella syndrome. Individual lesions were dark blue to magenta in color and flattened as they regressed, leaving dark red to pale gray macules. Extramedullary dermal erythropoiesis was demonstrated in these lesions on biopsy. Since the central nervous system may be extensively involved, severe

neurologic damage is not uncommon. These findings may be apparent in the immediate neonatal period or may take weeks or months to develop. Microcephaly, mental retardation and motor disability are the most frequent sequelae, but spastic diplegia, epilepsy, blindness and optic atrophy may also occur. Cerebral calcifications, often paraventricular in location, may be detectable on roentgenograms in some patients.

The cytomegalovirus often persists in the tissues for long periods, and its presence is indicated by intranuclear and intracytoplasmic inclusion bodies in the enlarged cells of many viscera. Since infected cells are intermittently exfoliated, they may be identified in the sediment of fresh urine or gastric contents with the use of Giemsa, hematoxylin and eosin or Papanicolaou stains. Re-examination at intervals may be required to demonstrate these cytomegalic cells. Direct isolation of the virus from the urine or from tissue obtained by liver biopsy is the diagnostic procedure of choice. Complement-fixation titers may provide confirmatory evidence for presence of the disease if the infant's titer persists or rises after the decline of passively acquired maternal antibody.

The differential diagnosis includes syphilis, sepsis, erythroblastosis fetalis, disseminated herpes simplex infection and toxoplasmosis, which can present with almost identical clinical findings. The prognosis for complete recovery is poor since neurologic sequelae are an almost inevitable outcome (Weller, 1962). No satisfactory treatment is available. Antibiotics, corticosteroids and gamma globulin have been administered without demonstrable benefit.

Rubella

Although it had long been appreciated that the classic triad of cataracts, deafness and congenital heart disease was a consequence of intrauterine infection with rubella virus, intensive investigation of large numbers of affected infants during recent years has led to an expanded concept of the rubella syndrome. Maternal infection prior to and during the first eight weeks of pregnancy is usually responsible for the anatomic malformations seen in this syndrome, whereas infection during both the early months and the subsequent period of gestation can result in widespread systemic disease. Permanent defects include cataracts, deafness, congenital heart disease (most frequently patent ductus arteriosus), microcephaly and mental retardation. Less commonly, cleft palate, dental anomalies, eye malformations, hypospadias and skeletal defects have been reported.

The infant with generalized disease may have a typical appearance at birth with growth retardation, hepatosplenomegaly, purpura and evidence of central nervous system involvement. Anemia, hepatitis, pneumonitis, encephalitis, otitis media, chronic rhinitis, diarrhea and congestive heart failure can complicate the course. Infected infants may secrete virus for many months and should be handled with caution by susceptible hospital personnel.

The most striking and characteristic cutaneous findings are the "blueberry muffin" lesions that are usually evident at birth. They may be scant or numerous but are generalized in distribution, at times involving even the palms and soles, and show a predilection for the face, neck and upper trunk. Some lesions are slightly raised and infiltrated, while others are macular. Variation in color ranges from dark blue to gray, purple or copper brown. The size of the individual lesions may vary from 2 to 8 mm. Bright red petechiae also have been reported, as well as purpuric lesions measuring several centimeters in diameter. New lesions rarely appear after two days of age and virtually all have disappeared by six weeks. Histopathologic studies have shown that the infiltrated lesions appear to result from islands of dermal erythropoiesis that are particularly prominent in the periadnexal tissue of the upper dermis (Brough, 1967). Dermal erythropoiesis has also been found in infants with cytomegalic inclusion disease.

In one study of 200 infants with rubella-associated defects, purpura was noted in 70, an incidence of 35 per cent (Cooper, 1965). Eighty-six per cent of infants with neonatal purpura also had some degree of thrombocytopenia. The highest attack rate of purpura occurred in infants infected during the fourth to eighth week of gestation.

Additional cutaneous findings have included persistent cutis marmorata, slate blue discoloration of dependent extremities, and flushing of the ears, cheeks, fingertips and toes on warming, probable manifestations of dermal vasomotor instability. In a series of 100 patients with the rubella syndrome (Desmond, 1967), hyperpigmentation of the navel, forehead and cheeks was noted in 39 per cent, seborrhea in 38 per cent, eczema in 8 per cent, recurrent urticaria in three infants and acne in one infant. The significance of this last set of findings in relation to viral infection is unknown.

FUNGAL INFECTIONS

Apart from candidiasis, (See Chap. 13) fungal infections are extremely uncommon during the first month of life (Fig. 14–3). Conceivably, with exposure to infected material from humans or animals, the neonate could acquire a dermatophyte (tinea or ringworm) infection (Jacobs, 1972). If the diagnosis is suspected, scales and hair should be treated with 15 per cent potassium hydroxide and examined under the microscope for hyphae and spores (see Chap. 4). The material should also be cultured on Sabouraud's or Mycosel agar.

SYSTEMIC

Deep fungal infections with cutaneous manifestations are also exceedingly rare during the first month of life. A premature infant with congenital *coccidioidomycosis* (Delta, 1969), born to a mother with asymptomatic disease, became ill at 13 days of age with increasing respiratory distress and generalized maculopapular eruption. A chest roentgenogram showed opacification of both lung fields and, at post mortem examination, disseminated coccidioidomycosis was demonstrated. The organism was recovered from maternal uterine tissue obtained by curettage. A few

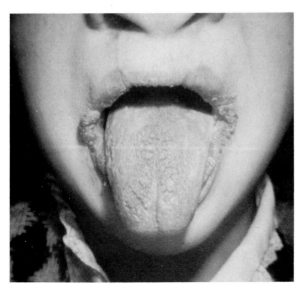

Figure 14–3. Candidiasis (patient with EEC syndrome). (Courtesy of Dr. Samuel Pruzansky.)

very young infants have been reported with acquired coccidioidomycosis but these patients have not had skin manifestations (Townsend, 1953).

Both primary and secondary *aspergillosis* have been documented in infants under one month of age. In one infant with primary disease (Allan, 1960), a nonspecific maculopapular rash on the second day of life was followed by a sparse eruption of crusted, 3 to 4 mm papules and vesico-pustules thought to be embolic lesions. A shallow serpigenous ulcer with a grey-yellow, granular base was also noted on the tongue. The infant deteriorated and died at 18 days; disseminated visceral caseous granulomas were found at post mortem examination.

CUTANEOUS PARASITIC INFESTATIONS

SCABIES

Although not usually considered a disease of young infants, scabies occasionally occurs during the first month of life (Madsen, 1970). Since the infecting mite, *Sarcoptes scabei*, is transmitted by sustained body contact, the infant almost always contracts the disease from his mother. Breast feeding provides an ideal opportunity for transfer of these parasites.

The distribution of lesions in the infant differs from that of the adult. Whereas the hands, wrists, elbows, axillary folds, buttocks and nipples are common sites of involvement in the mother, the infant often has lesions on the palms and soles, scalp, face and neck, as well as elsewhere on the body. (Fig. 14–4) The primary lesions consist of grey or skin-colored burrows that may be curved or S-shaped and vary in length up to 15 mm. Vesicles may mark the ends of the burrows and, in the infant, even bullae may occur, particularly on the palms and soles (Rook, 1968). Urticarial papules also develop and are thought to be due to an allergic sensitivity to mite antigens. Excoriations are almost always present because of the severe accompanying pruritus. Eczematous changes and impetiginzation may be extensive.

The female mite excavates her burrow in the stratum corneum and deposits her eggs along the tract. Emerging larvae remain on the skin, moult several times and copulate within a shallow depression in the host's skin, thus completing the reproductive cycle. In the adult, the mites avoid dense hair-bearing areas, thus no lesions are seen above the neck. In the infant, however, the mites may reside in these areas, cause exudation of serous material on the head and neck and then burrow in the crusts which have been formed (Madsen, 1970). To confirm the diagnosis, scrapings from burrows or crusts should be treated with 10 per cent potassium hydroxide and examined under the microscope (low power) for the presence of ova and mites.

Treatment with one of the available scabicides, such as gamma hexabenzene (Kwell), is

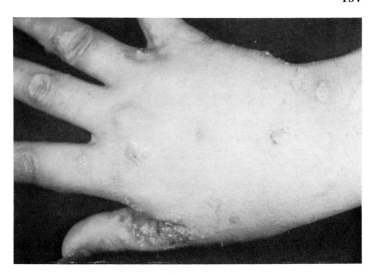

Figure 14–4. Scabies.

usually curative, but all infected family members must be treated. This compound can be somewhat irritating, and may be absorbed, so great care should be exercised in treating small infants. If the lesions are few in number and above the neck they may respond to thorough cleansing and simple mechanical removal of crusts.

MYIASIS

Cutaneous myiasis, or infestation by Diptera larvae, usually occurs on exposed surfaces. The burrowing larvae may produce a variety of lesions, depending on the causative species. The most characteristic lesions are pustules that may be single or grouped, but occasionally deeper and larger subcutaneous abscesses may form. Less commonly the resultant lesion is a serpiginous thread-like erythematous tract, often with a terminal vesicle. The authors have also seen infestation with maggots in the moist umbilical area of the very young (and often debilitated) infant. Such a situation can occur if the infant is left exposed for long periods of time out-of-doors or in a room unprotected by window screens.

The diagnosis is made by identification of larvae in the pustules or abscesses. In serpiginous lesions the larva is usually found in the normal skin, just ahead of the vesicle or termination of the tract. Larva on exposed surfaces, such as the umbilicus, must be removed with fine forceps. Pustules and nodules may have to be evacuated. Involved tissue should be thoroughly cleaned and antibiotics administered if necessary.

SYSTEMIC PARASITIC INFESTATIONS

TOXOPLASMOSIS

Toxoplasmosis is caused by an obligate intracellular parasite, *Toxoplasma gondii*, which is ubiquitous in the animal world. Large reservoirs of organisms exist, and the prevalence of subclinical infections in man, birds and animals is high. Congenital toxoplasmosis is the result of placentally transmitted maternal infection acquired during pregnancy and may result in a wide spectrum of clinical signs and symptoms of varying severity. Affected infants may be stillborn, born prematurely or at term. The infection can be manifest at birth or may not be apparent until several days thereafter. The clinical signs and symptoms include chlorioretinitis, cerebral calcifications, microcephaly, hydrocephaly, pneumonitis, hepatosplenomegaly, jaundice, anemia, lymphadenopathy, vomiting, diarrhea, fever and a maculopapular eruption.

The frequency of the eruption is difficult to determine; however, in a series of 150 cases tabulated by Eichenwald (1957), a rash occurred in 25 per cent of infants with generalized findings (patients with hepatosplenomegaly, anemia, fever and jaundice) in contrast to an incidence of 0.9 per cent in the group with predominantly central nervous system disease (Krugman, 1964). The maculopapular eruption is generalized,and tends to spare the palms, soles and scalp. The duration is variable, but it rarely lasts more than two weeks and, if severe, may be followed by desquamation or hyperpigmentation.

Abnormal laboratory findings include xanthochromic cerebrospinal fluid with elevated protein and pleocytosis of both red and white cells. The toxoplasma organism may be demonstrated on Wright or Giemsa-stained smears of the sediment. The organism may also be demonstrated and identified by inoculation of a laboratory mouse with fresh suspensions of tissue or sediment from body fluids.

A relatively reliable indicator of active infection in the Sabin dye test, which measures the level of neutralizing antibody in the serum. Antibody titers will rise within one to two weeks after onset of infection and remain at high levels for months, after which they tend to persist indefinitely at low levels. Complement-fixing antibody, on the other hand, appears later in the course of the disease, and eventually disappears completely. Although both types of antibodies are passively transferred via the placenta, they should no longer be present by four months of life if the infant is not infected. A positive dye test in the absence of complement-fixing antibody in an infant born to a mother with high titers of both types of antibody invariably signifies active disease (Krugman, 1964). A fluorescent antibody test for the detection of fetal IgM antibody to the toxoplasma organism has recently been developed and, although not without pitfalls, is a rapid means of confirming the diagnosis. The skin test for toxoplasmosis is somewhat unreliable and should not be used as the sole criterion for diagnosis.

Overt congenital infection may result in death within the first weeks of life or eventually become inactive, leaving serious deformities. In a large series of infants, Feldman (1958) reported the following incidence of serious sequelae: 94 per cent had chorioretinitis; 59 per cent had cerebral calcification; 45 per cent had psychomotor retardation; and 43 per cent had hydrocephalus or microcephaly. In another series (Couvreur, 1962), 25 per cent of the patients were found to be hydrocephalic or microcephalic, 76 per cent had ocular disorders, 33 per cent had intracranial calcifications and 52 per cent were affected by neurologic disorders.

The treatment of choice is a combination of pyrimethanine (Daraprim) and sulfadiazine. Since there is no evidence that these drugs affect intracellular or encysted organisms, therapy is useful only in that it will prevent further tissue damage (Feldman, 1968).

TREPONEMAL INFECTIONS

CONGENITAL SYPHILIS

Since the organism of syphilis is transmitted to the fetus via the placenta, the incidence of disease in infants is a reflection of the incidence of untreated maternal syphilis (Willcox, 1964). If maternal infection has been present for several years the offspring is less likely to be affected than if the infection had taken place shortly before or during pregnancy. Up to 80 per cent of infants born to untreated syphilitic mothers in an early stage of disease will be infected prior to delivery. Of these, approximately 25 per cent will die in utero and a high percentage of those infants born alive will be delivered prior to term (Rasmussen, 1968). Untreated maternal syph-

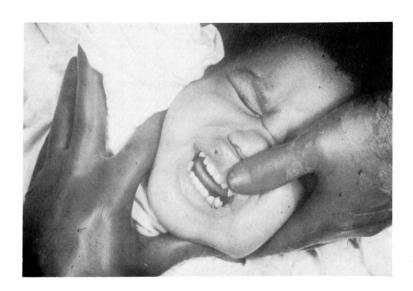

Figure 14–5. Syphilitic chancre of the lip. (Courtesy of Dr. Alan Lasser.)

ilis may therefore result in any of the following: (1) the child may remain uninfected; (2) spontaneous abortion may occur; (3) late death in utero may result in a stillborn macerated fetus; (4) clinical evidence of infection may be present at birth; (5) the infant may develop signs of early congenital syphilis in the first weeks or months of life; and (6) the manifestations of late congenital syphilis may emerge later in childhood or early adulthood. It is usually stated that infection prior to the 18th week of gestation is impossible due to the protection afforded by the Langhans layer of the chorion which allegedly serves as a barrier to treponemal invasion. This supposition implies that treatment of the mother prior to the 18th week prevents fetal infection while treatment after the 18th week will cure it. Silverstein (1964) has made the intriguing suggestion that the absence of pathologic evidence for syphilis in the first 18 weeks of life may, in fact, be due to the inability of the young fetus to marshall a plasma cell or immune response rather than the actual absence of *T. pallidum* in fetal tissue.

Fetal infection results in multiple system involvement (Table 14-1) and the findings may vary considerably. The common age of onset is from two to six weeks of life; however, signs and symptoms may be apparent before or after this period. At times a positive serologic test may be the only manifestation of infection. The classic combination of marasmus, senile facies, pseudoparalysis, pot belly and

Table 14–1. Signs of Early Congenital Syphilis

General: Marasmus, senile facies, jaundice, abdominal distention.

Mucous membranes: Snuffles, mucous patches.

Skin: Maculopapular, bullous, annular, polymorphous eruptions, condylomata lata; predilection for palms, soles, perioral and anogenital areas; nail deformities and paronychia, alopecia.

Bones: Osteochondritis, epiphysitis, pseudo-paralysis, periostitis, dactylitis.

Viscera: Hepatomegaly, splenomegaly, lymphadenopathy, pneumonia, nephritis.

Bone marrow: Hemolytic anemia, thrombocytopenia, leukocytosis.

Central nervous system: Meningitis, asymptomatic neurosyphilis.

Eyes: Iritis, chorioretinitis.

withered yellow-tan skin, is extremely unusual as it is seen only in the severely affected preterm infant and denotes a serious prognosis.

The cutaneous lesions may be extremely variable in morphology. A predilection for the perioral and anogenital areas and the palms and soles is characteristic (Fig. 14-6). The most common eruption consists of ovoid, ham-colored maculopapular lesions (Plate XV-A, page 95) which acquire a coppery-brown color as they age. Vesico-bullous hemorrhagic lesions are relatively rare but highly diagnostic, especially when they occur on the palms and soles. Commonly the palms and soles may be fissured, indurated, erythematous and have a polished appearance. The nails and paronychial tissue may also be involved. Scaling is not uncommon. Annular lesions comparable to those seen in adult secondary syphilis and less commonly, pustular and ulcerative lesions, have been observed. Petechial lesions are usually indicative of an accompanying thrombocytopenia. If left untreated the skin lesions will regress spontaneously in approximately 1 to 3 months, often leaving residual hyperpigmentation or hypopigmentation.

Mucous membrane lesions are usual and snuffles (syphilitic rhinitis) may be the first clinical manifestation of the disease. The nasal discharge is profuse, mucoid and highly infectious; later, it becomes blood-tinged from ulceration of the nasal mucous membranes. Interference with feeding because of nasal obstruction may occur. If ulceration is sufficiently deep, involvement of the nasal cartilages may alter the normal architecture of the nose and result in the well-known saddle deformity. Raised, flat moist lesions (condylomata lata), also highly infectious, may be prominent around the mucocutaneous junctions, the nares, at the angles of the mouth or in the anogenital region. Indurated lesions in these areas may lead to deep fissuring, radial to the orifices which, upon healing, result in fine scars (rhagades). Mucous patches may occur on the lips, tongue and palate.

Overt cutaneous manifestations may be absent in some infants and should not be considered necessary for the diagnosis of congenital syphilis (Oppenheimer, 1971). Any undiagnosed sick infant with suggestive signs and symptoms involving one or more organ systems should have a serologic test for syphilis (Wilkinson, 1971).

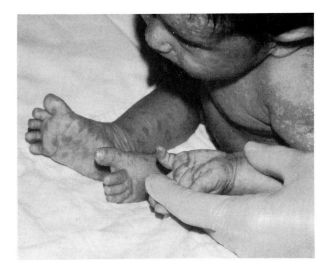

Figure 14–6. Congenital syphillis. Plantar papules. (Courtesy of Drs. David Fisher and John Paton.)

If skin or mucous membrane lesions are evident, a darkfield examination should be performed on material obtained from the lesions. The nasal discharge or preparations from moist periorifical lesions yields the most fruitful results. Material from intraoral lesions is not as useful because saprophytic spirochetes can be readily confused with *T. pallidum.** Skin lesions, if fresh, are often suitable for darkfield preparations; however, lesions on the palms and soles, unless vesicobullous, are difficult to study because of the relatively thick stratum corneum (see Chap. 5 and 13).

Serologic tests for syphilis should always be performed on both mother and infant if congenital syphilis is suspected. A routine VDRL is often sufficient, providing the physician is aware of its limitations. A serologic titer higher than the maternal titer is diagnostic; a titer equal to or lower than the maternal titer may simply reflect the transplacental passage of maternal antibody. If no other indications of active infection are evident, these infants should be closely followed without treatment and the serologic titers repeated at appropriate intervals. If a biologic false positive (BFP) reaction is suspected, a fluorescent, treponemal antibody absorption (FTA-ABS) test should be requested since it should be negative in BFP. Infants with a rising titer on repetition of the VDRL should be treated. Table 14–2 lists the conditions under which a specific diagnosis of congenital syphilis can be made. Rarely, a mother infected late in pregnancy will not have a reactive VDRL since it is too early for significant antibody production to have occurred. For this reason, if there is a suspicion of syphilis, the titer should be repeated at weekly intervals. The passively transferred maternal antibody (reagin) present in the infant declines progressively during the first three months of life. The passively transferred antibody measured by the FTA-ABS test declines more slowly and will not disappear until about six months of age. The serologic status in relation to active infection in the infant is outlined in Table 14–3.

The recently developed γ M FTA-ABS test may prove to be the diagnostic procedure of choice. Since maternal IgM antibody does not cross the placenta, this test will detect specific antitreponemal antibody produced by the fetus. Although it may not replace the more

Table 14–2. Diagnosis

Diagnosis of congenital syphilis can be made if:

(1) Darkfield examination of lesions is positive.

(2) Infant's serologic titer is higher than the maternal titer.

(3) Infant's titer is sustained during the first month of life.

(4) Infant has a confirmed reactive serological test after initial negative test.

(5) Infant has a confirmed reactive serological test at three months of age.

Serology should be repeated at one, two and three weeks, and one, two and three months of age.

---

*While less commonly found in the infant, it is best to avoid the possibility of confusing saprophytic spirochetes with *T. pallidum.* Anaerobic oral spirochetes, in fact, seldom are present before the eruption of teeth.

Table 14–3. Serologic Status

If reagin is passively transferred the serology will be *negative* in:

> 90% of intants at 1 month of age
> 98% of infants at 2 months of age
> 99% of infants at 3 months of age

If the infant is infected, the serology will be *positive* in:

> 85% of infants at 1 month of age
> 95% of infants at 2 months of age
> 100% of infants at 3 months of age

routine VDRL for screening purposes, a standardized test of this sort may provide a valuable addition to the pediatrician's armamentarium (Mamunes, 1970).

The criteria for treatment are listed in Table 14–4. The treatment of choice is intramuscular aqueous procaine penicillin in a dosage of 200,000 units/Kg divided over a 10-day period (20,000 units/Kg/day). Alternatively, if daily injections cannot be given, a single injection of benzathene penicillin G 100,000 units/Kg may be administered. The treated newborn *must* be followed with quantitative serologic titers every month for six months, and then every three months for a year to insure adequate treatment response. Serologic reversal may be expected within a year if treatment is early and adequate. Reporting the patient to the local Public Health authorities is mandatory so that proper epidemiologic information can be obtained. The necessity of more than one maternal serologic titer during gestation cannot be stressed enough. Infants born to mothers with no prenatal serologic studies or with only one obtained early in pregnancy, should have a VDRL drawn as a routine nursery procedure.

A syphilitic chancre may also occur as a result of primary infection during birth or soon thereafter (Fig. 14–5).

Table 14–4. Treatment

Treat:

(1) Any infant with a positive darkfield examination.

(2) Any infant of an untreated or inadequately treated mother with X-ray evidence of congenital syphilis.

(3) Any infant with a serologic titer higher than the maternal titer.

(4) Any infant with a sustained or rising serologic titer.

(5) Any infant with a positive serologic titer following a previously negative titer.

REFERENCES

Allan, G. W. and Anderson, D. H.: Generalized asperigillosis in an infant 18 days of age. Pediatrics *26*:432, 1960.

Brough, A. J., Jones, D., Page, R. H. and Mizokami, I.: Dermal erythropoiesis in neonatal infants. Pediatrics *40*:627, 1967.

Cooper, L. Z., Green, R. H., Krugman, S. et al.: Neonatal thrombocytopenic purpura and other manifestations of rubella contracted in utero. Amer. J. Dis. Child. *110*:416, 1965.

Couvreur, J. and Desmonts, G.: Congenital and maternal toxoplasmosis. A review of 300 congenital cases. Develop. Med. Child. Neurol. *4*:519, 1962.

Delta, B. G., Larwood, T. R., Poh, S. and Huntington, R. W., Jr.: Congenital coccidioidomycosis. Memoirs. XII International Congress of Pediatrics, Mexico City, December, 1968. Vol. III, pp. 123–124.

Desmond, M. M., Wilson, G. S., Melnick, J. L. et al.: Congenital rubella encephalitis. J. Pediat. *71*:311, 1967.

de Torregosa, M. V. and Ortiz, A.: Severe infections in children due to rare gram-negative bacilli (*Mima polymorpha* and *Bacillus anitratum*). J. Pediat. *59*:35, 1961.

Dexter, H. L. T., Glacy, J., Leonard, J., Dexter, M. W. and Lawton, A.: A skin disease due to *Mima polymorpha*. Arch. Derm. 77:109, 1958.

Dillon, H. C., Jr.: Group A type 12 streptococcal infection in a newborn nursery. Amer. J. Dis. Child. *112*:177, 1966.

Dincsoy, M. Y., Booker, C. R. and Scott, R. B.: Skin manifestations in listeria infection. J. Nat. Med. Ass. 57:290, 1965.

Eichenwald, H. F.: Congenital toxoplasmosis. Am. J. Dis. Child. *94*:411, 1957.

Eickhoff, T. C. et al.: Neonatal sepsis and other infections due to group B beta-hemolytic streptococci. New Eng. J. Med. 271:1221, 1964.

Erdmann, G.: Pediatric problems in listeriosis research. Gray, M. L. (ed.): Symposium on Listeric Infection. 1962, p. 267.

Feldman, H. A.: Toxoplasmosis. New Eng. J. Med. *279*:1370, 1431, 1968.

Feldman, H. A.: Toxoplasmosis. Pediatrics *22*:559, 1958.

Geil, C. C., Castle, W. K. and Mortimer, E. A., Jr.: Group A streptococcal infections in newborn nurseries. Pediatrics *46*:849, 1970.

Hanshaw, J. F.: Congenital and acquired cytomegalovirus infection. Pediat. Clin. N. Amer. *13*:279, 1966.

Hood, M.: Listeriosis as an infection of pregnancy manifested in the newborn. Pediatrics *27*:390, 1961.

Hood, M., Janny, A. and Dameron, G.: Beta hemolytic streptococcus group B associated with problems of the perinatal period. Amer. J. Obstet. Gynec. *82*:809, 1961.

Jacobs, A. H., Jacobs, P. H. and Moore, N.: Tinea facie due to microsporum canis in an eight-day-old infant. JAMA. *219*:1476, 1972.

Krugman, S. and Ward, R.: Infectious Diseases of Children. St. Louis, C. V. Mosby Co., 1964.

Lynch, P. J. and Minkin, W.: Molluscum contagiosum of the adult. Arch. Derm. *98*:141, 1968.

Madsen, A.: Mite burrows in crusts from young infants. Acta Dermatovener. *50*:391, 1970.

Mamunes, P., Cave, V. G., Budell, J. W., Anderson, J. A. and Steward, R. E.: Early diagnosis of neonatal syphilis. Evaulation of a gamma M; fluorescent treponemal antibody test. Amer. J. Dis. Child. *120*:17, 1970.

Mandel, M. J. and Lewis, R. J.: Molluscum contagiosum of the newborn. Brit. J. Derm. *84*:370, 1970.

Nichols, W., Jr. and Woolley, P. V., Jr.: *Listeria monocytogenes* meningitis. J. Pediat. *61*:337, 1962.

Oppenheimer, E. H. and Hardy, J. B.: Congenital syphilis in the newborn infant: Clinical and pathological observations in recent cases. Johns Hopkins Med. J. *129*:63, 1971.

Platt, M. S.: Neonatal *Hemophilus vaginalis (Corynebacterium vaginalis)* infection. Clin. Pediat. *10*:513, 1971.

Rasmussen, D. M.: Syphilis in the fetus. *In* Barnes, A. C. (ed.): Intrauterine Development. Philadelphia, Lea and Febiger, 1968, pp. 419.

Ribble, J. C.: Nursery infections with group B hemolytic streptococci. Amer. Ped. Soc. 1967. (abstract).

Rook, A., Wilkinson, D. S. and Ebling, F. J. G.: Textbook of Dermatology. Philadelphia, F. A. Davis Co., 1968.

Schaffner, W., Lefkowitz, L. B., Goodman, J. S. and Loenig, M. G.: Hospital outbreak of infections with group A streptococci traced to an asymptomatic anal carrier. New Eng. J. Med. *280*:1224, 1969.

Silverstein, A.: Ontogeny of the immune response. The development of immunologic responses by the fetus has interesting pathobiologic implications. Science *144*:1423, 1964.

Towsend, T. E. and McKey, R. W.: Coccidioidomycosis in infants. AMA Amer. J. Dis. Child. *86*:51, 1953.

Weller, T. H. and Hanshaw, J. B.: Virologic and clinical observations on cytomegalic inclusion disease. New Eng. J. Med. *266*:1233, 1962.

Wilkinson, R. H. and Hiller, R. M.: Congenital syphilis: Resurgence of an old problem. Pediatrics *47*:27, 1971.

Willcox, R. R.: Textbook of Venereal Diseases and Treponematoses. Springfield, Ill., Charles C Thomas, 1964.

Young, W. J.: Molluscum contagiosum with unusual distribution. Kentucky Med. J. *24*:467, 1926.

Chapter Fifteen

INFILTRATIVE
DISEASES

Although at first glance the diseases in this chapter may seem dissimilar, all have skin lesions that are either characterized by infiltrates of a specific cell type or, alternatively, have an abnormal accumulation of a histochemically identifiable substance. Some entities, such as the mucopolysaccharidoses, are heritable, but the infiltrative nature of the disease process is their outstanding feature; thus, we will discuss them here. Other diseases considered in this chapter have a number of morphologic variants; therefore, they have been mentioned briefly elsewhere. Despite their clinical diversity, we feel that these entities may be appropriately collected in one chapter.

LUPUS ERYTHEMATOSUS

It is well known that the LE cell factor can be transmitted via the placenta to infants born of mothers with acute and subacute systemic lupus erythematosus (Bridge, 1954). The maternal antibodies generally disappear and the LE test reverts to negative within the first four months of life, but in rare cases the infant may manifest transient hematologic abnormalities (Seip, 1960; Nathan, 1958). Congenital disseminated lupus erythematosus has also been reported in offspring of both affected and unaffected mothers (Nice, Jr., 1962). The infants with generalized disease are usually acutely ill and have no skin lesions other than petechiae and purpura secondary to thrombocytopenia. Rarely, however, a newborn infant may present with typical localized lesions of discoid lupus erythematosus and no evidence of systemic involvement. All the reported cases have had a family history of "collagen" disease in the mother or in maternal relatives (Epstein, 1951; McCuiston, 1954; Jackson, 1964; Reed, 1967). Only two have had serologic evidence of lupus erythematosus (Jackson, 1964; Reed, 1967).

The skin lesions are usually confined to the scalp and face but may extend onto the neck and upper back. They are erythematous, depressed areas of variable size, with sharply demarcated borders that may be irregular in outline (Plate XV–B, page 95). The skin within the lesion is atrophic, telangiectatic and scaly, often with conspicuous follicular plugging ("carpet-tack" scale). Areas of scalp involvement are associated with alopecia, and lanugo hair may be noticeably absent in plaques on the face and neck. The lesions heal with scarring and, on the scalp, result in permanent hair loss.

If lupus erythematosus is suspected a biopsy should be obtained from a typical and active lesion; if possible, it is preferable to biopsy a cosmetically inconspicuous area or one which can be covered by hair. A second biopsy, or part of the first if it is large enough, can be snap-frozen for immunofluorescent studies (see Chap. 4). A characteristic section will show hyperkeratosis, plugging of the follicles and epidermal atrophy with degeneration of the basal layer. A lymphocytic dermal infiltrate is concentrated in the perivascular and periappendageal areas. When the histologic picture is less characteristic, the additional information provided by immunofluorescent studies of the skin biopsy

163

can be extremely helpful. If the immunofluorescent test is positive, the skin specimen will show basement membrane staining using a direct staining technique (patient's skin plus fluorescein-conjugated antihuman globulin). The positive fluorescence is due to the deposition of globulin, most often IgG, in the basement membrane zone. Complement is also fixed in this region and may be identified by staining with a fluorescein-labeled preparation of antihuman B_1C. Staining is present in the skin lesions of approximately 90 per cent of patients with lupus erythematosus. Basement membrane staining of unaffected skin can be demonstrated in approximately 50 per cent of patients with systemic lupus erythematosus.

Subsequent laboratory investigations should include: a complete blood and platelet count; LE cell tests; serum titers for antinuclear antibody, rheumatoid factors, and syphilis; a serum protein level and immunoelectrophoresis; erythrocyte sedimentation rate; urinalysis; B_1C level; and a serum urea nitrogen. Appropriate tests for "collagen" disease should also be performed on the mother.

The skin of the infant should be protected from direct sunlight, physical trauma and irritating substances. The use of a sunscreen is indicated when the infant is taken outside, particularly during the spring and summer months. Local treatment with a fluorinated corticosteroid cream is usually the most effective form of therapy for the lesions. Low-dosage antimalarial therapy has been used with some success (Epstein, 1961), but is rarely indicated because of the hazard of serious toxicity. The paucity of information on long-term follow-up of these infants makes it difficult to predict the natural course of the disease.

JUVENILE XANTHOGRANULOMA

Juvenile xanthogranuloma is a benign, self-limited disorder which usually has its onset during the first two years of life, and remains confined to the skin in the majority of cases. In one series of 53 patients, 20 per cent were affected at birth (Helwig, 1954), while in another group of 42 cases, two-thirds had onset before six months of age (Nomland, 1959). There was no predilection for race or sex, and no familial predisposition has been noted.

The skin lesions are often restricted to the head, neck and upper trunk (although they may occur elsewhere), and vary in size from a few millimeters to several centimeters in diameter (Fig. 15–1). The typical lesion is a firm, reddish-yellow papule which may rapidly enlarge and become bright yellow as it matures. Macules and nodules are less commonly observed and, rarely, the eruption becomes confluent and reticulated in appearance (Esterly, 1972). Lesions may be solitary, few or numerous, widely scattered or closely grouped in one area. The course is indolent with spontaneous regression usually occurring within six to 12 months of onset (Nomland, 1959). A flat atrophic scar or an area of altered pigmentation may remain after involution of the lesions.

Affected infants are healthy otherwise, with no consistently abnormal laboratory findings. Serum lipids are normal, distinguishing this disorder from a xanthomatous process secondary to hyperlipidemia. A skin biopsy is indicated and may be diagnostic. In early lesions a dense infiltrate of histiocytic cells may be present throughout the dermis, but in mature lesions Touton giant cells are almost always evident. These giant cells are characteristic for juvenile xanthogranuloma and are

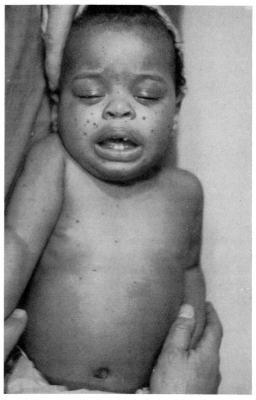

Figure 15–1. Juvenile xanthogranuloma.

identified by multiple nuclei surrounded by a rim of foamy cytoplasm. A few foreign-body giant cells, lymphocytes and eosinophils may be found interspersed throughout lesions of any age. Lipid deposition increases as the lesion matures and may be demonstrated by fat stains such as oil-red-O.

Ocular lesions represent the most frequent systemic complication of juvenile xanthogranuloma, although in very rare cases involvement of other tissues, such as lung, testes and pericardium, has been observed (Helwig, 1954; Lottsfeldt, 1964; Webster, 1966). Ocular infiltrates can arise in the iris, ciliary body, episclera or orbit, and may present as: a localized or diffuse tumor of the iris; unilateral glaucoma; spontaneous and recurrent hyphema; uveitis; congenital or acquired heterochromia iridum; and severe and sudden proptosis (Zimmerman, 1965; Gaynes, 1967). Infants with such ocular lesions should be thoroughly examined for skin tumors since the diagnosis of xanthogranuloma can be made by skin biopsy, often sparing the patient a major ophthalmological procedure. Eye involvement may occur in the absence of lesions or may predate the appearance of skin nodules. In contrast to the cutaneous lesions, ocular tumors usually require treatment if extensive damage from secondary glaucoma is to be avoided. Accepted therapeutic modalities include low doses of X-irradiation and topically or systemically administered corticosteroids (Gaynes, 1967; Smith, 1968).

The etiology of juvenile xanthogranuloma is unknown. Some authors have included this disorder in the group of reticulendothelioses; however, these patients do not have the systemic findings of histiocytosis X. Furthermore, the characteristic microsomal granules of the histiocytosis X cell (Langerhans granules) are not found in juvenile xanthogranuloma histiocytes (Gonzales-Crussi, 1970; Esterly, 1972). (See following section.)

Although individual lesions may be surgically removed, anticipatory observation is the management of choice. Xanthomas secondary to the hyperlipidemia states do not occur during the neonatal period.

HISTIOCYTOSIS X

The nonlipid reticuloendothelioses, collectively known as histiocytosis X, include Letterer-Siwe disease, Hand-Schuller-Christian disease and eosinophilic granuloma of the bone. Only the Letterer-Siwe variant has been seen at birth or during the neonatal period. Infants affected in utero may be stillborn or die immediately after delivery (Ahnquist, 1960; Cohen, 1966) and are found at autopsy to have extensive histiocytic infiltrates in several organ systems.

Cutaneous manifestations, which may precede systemic signs, can be a valuable early clue to the diagnosis. It should be remembered that petechiae and purpura are not a sine qua non of this disease, nor will the lesions necessarily conform to the classic description of an eczematous, seborrheic eruption. Initial lesions are most often papular and scaly, but maculopapules, pustules, purpura, widespread erythema and scaling have all been observed (Plate XIII--B, page 93). Rarely, vesicular lesions may be the presenting sign (Jones, 1967). Discrete nodules, some measuring up to 3 cm in diameter, have been seen in occasional patients (Cohen, 1966) and, if purpuric, may be readily mistaken for vascular tumors. The usual areas of predilection are the scalp, neck, axillae and groin, but generalized eruptions are not unusual. Papular, vesicular and nodular lesions can occur on the palms and soles or there may be only diffuse erythema and scaling (Plate XV--C, page 95). Nodules and ulcerations may appear on the mucous membranes of the mouth and vagina.

Since the proliferating cell is of the same type in all affected organs, a skin biopsy of suspicious or persistent lesions may provide useful diagnostic information. All types of skin lesions show a similar histologic picture. The upper and papillary dermis is infiltrated by masses of peculiar histiocytes with abundant, pale-staining cytoplasm. Extravasated erythrocytes are seen in petechial or purpuric lesions admixed with a few eosinophils, lymphocytes and polymorphonuclear leukocytes. Frequently the epidermis is invaded and replaced by the histiocytes, resulting in the clinical features of ulceration and crusting. On electron microscopy, the abnormal histiocyte has been shown to contain characteristic cytoplasmic inclusions (Shamoto, 1971). These inclusions are racket-shaped organelles identical to those normally present in the epidermal Langerhans' cell (Langerhans' granules). The significance and function of these granules and the origin of the histiocyte in Letterer-Siwe disease are as yet unknown. Of particular interest, however, is the evidence for the influence of genetic factors (concordance of the disease in monozygous twins and multiple cases within sibships) in the incidence of this disease (Juberg, 1970).

Affected infants may appear relatively well or acutely ill (Jones, 1967). Systemic signs and symptoms include fever, bleeding, pallor, dyspnea, irritability, pain on motion, maramus, lymphadenopathy, hepatosplenomegaly and destructive bone tumors. Such infants should be carefully evaluated to assess the extent of the disease. Complete hematologic studies, bone marrow examination, roentgenograms of the skull, chest and long bones, and biopsies of skin, oral mucous membrane, lymph node and liver may all be indicated. Suppurative ear involvement is common and an otologist should be consulted.

Therapeutic regimens have varied widely; however, the most frequently used modalities, administered either singly or in combination, are systemic corticosteroids, antimitotic agents and irradiation (Doede, 1967). With judicious therapy the outcome may be favorable, even in the very young infant (Hertz, 1968).

Eczematized or ulcerated skin lesions should be treated with cool water compresses and a corticosteroid cream. If bacterial infection is present either topical or systemic antibiotic therapy should be instituted, depending on the extent of involvement and the organism obtained on culture. Secondary yeast infection may occur and should be treated topically with anticandidal agents, such as nystatin or amphotericin B. Systemic infestation with yeast or other organisms may be a terminal complication in debilitated infants.

CHRONIC GRANULOMATOUS DISEASE
(CGD)

Chronic granulomatous disease is an inherited disorder which usually affects only males and is transmitted by an X-linked gene (Good, 1968). A few families have been described in which only female siblings were affected, probably on the basis of an autosomal recessive type of inheritance (Holmes, 1970). Patients with CGD are extremely susceptible to infection by certain organisms, most of which are considered to be of low virulence in other circumstances.

One of the first manifestations of the disorder occurs in early infancy with an infectious eczematoid eruption that may resemble seborrhea or folliculitis. Areas of predilection are the nares, the postauricular and periorbital skin, the scalp, the axillae and the inguinal region. A chronic draining lymphadenitis, particularly in the cervical and inguinal areas, is another common feature of the disease, but one which usually occurs after the neonatal period. Aphthous stomatitis, paronychiae, recurrent impetiginization around the nares, indolent firm papules on the central face, deeply infiltrated plaques, nodules, and ulcerating, necrotic lesions on the lower legs, have all been observed during childhood (Windhorst, 1971).

Other organs that are frequently affected are the liver, spleen, lungs, bone marrow, gastrointestinal tract and pericardium. The histologic pattern consists of a granulomatous reaction with proliferation of all types of inflammatory cells, including plasmacytes. Pigmented lipid-filled histiocytes dispersed throughout the tissue are a frequent finding. Other clinical manifestations include pyoderma, suppurative adenitis, stomatitis, conjunctivitis, osteomyelitis, meningitis, pneumonia, enteritis, peritonitis and septicemia. The infecting organisms are catalase positive and include coagulase positive and negative staphylococci, *Klebsiella*, *Aerobacter*, *E. coli* and *Serratia marcescens*, although other types of bacteria may be involved (Johnston, 1971). Some patients have had terminal infections with actinomycetes or *Aspergillus*; however, viral and candidal infections are usually not particularly troublesome. A report of twin boys with the presumptive diagnosis of CGD and disseminated BCG infection (following inoculation at birth) perhaps indicates an inability to handle this organism as well (Esterly, 1971). On laboratory examination, anemia, leukocytosis, elevated erythrocyte sedimentation rate, hypergammaglobulinemia, normal complement levels and intact cellular immunity are typical findings.

The underlying defect in CGD is the impaired capacity of the peripheral leukocytes, both neutrophils and monocytes, to kill particular organisms. Phagocytosis proceeds normally, but intracellular destruction of these organisms does not occur. In metabolic studies of the leukocytes from such patients it has been demonstrated that the intracellular burst of oxidative metabolism and hydrogen peroxide production which ordinarily follows ingestion of particles, fails to occur in the abnormal cells. The mechanisms involved in the pathogenesis of this disease have been discussed extensively (Johnston, 1971).

The leukocyte defect is detectable by use of the nitro-blue tetrazolium (NBT) slide test. White cells from normal individuals reduce nitroblue tetrazolium dye during phagocytosis, whereas cells from CGD patients have a marked decrease or inability to reduce the dye. Heterozygote carriers may have both normal and abnormal cells. (This test should be employed for screening only; quantitative NBT assays or phagocytic bactericidal assays using several test organisms are required for confirmation of the diagnosis [Johnston, 1971]).

Treatment with systemically administered antibacterials should be based on careful identification and antibiotic sensitivities of the infecting organism. Prolonged courses of antibiotic therapy may be necessary to eradicate the infection.

Job's syndrome, a variant of chronic granulomatous disease, is characterized by cold staphylococcal abscesses recurring from the time of birth. The disease is usually seen in red-haired, fair-skinned girls and is thought to be inherited in an autosomal recessive manner. Defective NBT reduction and impaired bactericidal acitivity against staphylococci have been demonstrated in leukocytes from one child with this disorder (Bannatyne, 1969); however, another patient was believed to have impaired chemotaxis for neutrophilic granulocytes (Pabst, 1971).

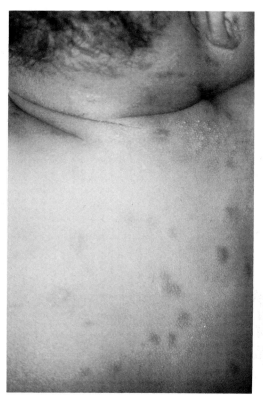

Figure 15–2. Urticaria pigmentosa (mastocytosis).

MASTOCYTOSIS
(Urticaria pigmentosa)

Mast cell disease in infancy has a variable appearance. It may occur as a solitary tumor (mastocytoma), a disseminated maculopapular or nodular eruption, a predominantly bullous eruption (see Chap. 13) or as a diffuse infiltration of the skin. All forms may be associated with systemic signs and symptoms, and the disseminated forms of the disorder may be complicated by mast cell infiltrates in organs other than the skin (Fig. 15–2).

The solitary tumor is often present at birth or may appear during the early months of life (Caplan, 1963). These lesions represent approximately 10 to 15 per cent of all cases of mastocytosis. Typical mastocytomas are oval or round, of a pink-yellow to tan hue and rarely exceed 6 cm in diameter. Many have a pebbly texture and a thickened or rubbery consistency. Although they occur with greatest frequency on the wrist, they may appear anywhere on the body surface. Mastocytomas usually urticate when traumatized and may develop vesicles or bullae on the surface, particularly during the first few months of life. Solitary lesions are generally of no consequence and involute spontaneously within months or years after onset. Rarely, pruritus and flushing attacks secondary to release of histamine from mast cell granules may be troublesome. Although most lesions remain solitary, in a few instances a disseminated cutaneous eruption follows the appearance of the lesion after a delay of several weeks (Sagher, 1967).

Maculopapular and nodular forms are present in a small proportion of patients at birth, but more commonly have their onset during late infancy or early childhood. Lesions may be sparse, or numerous and widely dispersed, but they often spare the palms, soles, face and scalp. The efflorescence of lesions can span a period of several months. Episodes of urticaria may precede the more prominent pigmented lesions, and bullous or vesicular lesions are frequently seen in early infancy either superimposed on pigmented lesions, or at times, as the first manifestation of the disorder.

Rarely, a hemorrhagic component is present. Darier's sign (whealing of the lesions on rubbing) is a useful diagnostic marker; however, it is absent in an occasional patient.

Dermographism may also be elicited on normal areas of skin.

Individual lesions may vary tremendously in size from a few millimeters to several centimeters, may be firm or soft in consistency and sharply or poorly defined. The color may range from that of normal skin to deep chocolate brown. In the diffuse infiltrative type of disease, the skin may have a yellow, tan or ivory hue, a doughy consistency and a Scotch-gained texture with accented cutaneous markings, particularly in the skin folds (Burgoon, 1968). One patient has been reported with severe dermographism and pressure urticaria from birth, but with no pigmented skin lesions or alterations in skin texture (Sahihi, 1972). In all types of the disease a dermal mast cell infiltrate is demonstrable in histologic sections stained with Giemsa.

Symptoms are due to the release of massive amounts of histamine from mast cell granules. Pruritus can be mild or extremely severe. Episodic flushing attacks may occur in all forms of the disease but are more usual in the widely disseminated types and may be accompanied by dizziness, irritability, tachycardia, respiratory distress and hypotension. Flushing can occur spontaneously or follow rubbing of the lesions, emotional stimuli, alterations in ambient temperature or exercise. Gastrointestinal symptoms include nausea, vomiting, abdominal pain and diarrhea. Bone pain may result from skeletal lesions.

Affected individuals can have elevated urinary histamine levels as well as increased urinary hyaluronic acid and other mucopolysaccharides (Demis, 1963). Peripheral eosinophilia and increased numbers of mature eosinophils in bone marrow preparations have also been noted. Coagulation defects and a bleeding diathesis are infrequent findings; however, the prothrombin time may be prolonged. Internal involvement, although rare in infancy, most often occurs with the diffuse type of disease. The organs that can be affected include the liver, spleen, lymph nodes, bones, bone marrow and gastrointestinal tract (Sagher, 1967). If bony changes occur, they are readily demonstrable on roentgenograms and consist of cystic osteoporosis, thickening of bony traveculae, stippling and osteosclerosis. Abnormal mucosal patterns, disturbances of motility and even frank peptic ulcers have been detected on gastrointestinal roentgenograms.

Treatment is difficult, particularly in severe cases, but cyproheptadine hydrochloride in regular doses is the safest medication for infants and may offer some relief for the more distressing symptoms. Mothers should be advised to avoid toweling the child vigorously after baths and not to use hot water for bathing. Drugs such as aspirin, codeine, procaine and polymyxin B are contraindicated since they may precipitate severe reactions due to histamine release from mast cell granules. Although there are many reports of pedigrees with more than one affected family member, the genetics of this condition remain unclear (Selmanowitz, 1970; Gay, 1970).

MUCOLIPIDOSES
(MLS)

The mucolipidoses (Table 15–1) are a group of storage diseases related to both the mucopolysaccharidoses and the sphingolipidoses. They are characterized by an accumulation of acid mucopolysaccharides, sphingolipids or glycolipids in the visceral and mesenchymal cells (Spranger, 1970). Clinically, the affected patients have many of the salient features of the mucopolysaccharidoses; however, all (with the exception of juvenile sulfatidosis, Austin type) have normal excretion of mucopolysaccharides in the urine. Only three, GM_1, gangliosidosis I, mannosidosis and mucolipidosis II (I-cell disease), are evident during the neonatal period. Of these, only the last has prominent cutaneous changes.

I-Cell Disease
(MLS II)

MLS II, or I-cell disease, is a rare progressive disorder inherited as an autosomal reces-

Table 15–1.   The Mucolipidoses

Generalized gangliosidosis
   (Gm_1 – gangliosidosis I and II)

Fucosidosis

Mannosidosis

Juvenile sulfatidosis, Austin type

MLS I (lipomucopolysaccharidosis)

MLS II (I-cell disease)

MLS III (pseudo-Hurler polydystrophy)

Farber's disease (Lipogranulomatosis)

Sea-blue histiocyte syndrome

---

sive trait. Affected infants show marked growth deficiency, severe psychomotor retardation, generalized hypotonia, mild hepatomegaly, Hurler-like facies with striking gingival hyperplasia, hernias, recurrent infections, persistent nasal discharge and skeletal dysplasia with restricted joint mobility, dorsolumbar kyphosis and broadening of the wrists and fingers. Symmetrically enlarged corneas and fine granularity of the corneal stroma have also been described (Kenyon, 1971). The skin is thickened and tight over the entire body and cannot be compressed into folds. Small cavernous hemangiomas have also been noted in some patients, as well as prominent subcutaneous veins around the eyes and telangiectatic vessels on the cheeks (Leroy, 1971).

Circulating lymphocytes from these patients have a vacuolated appearance. Cultured fibroblasts possess refractile cytoplasmic inclusions that are reactive with periodic acid-Schiff and Sudan black stains. Following incubation with chloroform-methanol, the inclusions become metachromatic when exposed to toluidine blue, thus indicating storage of both acid mucopolysaccharide and glycolipid. Urinary mucopolysaccharide excretion is normal (Leroy, 1969).

The enzyme defect has not been unequivocably established, but a disorder of the lysosomes has been implicated since deficient activity of several major hydrolytic enzymes has been demonstrated. Electron microscopic studies of skin and conjunctiva have confirmed the presence of storage vacuoles in connective tissue histiocytes and fibroblasts, as well as in Schwann cells, axonal processes of peripheral nerves and vascular perithelial cells. These vacuoles appear to be derived from lysosomes containing excessive amounts of acid mucopolysaccharides and glycolipid (Kenyon, 1971).

Farber's Disease
(Lipogranulomatosis)

This is another rare disorder which has been thoroughly documented in only a few infants. The earliest manifestations, usually noted soon after birth, are irritability, pain on motion and a hoarse, weak cry. Subsequent signs and symptoms include: difficulty in feeding; poor weight gain; laryngeal stridor; aphonia; pulmonary infiltrates; hepatomegaly; febrile episodes; periarticular swelling, particularly in the fingers, wrists, elbows, knees and toes; and cutaneous and subcutaneous nodules which may be widespread but are most prominent over areas of pressure. The nodular lesions are yellow in color, firm, rubbery and nonpitting, and most noticeable over the joints of the hands, which are deformed and exquisitely tender. Similar nodules have been found on the abdomen and thorax (Farber, 1957), on the infraorbital ridges, on the scalp, on the heels and over the lumbosacral region of the spine. The nodules vary in size from 1 to 2 cm, but in some areas may coalesce to form confluent plaques as large as 10 cm (Abul-Haj, 1962).

Roentgenograms of the joints show soft tissue swelling, erosion of bone and soft tissue calcification. Histologically, the skin lesions consist of a polymorphous granulomatous infiltrate containing sheets of large histiocytic and foam cells. Late lesions show dense hyaline fibrosis with sparse, foamy, degenerated histiocytes. Periodic acid-Schiff reactive, diastase-resistant material is abundant in histiocytes of early lesions; this substance also stains with colloidal iron and Alcian blue. At necropsy wide-spread involvement of all viscera has been noted, but the joints, the skin over pressure areas, the vocal cords and the pleura are the most severely affected tissues. An increase in ceremide and ganglioside content of involved tissues has been reported. The disease is progressive and the usual outcome is death before the third year of life.

THE MUCOPOLYSACCHARIDOSES
(MPS)

Six distinct types of generalized mucopolysaccharidosis can be delineated by virtue of their clinical, biochemical and genetic patterns (Table 15–2). In addition, a few patients have been described who appear to have a more focal disorder of mucopolysaccharide metabolism (Esterly, 1971; Spranger, 1971). In all but one of the focal types—geleophysic dwarfism—cutaneous abnormalities are a minor, but consistent, component of the picture.

Two basic types of cutaneous lesions have been described in generalized MPS. Thickened, inelastic, roughened skin, the first type of lesion, is the most universal and has been observed in all six of the MPS syndromes (McKusick, 1965; Scheie, 1962; Hambrick, 1966; Greaves, 1969; Spranger, 1970; Haust,

Table 15–2. The Genetic Mucopolysaccharidoses

Generalized	Inheritance	Clinical Findings	Skin Findings	Urinary AMPS Excretion
(1) Hurler's syndrome	Autosomal recessive	Clouded cornea Skeletal deformities Joint contractures Dwarfism Abnormal facies Deafness Hernias Hepatosplenomegaly Cardiomegaly Hydrocephalus Mental retardation	Hirsutism Thickened, inelastic, rough skin on extremities Eczema (inconstant)	Dermatan sulfate Heparan sulfate
(2) Hunter's syndrome	X-linked recessive	Similar to (1) but milder course No corneal clouding or lumbar gibbus Atypical retinitis pigmentosa	Hirsutism Thickened, inelastic, rough skin on extremities Pale nodules and plaques with orange peel texture, on upper trunk, arms and thighs	Dermatan sulfate Heparan sulfate
(3) Sanfilippo syndrome	Autosomal recessive	Mental retardation Frequent seizures Mild to moderate dwarfing and joint stiffness	Hirsutism Dry, coarse skin	Heparan sulfate
(4) Morquio syndrome	Autosomal recessive	Cloudy cornea Intelligence ↓ ± Severe bone changes of distinctive types Hernias Neurologic symptoms Aortic regurgitation Dwarfism	Thickened, inelastic, rough skin particularly on extremities Generalized telangiectasia (inconstant)	Keratosulfate
(5) Scheie syndrome	Autosomal recessive	Cloudy cornea Retinitis pigmentosa Intellect ↓ ± Coarse facies Stiff joints Aortic regurgitation	Hirsutism Thickened, inelastic, rough skin on extremities Telangiectasia (inconstant)	Dermatan sulfate
(6) Maroteaux-Lamy syndrome	Autosomal recessive	Normal intellect Severe osseous changes Corneal clouding Coarse facies Hepatosplenomegaly Frequent hernias Cardiac involvement	Dry, tight skin Thickened skin on volar surface of fingers Hypertrichosis	Dermatan sulfate
Focal				
Stiff skin syndrome	? Autosomal dominant	Limited mobility in a variable number of joints	Rock-hard skin most marked over buttocks and thighs	Normal
Geleophysic dwarfism	? Autosomal recessive	Dwarfism Joint contractures Bony abnormalities Hepatomegaly Cardiomegaly Abnormal facies	None	Normal

1971). The skin is taut and feels bound to the underlying structures. These changes are usually limited to the extremities but occasionally have been noted over other areas, such as the face and trunk (Greaves, 1969).

The second, and perhaps more striking cutaneous abnormality, is frequently found on the upper trunk, arms and thighs of patients with Hunter's syndrome. The lesions in these patients consist of isolated nodules or plaques of papules and nodules, lighter in color than the surrounding skin, firm in consistency, and with a surface texture resembling orange peel or corrugated cardboard. They may vary in size from a few millimeters to greater than a centimeter when coalescence of individual papules occurs (Levin, 1960).

Patients with an apparent focal mucopolysaccharide disorder, *stiff skin syndrome*, have localized cutaneous involvement that is usually present from birth. The skin is stony hard to palpation and cannot be compressed between the fingers nor indented with pressure. There is no atrophy, telangiectasia or pigmentary change to distinguish normal from abnormal tissue nor any alteration in temperature or surface texture. The most severely involved areas are the buttocks and thighs, but the skin of the abdomen, lumbar area and arms may also be firmer than normal (Esterly, 1971).

Hirsutism, particularly of the trunk and extremities, is a regular feature of most of the MPS, but often is not pronounced until after two years of life. The reason for the increased hairiness in these disorders is unknown. In addition, telangiectasia on the face, forearms, trunk and legs has been noted in some individuals with Scheie and Morquio syndromes (Scheie, 1952; Greaves, 1969).

Skin biopsies taken from both thickened rough areas and nodular lesions show diffuse vacuolization of the epidermal cells with occasional solitary swollen cells at all levels of the epidermis. The dermis is thickened, with some fragmentation and separation of collagen fibers. Large vacuolated mononuclear cells ("gargoyle" cells) are present just beneath the basement membrane, as well as in periappendageal and perivascular areas. With special stains for mucins abnormally high, reactivity can be demonstrated in the epidermis, in the vacuolated mononuclear cells and throughout the dermis, but particularly in tissue contiguous to the "gargoyle" cells, where large amounts of granular material appear to be deposited. In the stiff skin syndrome there are no epidermal changes or vacuolated cells, but only large amounts of an acid mucopolysaccharide in the dermis. On the basis of its staining characteristics, this MPS is most likely hyaluronic acid.

With the Rebuck skin window technique (see chap. 4), and using toluidine blue or Wright-Giemsa stain, metachromatic granules can be demonstrated in the macrophages from patients with generalized MPS. Metachromatic granules are also identifiable in circulating polymorphonuclear leukocytes and bone marrow cells (McKusick, 1965). Similarly, cultured skin fibroblasts from patients with generalized mucopolysaccharidoses contain cytoplasmic metachromatic granules when stained with toluidine blue O or alcian blue (Danes, 1966).

REFERENCES

Abul-Haj, S. K., Martz, D. G., Douglas, W. F. and Geppert, L. J.: Farber's disease. J. Pediat. *61*:221, 1962.

Ahnquist, G. and Holyoke, J. B.: Congenital Letterer-Siwe disease (reticulo-endotheliosis) in a term stillborn infant. J. Pediat. *57*:897, 1960.

Bannatyne, R. M., Skowron, P. N. and Weber, J. L.: Job's syndrome — A variant of chronic granulomatous disease. J. Pediat. *75*:236, 1969.

Bridge, R. G. and Foley, F. E.: Placental transmission of the lupus erythematosus factor. Amer. J. Med. Sci. *227*:1, 1954.

Burgoon, C. F., Graham, J. H. and McCaffere, D. L.: Mast cell disease. A cutaneous variant with multisystem involvement. Arch. Derm. *98*:590, 1968.

Caplan, R. M.: The natural course of urticaria pigmentosa. Arch. Derm. *87*:146, 1963.

Cohen, D. M., Mitchell, C. B. and Alexander, J. W.: Letterer-Siwe disease in a newborn. Arch. Path. *81*:347, 1966.

Danes, B. S. and Bean, A. G.: Hurler's syndrome.: A genetic study in cell culture. J. Exp. Med. *123*:1, 1966.

Demis, D. J.: The mastocytosis syndrome, clinical and biological studies. Ann. Intern. Med. *59*:194, 1963.

Doede, R. G. and Rappaport, H.: Long-term survival of patients with acute differentiated histiocytosis (Letterer-Siwe disease). Cancer *20*:1782, 1967.

Epstein, H. C. and Litt, J. Z.: Discoid lupus erythematosus in a newborn infant. New Eng. J. Med. *265*:1106, 1961.

Esterly, N. B. and McKusick, V. A.: Stiff skin syndrome. Pediatrics *47*:360, 1971.

Esterly, N. B., Sahihi, T. and Medenica, M.: Juvenile xanthogranuloma: An atypical case with study of ultrastructure. Arch. Derm. *105*:99, 1972.

Esterly, J. R., Sturner, W. A., Esterly, N. B. and Windhorst, D. B.: Disseminated BCG in twin boys with presumed chronic granulomatous disease of childhood. Pediatrics *48*:141, 1971.

Farber, S., Cohen, J. and Uzman, L. L.: Lipogranulomatosis. A new lipoglycoprotein "storage" disease. J. Mt. Sinai Hosp. *24*:816, 1957.

Gay, M. W., Noojin, R. O. and Finley, W. H.: Urticaria pigmentosa discordant in identical twins. Arch. Derm. *102*:29, 1970.

Gaynes, P. M. and Cohen, G. S.: Juvenile xanthogranuloma of the orbit. Amer. J. Ophthal. *63*:755, 1967.

Gonzales-Crussi, F. and Campbell, R. J.: Juvenile xanthogranuloma, ultrastructural study. Arch. Path. *89*:65, 1970.

Good, R. A., Quie, P. G., Windhorst, D. B., Page, A. R., Rodey, G. E., White, J., Wolfson, J. J. and Holmes, B. H.: Fatal (chronic) granulomatous disease of childhood: A hereditary defect of leukocyte function. Sem. Hemat. 5:215, 1968.

Greaves, M. W. and Inman, P. M.: Cutaneous changes in the Morquio syndrome. Brit. J. Derm. *81*:29, 1969.

Hambrick, G. W., Jr. and Scheie, H. G.: Studies of the skin in Hurler's syndrome. Arch. Derm. *85*:455, 1962.

Haust, M. D., Gordon, B. A., Bryans, A. M., Wollin, D. G. and Bennington, V.: Hepasulfate mucopolysaccharidosis (Sanfilippo disease): A case study with ultrastructural, biochemical and radiological findings. Pediat. Res. 5:137, 1971.

Helwig, E. B. and Hackney, V. C.: Juvenile xanthogranuloma. Amer. J. Path. *30*:625, 1954.

Hertz, C. B. and Hambrick, G. W.: Congenital Letterer-Siwe disease. Amer. J. Dis. Child. *116*:553, 1968.

Holmes, B., Park, B. H., Malawista, S. E., Quie, P. G., Nelson, D. L. and Good, R. A.: Chronic granulomatous disease in females. A deficiency of leukocyte glutathione peroxidase. New Eng. J. Med. *283*:217, 1970.

Jackson, R.: Discoid lupus in a newborn infant of a mother with lupus erythematosus. Pediatrics *33*:425, 1964.

Johnston, R. B., Jr. and Bachner, R.: Chronic granulomatous disease: Correlation between pathogenesis and clinical findings. Pediatrics *48*:730, 1971.

Jones, B., Welton, W. A. and Gilbert, E. F.: Congenital Letterer-Siwe disease. Cutis 3:750, 1967.

Juberg, R. C., Kloepfer, H. W. and Oberman, H. A.: Genetic determination of acute disseminated histiocytosis X (Letterer-Siwe syndrome). Pediatrics *45*:753, 1970.

Kenyon, K. R. and Sensenbrenner, J. A.: Mucolipidosis II (I-cell disease); Ultrastructural observations of conjunctiva and skin. Invest. Ophthal. *10*:555, 1971.

Leroy, J. G., Spranger, J. W., Feingold, M., Opitz, J. M. and Crocker, A. C.: I-cell disease: A clinical picture. J. Pediat. *79*:360, 1971.

Levin, S.: A specific skin lesion in gargoylism. AMA J. Dis. Child. *99*:444, 1960.

Lottsfeldt, F. J. and Good, R. A.: Juvenile xanthogranuloma with pulmonary lesions. Pediatrics *33*:233, 1964.

McCuiston, C. H. and Schoch, E. P., Jr.: Possible discoid lupus erythematosus in newborn infant: Report of a case with subsequent development of acute systemic lupus erythematosus in mother. Arch. Derm. *70*:782, 1954.

McKusick, V. A., Kaplan, D., Wise, D., Hanley, W. B., Suddarth, S. B., Sevick, M. E. and Maumanee, A. E.: The genetic mucopolysaccharidoses. Medicine *44*:1, 1965.

Nathan, D. J. and Snapper, I.: Simultaneous placental transfer of factors responsible for LE cell formation and thrombocytopenia. Amer. J. Med. *25*:647, 1958.

Nice, C. M., Jr.: Congenital disseminated lupus erythematosus. Amer. J. Roent. *88*:585, 1962.

Nomland, R.: Nevonxanthoendothelioma. J. Invest. Derm. *22*:207, 1959.

Pabst, H. F., Holmes, B., Quie, P. G., Gewurz, H., Rodey, G. and Good, R. A.: Immunological abnormalities in Job's syndrome. Soc. Ped. Res. 1971. (abstract).

Reed, W. B., May, S. B. and Tuffanelli, D. L.: Discoid lupus erythematosus in a newborn. Arch. Derm. *96*:64, 1967.

Sagher, F. and Even-Paz, Z.: Mastocytosis and the Mast Cell. Chicago, Year Book Medical Publishers, Inc., 1967.

Sahihi, T. and Esterly, N. B.: Atypical diffuse cutaneous mastocytosis. Amer. J. Dis. Child. *124*:133, 1972.

Scheie, H. G., Hambrick, G. W., Jr. and Barness, L. A.: A newly recognized forme fruste of Hurler's disease (gargoylism). Amer. J. Ophthal. *53*:753, 1962.

Seip, M.: Systemic lupus erythematosus in pregnancy with haemolytic anaemia, leucopenia and thrombocytopenia in the mother and her newborn infant. Arch. Dis. Child. *35*:364, 1960.

Selmanowitz, V. J., Orentreich, N., Tiangco, C. C. and Demis, D. J.: Uniovular twins discordant for cutaneous mastocytosis. Arch. Derm. *102*:34, 1970.

Shamoto, M.: Langerhans cell granule in Letterer-Siwe disease. Cancer *26*:1102, 1970.

Smith, J. L. S. and Ingram, R. M.: Juvenile oculodermal xanthogranuloma. Brit. J. Ophthal. *52*:696, 1968.

Spranger, J. W., Gilbert, E. F., Tuffli, G. A., Rossiter, F. P. and Opitz, J. M.: Geleophysic dwarfism—A "focal" mucopolysaccharidosis? Lancet *2*:97, 1971.

Spranger, J. R., Koch, F., McKusick, V. A., Natzschka, J., Wiedermann, H. -R. and Zellweger, H.: Mucopolysaccharidosis. VI (Maroteaux-Lamy disease). Helv. Paediat. Acta *25*:337, 1970.

Springer, J. W. and Wiedemann, H. -R.: The genetic mucolipidoses. Diagnosis and differential diagnosis. Humangenetik *9*:113, 1970.

Webster, S. B., Reister, H. C. and Harman, L. E., Jr.: Juvenile xanthogranuloma with extracutaneous lesions. Arch. Derm. *93*:71, 1966.

Windhorst, D. B. and Good, R. A.: Dermatologic manifestations of fatal granulomatous disease of childhood. Arch. Derm. *103*:351, 1971.

Zimmerman, L. C.: Ocular lesions of juvenile xanthogranuloma. Amer. J. Ophthal. *60*:1011, 1965.

Chapter Sixteen

MISCELLANEOUS HEREDITARY DISEASES

Most of the genetically determined dermatoses manifested in the newborn period have been considered in other chapters, classified according to their presenting sign or symptom. A number of entities having unusual clinical features remain, and we will discuss these here.

DEFECTS IN CUTANEOUS ELASTICITY

The skin is an elastic organ with the properties of stretch and recoil. More accurately, the elasticity of skin results from the stretch properties of its components, one of which is elastic tissue. The definition of hyperelasticity (excessive stretch and recoil) remains an imprecise clinical term. Stress-strain studies on strips of skin *in vitro*, light microscopy of specifically stained skin sections, studies of hydroxyproline and lysine metabolism *in vivo* and ultrastructural examination of the fibrous structure of the dermis have increased our understanding of diseases affecting cutaneous elasticity and have further delineated their classification. (Skin elasticity is *decreased* in a number of diseases which result in an infiltrate in the dermis, such as the mucopolysaccharidoses [see Chap. 15].)

Increased elasticity is found in the *Ehlers-Danlos syndrome, Turner's syndrome, Trisomy 21* and *Pseudoxanthoma elasticum.* The most spectacular changes are found in the Ehlers-Danlos syndrome. In this disease the skin may be stretched to excess but recoils to its normal shape after it is released. Another disease, the result of a quantitative deficiency of elastic tissue, has unfortunately been called "cutis laxa." In this disorder the skin hangs in loose folds and does not recoil (see following section). Certainly, a fulcrum for confusion was created by double use of the term cutis laxa, since both Ehlers (1901) and Danlos (1890) used it to describe the disease which is today called "cutis hyperelastica." Perhaps the syndrome caused by a decrease in elastic tissue should have been called "cutis anelastica."

CUTIS LAXA

(Dermatomegaly, Generalized Elastolysis)

In cutis laxa (Fig. 16–1), the cutaneous elasticity has been lost so that gravity causes sagging of the skin, and it hangs in doughy folds about the neck, ears, wrists, knees, ankles, chest wall and abdomen (Goltz, 1965). The patient has a sad, bloodhound appearance. This is accompanied by ectropion and systemic manifestations including: inguinal and ventral hernias; diaphragmatic atony; intestinal and urogenital diverticula; cardiopulmonary disease (Hajjar, 1968); emphysema (Maxwell, 1969); tracheobronchiomegaly (Wanderer, 1969); and growth retardation (Reisner, 1971). The joints are not hyperextensible.

173

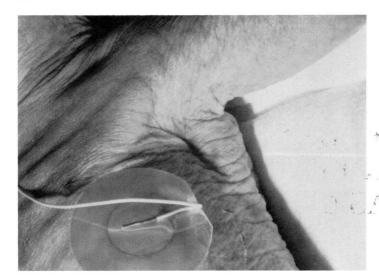

Figure 16–1. Cutis laxa.

Cutis laxa is extremely rare. It has two types of inheritance and may be acquired in childhood or as an adult. One form may be transmitted by an autosomal recessive gene; the other by an autosomal dominant gene (Grahame, 1971).

The diagnosis may be made at birth by skin biopsy. On histological examination of skin sections stained for elastic tissue, the fibers are found to be reduced in size and number, with the greatest decrease apparent in the papillary portion of the dermis. Goltz (1965) observed that the elastic fibers were swollen and had inconsistent and variable osmiophilia on electron microscopy. The histological features of elastolysis were also seen in the internal organs on post mortem examination.

Grahame and Beighton (1971) studied the physical properties of the skin in cutis laxa. They found that the tensile strength of the skin was normal and concluded that this finding was further evidence for an elastin deficiency rather than an abnormality of collagen.

The cosmetic defect may be ameliorated by plastic repair but the prognosis of this disease is grave.

EHLERS-DANLOS SYNDROME
(Cutis hyperelastica)

Ehlers-Danlos syndrome is more common than cutis laxa and is transmitted by an autosomal dominant gene. It results in a spectacular increase in cutaneous elasticity, permitting excessive stretching of the skin. The hyperelastic state allows recoil of the stretched skin so that it snaps back and is of normal appearance. If the integrity of the skin is breeched, there is a tendency to form scars that characteristically accumulate over the elbows and knees. The scars are usually wide, flat and have a "cigarette paper" surface texture, or they may form soft tumors. A small wound results in a widely gaping aperture.

Patients with Ehlers-Danlos syndrome tend to bruise easily, forming subcutaneous hematomas which may calcify and result in small (under 1 cm), persistent, oval, intradermal calcifications. Associated anomalies include: frontal bossing; hypertelorism; prognathism; flat feet; myopia; large floppy ears; and, most typically, hyperextensible joints. This last clinical finding is found so frequently that it should suggest the diagnosis to the alert physician. Herniation of the diaphragm and gastrointestinal tract diverticulae can develop with aging. Hemetemesis and lower intestinal bleeding are common. Aortic aneurysms, arteriovenous fistulae, blue sclerae, retinal detachments and lenticular abnormalities have also been described in some cases (Pemberton, 1966; Maxwell, 1969; Lynch, 1965). The skeleton is affected in many patients. In a recent series, Beighton (1969) found kyphosis or scoliosis, subluxation of joints, pes planus and genu recurvatum in significant numbers of patients with Ehlers-Danlos syndrome.

The interpretation of the histologic findings in Ehlers-Danlos syndrome has been controversial at times. Goltz and Hult (1965) found increased numbers of elastic fibers in the dermis and in other organs, but Fischer and Wechsler (1971) noted no such abnormality. Jansen (1955) postulated a deficiency of cross-collagen fiber linkage and Barabas (1967) suggested a defective "wicker-work" of cutaneous collagen. In contrast, others have found no consistent qualitative changes in the collagen. The dermis appears thin, and additional evidence (Varadi, 1965; Mason, 1965; Strauss, 1966) supports the postulate that there is a quantitative deficiency of dermal collagen in Ehlers-Danlos syndrome, making the elastic tissue appear excessive (Fisher, 1971). The management of patients with Ehlers-Danlos syndrome should include informed genetic counseling of the parents, expectation of premature birth (Barabas, 1966) and protective measures to prevent trauma to the skin of affected children. Skeletal examination by radiography is advised after puberty and when clinical findings suggest possible abnormalities. Ophthalmologic examination should be performed yearly during the growth period.

HYPOPLASIAS

FOCAL DERMAL HYPOPLASIA
(Goltz' syndrome)

Focal dermal hypoplasia is a hereditary disease affecting both mesodermal and ectodermal structures in the skin and internal organs. Although there are about 50 reported cases to date, the syndrome is well-established and the clinical findings have been reviewed by Goltz and his colleagues (1970). The preponderance of affected individuals are female, although some severely affected males have been reported (Hook, 1968), suggesting that the mode of inheritance may be X-linked dominant or sex-limited autosomal dominant.

The cutaneous findings are striking. The most characteristic lesions are linear areas of thinning or absence of the dermis, allowing herniation of fat through the surrounding skin. Since the thinned areas are covered by the epidermis, the overall appearance is that of linear or patchy lesions resembling red or yellow-brown deflated balloons. Other areas look like atrophic scars. Red papillomas also occur around the mouth, anus, vulva, gingiva and tongue. Telangiectasia may be prominent in some areas. The vascular tone is unstable, resulting in intense whealing when the skin is stroked. In some cases the skin may be enitrely absent in different areas at birth, or blisters may form which heal by crusting. Hyperkeratotic lesions may also occur. Most often there are reticular areas of hypo- or hyperpigmentation. The nails and eccrine glands may be abnormal or absent, but not uniformly so. Alopecia or patchy areas of brittle, frizzy hair are common occurrences. Skeletal anomalies include rounded microcrania, kyphoscoliosis, vertebral anomalies, skeletal asymmetry, and rib, scapular and pelvic abnormalities. Anomalies of the limbs are extremely common and are usually manifested as hypoplasia or absence of fingers, hands, a greater part of a limb, syndactyly, polydactyly or camptodactyly.

A host of anomalies affecting all or any of the structures in the eye, ranging from anophthalmia to heterochromia iridum, may also occur in this syndrome. The teeth are dysplastic, and jaw, lips, palate and tongue may have hypoplasia or clefts. The nervous system is also involved and the patients may be mentally retarded or deaf. One of our patients with Goltz' syndrome has most of the anomalies described, as well as a renal malformation resulting in a horseshoe kidney. The constellation of findings indicates that malformations take place early (prior to the eighth week) in embryonic development.

The diagnosis is usually quite obvious and may be confirmed by biopsy of an affected area of skin, which will show a thin to almost absent dermis with fat lying just beneath the epidermis.

DERMAL HYPOPLASIA, OSSEOUS DYSPLASIA AND MENTAL DEFICIENCY

A familial syndrome with "hypoplastic" skin lesions and eczema was reported by Ruvalcaba, Reichert and Smith (1971). The two male siblings were both mentally retarded and microcephalic with a narrow thoracic cage, hypoplastic genitalia, short metatarsals, metacarpals and phalanges, as well as epiphysitis of the spine. Since no cutaneous biopsy was reported, the significance of the "hypoplastic" skin lesions is not clear. The disease seems to be inherited but the mechanism of inheritance cannot be deduced from the data available.

THE NAIL-PATELLA SYNDROME

This peculiar hereditary syndrome (Lucas, 1966; Warkany, 1971), which is characterized by anomalies of the thumb nails and absence of the patella, has been known for about 150 years (Little, 1897). A fuller description of the syndrome includes deformity of the elbow resulting from hypoplasia of the radial and humeral heads, osseous horns on the iliac crest and, occasionally, mental retardation. Renal dysplasia, which may eventuate in a nephrotic syndrome, has been noted as a more recent finding in a significant number of these patients (Hawkins, 1950). The disorder is inherited as an autosomal dominant trait, although somatic mutation is also possible. The loci for the ABO blood groups and erythrocyte adenylate kinase are closely linked with that of the nail-patella syndrome (Sobel, 1971); however, not all patients with nail-patella syndrome have the same blood groups.

The nail changes consist of spooning, softening, discoloration, central grooving, splitting and cracking, narrowing, or, less commonly, thickening. Most often there is severe hypoplasia or total absence of the thumb nail and index finger nail. The other nails can show minimal changes, and the toenails are normal in most affected individuals.

Nail and patellar abnormalities may be found in the affected neonate and the nephrotic syndrome may also be present during this period (Simila, 1970). Angiomas, ichthyotic changes, palmar keratoses, hypertrichosis, alopecia, polydactyly and cleft palate are occasional cutaneous findings in this syndrome. Skeletal exostoses and other malformations have been found in isolated cases.

The prognosis is guarded for those patients with glomerular and renal tubular lesions resulting in albuminuria and reduced renal clearance.

METABOLIC DEFECTS

XERODERMA PIGMENTOSUM

Xeroderma pigmentosum is a serious, life-limiting disorder resulting in photosensitivity and pigmentary changes (Fig. 16–2), accompanied by a propensity for formation of cutaneous malignancies which cause awesome suffering and mutilation of the unfortunate victims, the majority of whom usually die before 20 years of age (Reed, 1965; Rook, 1969). The disease is inherited in an autosomal recessive fashion. The earliest signs of xeroderma pigmentosum are photophobia and conjunctivitis, and these are often apparent during the first month of life. Within a variable period (depending on the severity of the disease) a reaction resembling sunburn with redness and scaling is noticeable in light-exposed areas. The erythema is followed by freckling and white spots. Blepharitis, symblepharon and crusting of the lid margins are also characteristic. In 75 per cent of cases the latter symptoms are noted first between the sixth month and third year of life. The skin of the face, hands and often the legs, becomes atrophic and telangiectatic. Vesicobullous lesions, crusts, keratoses and scars supervene, while self-healing epitheliomata (keratoacanthomas) develop even in mild cases. After six years of age or so, basal cell epitheliomas, squamous cell cancer and malignant melanomas cause considerable destruction of tissue, and ultimately metastatic disease presages the demise of the child.

Associated anomalies include some degree of mental retardation and dwarfism. The combination of xeroderma pigmentosum

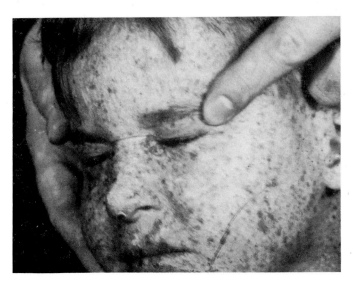

Figure 16–2. Xeroderma pigmentosum.

with mental retardation, microcephaly, hypogonadism and dwarfism is called the *de Sanctis-Cacchione syndrome* (Reed, 1965).

The diagnosis of xeroderma pigmentosum is not difficult and can be confirmed by demonstration of an enzymatic aberration in fibroblasts cultured from the patient's skin. One of the most exciting biological discoveries in recent years has disclosed the basic abnormality in xeroderma pigmentosum (Cleaver, 1968). Ultraviolet light causes damage to DNA in epidermal and dermal cells. In normal individuals, an endonuclease excises the defective thymine dimer and the DNA is then repaired by a polynucleotide ligase. In xeroderma pigmentosum the endonuclease is defective, so repair of ultraviolet-damaged DNA is not achieved (Cleaver, 1970). The defect is specific for UV light, since DNA damaged by X-ray can undergo replication repair. In X-ray-induced trauma to DNA the chain is broken, allowing release of the damaged portion. Since the repair mechanism for a broken DNA chain does not require a functional endonuclease, only ligase, patients with xeroderma pigmentosum (who have adequate polynucleotide ligase activity) have no difficulty repairing these broken DNA chains. The intriguing possibility that an endonuclease defect is responsible for cancer has been explored. Although it may play a role in mutation, there is no endonuclease deficiency in skin cancer except in xeroderma pigmentosum.

The treatment and prevention of xeroderma pigmentosum can be approached in several different ways: (1) through genetic counseling; (2) interruption of pregnancy if the defect is identified in cultured amniotic fluid cells; (3) rigorous protection of an affected infant from exposure to UV light; (4) application of opaque sun screens to the skin; (5) early excision of small cutaneous malignancies; (6) excision of larger areas of skin that are studded by malignancies and their replacement by autografts from cutaneous areas less exposed to UV light (such as the buttocks); and (7) use of topical antimitotic agents such as 5 fluoro-uracil.

LOWE'S SYNDROME
(Oculo-cerebro-renal syndrome)

Congenital cataract, corneal dystrophy, and fine friable or frizzy hair may be the first signs of Lowe's syndrome (Lowe, 1952; Warkany, 1971). After age six months, the infant (almost always male) becomes increasingly hypotonic and shows signs of mental retardation, osteoporosis and rickets. The underlying defect, which may be due to an X-linked mutant gene, results in aminoaciduria, proteinuria, decreased ability to excrete ammonia and hydrogen ions, and metabolic acidosis. Renal tubular hyalinization and sclerosis may be a fatal complication, but several patients have managed to survive with adequate metabolic management. In a patient seen by us, the hair changes were most striking. The scalp hair was thin, of very fine caliber and vellus in character.

FAMILIAL DYSAUTONOMIA
(Riley-Day syndrome)

Familial dysautonomia occurs primarily among Ashkenazic Jews of southeastern European origin (Riley, 1949; Brunt, 1970). The disease is transmitted by an autosomal recessive gene, and consanguinity exists in many of the affected families. Affected infants have a wide variety of symptoms (Table 16–2), some of which may be found within a few hours after birth (Table 16–1).

Of particular interest are the changes relating to the skin, including the following: an absence of lingual fungiform papillae; vasomotor lability resulting in blotching; episodes of profuse sweating; and, abnormal vascular responses to histamine. When histamine is injected into normal skin (or, when the skin is stroked firmly with a blunt object) the response should consist of: (1) vasodilation (erythema) at the site of stroking; (2) a wheal (exudation of serum); and (3) a red flare around the area (the axon reflex). In familial dysautonomia the flare reaction does not occur, suggesting a defect in either peripheral sensory nerve conduction or the insympathetic nerves in the skin.

When methacholine is instilled in the conjunctival sac, miosis is induced in these infants. Although these tests have been positive in a significant number of dysautonomic children, they are not pathognomic, since 2.5 per cent of normal infants give a miotic response to methacholine. Infants with atopic eczema may also lack the normal flare in response to scratching or injection of histamine, and eczema may also be present in familial dysautonomia (Felner, 1964). Winkelmann (1966) has studied the peripheral nerves in the skin of patients with familial dysautonomia and found no anatomical abnormality.

Another interesting, albeit inconsistent finding is the abnormality in catecholamine

Table 16–1. Symptoms of Familial Dysautonomia*

Symptoms	Age at Onset or Recognition
Autonomic nervous system:	
Skin blotching	5 hr.
Coldness of extremities	5 hr.
Vacillation of temperature	24 hr.
Incoordination of suck and swallow	24 hr.
Bowel irregularities	2 wk.
Labile hypertension	1 mo.
Postural hypotension	1 mo.
Reduced or absent tear and resulting corneal abrasions	6 wk.
Drooling	—
Neuromuscular system:	
Diminished deep tendon reflexes	Birth
Hypotonia	Birth
Poor muscular coordination	24 hr.
Small stature	2 mo.
Dysarthria	—
Scoliosis	—
Sensory disturbance:	
Indifferent response to pain	Birth
Corneal anesthesia	6 wk.
Central nervous system:	
Motor-skill retardation	6 wk.
Breath holding	2 mo.
Behavior disturbance	6 mo.
Periodic vomiting	—
Mental retardation	?
Convulsions	?
Biochemical studies:	
Positive methacholine test	2 wk.
Positive histamine test	2 wk.
Elevated HVA	3 wk.
Depressed VMA	3 wk.

*Courtesy of Geltzer, A. I., Gluck, L., Talner, N. S. et al.: New England J. Med., *271*:436, 1964.

metabolism in these patients (Smith, 1963). As early as three weeks they show a decrease in secretion of vanylmandellic acid (VMA) and elevation in homovanillic acid (HMA) (Geltzer, 1964) and a deficiency of dopamine β-oxidase in the serum. The interpretation of these findings has led to many theories concerning the basic defect in familial dysautonomia; but, because of inconsistencies in the findings as well as considerable gaps in our knowledge about storage and release of neurotransmitters, a complete explanation of the enzyme abnormality is still awaited.

In 1968 Esterly et al. reported a three year old black girl with papillotonia, hyporeflexia and segmental hypohidrosis (*Holmes-Adie syndrome*). Most intriguing was the similarity of the syndrome to familial dysautonomia, as the patient apparently also lacked fungiform papillae of the tongue and failed to produce

Table 16–2. Frequency of Clinical Features in the Series

Feature	%
Absence of fungiform papillae*	100
Absence of overflow tears	100
Vasomotor disturbance (blotching)	98
Abnormal sweating	97
Episodic fever	92
Incoordination and unsteadiness	90
Swallowing difficulty in infancy	85
Physical retardation	78
Episodic vomiting	67
Breath-holding attacks	66
Marked emotional instability	65
Scoliosis*	55
Bowel disturbance	49

*In those examined only.
Courtesy of Brunt, P. W. and McKusik, V. A.: Medicine *49*:351, 1970.

overflow tears. Since early feeding difficulty, postural hypotension, and emotional lability were lacking, and corneal reflexes and sensitivity to pain were present, the "essential" diagnostic criteria for familial dysautonomia were not fulfilled. In addition, the cutaneous response to intradermal injection of histamine was normal in the patient.

HARTNUP DISEASE

Hartnup disease (appropriately bearing the name of the first patient so described) is a light-sensitive disorder which is inherited in an autosomal recessive manner and is associated with a characteristic aminoaciduria (Baron, 1956; Efron, 1971). About 20 per cent of affected individuals are mentally retarded, while others show signs of emotional instability and episodic cerebellar ataxia.

The earliest manifestations may occur in the first months of life. There is an intermittent eczematous, and occasionally vesicobullous eruption localized to the light-exposed areas that may progress to hyperkeratosis, hyperpigmentation and atrophic (poikilodermatous) changes. In sum, the clinical picture is extremely similar to that of pellagra in the adult. A nicotinic acid deficiency due to poor absorption of tryptophan has been postulated as the basic defect.

The differential diagnosis includes erythropoietic porphyria and xeroderma pigmentosum. There is no porphyrinuria, and cultured fibroblasts show no defect of replication repair of UV damage to DNA. The demonstration of a generalized aminoaciduria with large amounts of indican and an absence of proline, methionine and arginine in the urine, confirms the diagnosis of Hartnup disease.

Treatment should include protection from light and prevention of the neurologic and central nervous system by administration of nicotinic acid. Fortunately, Hartnup disease is extremely rare in the United States.

HEREDITARY ANGIONEUROTIC EDEMA

Hereditary angioneurotic edema is a rare disease transmitted by an autosomal dominant gene (Donaldson, 1966; Dennehy, 1970). It results from deficiency of an inhibitor of the first component of the serum complement cascade (C′1 esterase inhibitor). The clinical effect of a highly labile complement system in these patients is angio-edema affecting the hollow viscera, the skin and larynx. The edema does not respond to epinephrine; laryngeal swelling may necessitate tracheostomy or will result in death. Allergy has little to do with hereditary angioneurotic edema. Instead, the attacks may be precipitated by emotional stress, minor trauma or upper respiratory infections. The clinical mediator of the swelling is a polypeptide resembling kinin in its activity. Histamine plays a very minor part, or no role at all, in the etiology of the process. Although the onset of symptoms most frequently occurs in the adolescent years, it occurs very rarely during infancy.

The diagnosis may be confirmed in symptomless children of an affected family by finding a deficient level of C′1 esterase inhibitor in the serum.

REFERENCES

Barabas, A. P.: Ehlers-Danlos syndrome: Associated with prematurity and premature rupture of foetal membranes; possible increase in incidence. Brit. Med. J. 2:682, 1966.

Barabas, A. P.: Heterogeneity of the Ehlers-Danlos syndrome: Description of three clinical types of hypothesis to explain the basic defect(s). Brit. Med. J. 2:612, 1967.

Baron, D. N., Dent, C. E., Harris, H., Hart, E. W. and Jepson, J. B.: Hereditary pellagra-like skin rash with temporary cerebellar ataxia, constant renal aminoaciduria, and other bizarre chemical features. Lancet 2:421, 1956.

Beighton, P. and Thomas, M. L.: Radiology of the Ehlers-Danlos syndrome. Clin. Radiol. 20:354, 1969.

Brunt, P. W. and McKusick, V. A.: Familial dysautonomia. Medicine 49:343, 1970.

Cleaver, J. E.: Defective repair replication of DNA in xeroderma pigmentosum. Nature 218:653, 1968.

Cleaver, J. E.: DNA damage and repair in light-sensitive human skin disease. J. Invest. Derm. 54:181, 1970.

Danlos, M.: Un cas de cutis laxa avec tumeurs par contusion chronique des coudes et des genoux. Bull. Soc. Franc. Derm. Syph. 19:70, 1908.

Dennehy, J. J.: Hereditary angioneurotic edema. Ann. of Int. Med. 73:55, 1970.

Donaldson, V. H. and Rosen, F. S.: Hereditary angioneurotic edema: a clinical survey. Pediatrics 37: 1017, 1966.

Efron, M. L. and Gallagher, W. F.: Cutaneous changes in errors of amino acid metabolism. In Fitzpatrick, T. B., Arndt, K. A., Clark, W. H., Eisen, A. Z., Van Scott, E. G. and Vaughan, J. H. (eds.): Dermatology in General Medicine. New York, McGraw-Hill, 1971, p. 1098.

Ehlers, E.: Cutis laxa. Neigung zu Haemorrhagien in der Haut, Lockerung Mehrerer Artikulationen. Derm. Zeit. 8:173, 1901.

Esterly, N. B., Cantolino, S. J., Alter, B. P. and Brusilow, S. W.: Pupillotonia, hyporeflexia and segmental hypohidrosis: autonomic dysfunction in a child. J. Pediat. 73:852, 1968.

Fellner, M. J.: Manifestations of familial autonomic dysautonomia. Arch. Derm. *89*:190, 1964.

Fisher, E. R. and Wechsler, H. L.: The so-called collagen diseases and elastoses of skin. *In* Helwig, E. G. and Mostofi, F. K. (eds.): The Skin. Baltimore, Williams and Wilkins Co., 1971, pp. 366–403.

Geltzer, A. I., Gluck, L., Talner, N. S. and Plesky, H. F.: Familial dysautonomia. Studies in a newborn infant. New Eng. J. Med. *271*:436, 1964.

Goltz, R. W., Henderson, R. R., Hitch, J. M. and Ott, J. E.: Focal dermal hypoplasia syndrome. Arch. Derm. *101*:1, 1970.

Goltz, R. W., Hult, A. M., Goldfarb, M. and Gorlin, R. J.: Cutis Laxa. Arch. Derm. *92*:373, 1965.

Grahame, R. and Beighton, P.: The physical properties of skin in cutis laxa. Brit. J. Derm. *84*:326, 1971.

Hajjar, B. A. and Joyner, E. N., III: Congenital cutis laxa with advanced cardiopulmonary disease. J. Ped. *73*:116, 1968.

Hawkins, C. F. and Smith, O. E.: Renal dysplasia in a family with multiple hereditary abnormaliteis including iliac horns. Lancet *1*:803, 1950.

Hook, E. B.: Asymmetric manifestations of an apparently new syndrome: Depressed and pitted skin, facial tumors, syndactyly and other congenital defects. J. Pediatrics. *73*:913, 1968.

Jansen, L. H.: The structure of connective tissue: Explanation of symptoms of Ehlers-Danlos syndrome. Dermatologica *110*:108, 1955.

Little, W. M.: Congenital absence or delayed development of the patella. Lancet *2*:781, 1897.

Lowe, C. C., Terrey, M. and MacLachland, E. A.: Organic aciduria, decreased renal ammonia production, hydrophthalmos, and mental retardation. Am. J. Dis. Child. *83*:164, 1962.

Lucas, G. L. and Opitz, J. M.: The nail-patella syndrome. J. Pediat. *68*:273, 1966.

Lynch, H. T., Larsen, A. L., Wilson, R. and Magnuson, C.: Ehlers-Danlos syndrome and "congenital" arteriovenous fistulae. JAMA *194*:1011, 1965.

Mason, P. and Rigby, B. J.: Ehlers-Danlos syndrome. Arch. Path. *80*:363, 1965.

Maxwell, E. and Esterly, N. B.: Cutis laxa. Am. J. Dis. Child. *117*:479, 1969.

Pemberton, J. W., Freeman, H. M. and Schepens, C.: Familial retinal detachment and the Ehlers-Danlos syndrome. Arch. Ophthal. *76*:817, 1966.

Reed, W. B., May, S. B. and Nickel, W. R.: Xeroderma pigmentosum with neurological complications. Arch. Derm. *91*:224, 1965.

Reisner, S. H., Seelenfreund, M. and Ben-Bassat, M.: Cutis laxa associated with severe intrauterine growth retardation and congenital dislocation of the hip. Acta Paediat. Scand. *60*:357, 1971.

Riley, C. M., Day, R. L., Greeley, D. M. and Langford, W. S.: Central autonomic dysfunction with defective lacrimation. Report of five cases. Pediatrics *3*:468, 1949.

Rook, A. and Wells, R. S.: Genetics in dermatology. *In* Rook, A., Wilkinson, D. S. and Ebling, F. J. G. (eds.): Textbook of Dermatology. Philadelphia, F. A. Davis Co., 1968, p. 62.

Ruvalcaba, R. H. A., Reichert, A. and Smith, D. W.: A new familial syndrome with osseous dysplasia and mental deficiency. J. Pediat. *79*:450, 1971.

Similä, S., Vesa, L. and Wasz-Höckert, O.: Hereditary onycho-osteodysplasia (the nail-patella syndrome) with nephrosis-like renal disease in a newborn boy. Pediatrics *46*:61, 1970.

Smith, A. A., Taylor, T. and Wortis, S. B.: Abnormal catecholamine metabolism in familial dysautonomia. New Eng. J. Med. *268*:705, 1963.

Sobel, R. S., Tiger, A. and Gerald, P. S.: A second family with the nail-patella allele and the adenylate kinase allele in coupling. Am. J. Hum. Genet. *23*:146, 1971.

Strauss, B. and Tejaratchi, N.: Biochemical abnormalities in Ehlers-Danlos syndrome. Arch. Intern. Med. *118*:461, 1966.

Varadi, D. P. and Hall, D. A.: Cutaneous elastin in Ehlers-Danlos syndrome. Nature *208*:1224, 1965.

Wanderer, A. A., Ellis, E. F., Goltz, R. W. and Cotton, E. K.: Tracheobronchiomegaly and acquired cutis laxa in a child. Pediatrics *44*:709, 1969.

Warkany, J.: Lowe's syndrome. *In* Congenital Malformations. Chicago, Year Book Medical Publishers Inc., 1971, p.389.

Warkany, J.: Osteo-onycho dysplasia. *In* Congenital Malformations. Chicago, Year Book Medical Publishers, Inc., 1971, p. 1016.

Winkelmann, R. K., Bourland, A. and Smith, A. A.: Nerves in the skin of a patient with familial dysautonomia (Riley-Day syndrome). Pediatrics *38*:1060, 1966.

Chapter Seventeen

DISORDERS OF THE APPENDAGEAL STRUCTURES

Abnormalities of the appendageal structures—the glands, hair and nails—occur in a wide spectrum of disorders. Although a few of these diseases are limited to the appendages, the overwhelming majority are multisystem disorders with cutaneous features that are useful as indicators but are of minor importance to general health. Unfortunately, the conditions that are not congenital, progressive or permanent (e.g., acne neonatorum and miliaria) are also those that are most amenable to therapy. Much remains

to be learned about the etiology and pathogenesis of many of these disorders before rational preventative or therapeutic measures can be instituted.

The limitations of space preclude a full discussion of all the disease entities. Predominantly non-cutaneous disorders are listed only in the Tables at the end of the chapter; other sources should be consulted for more descriptive information. Some diseases seemed to fit more appropriately under other chapter headings and the Tables indicate

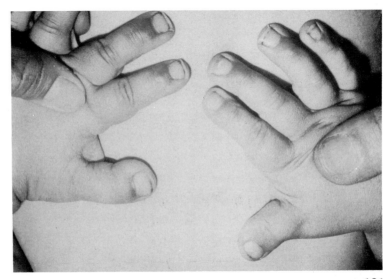

Figure 17–1. Broad thumbs: Rubenstein-Taybi syndrome.

where they may be found. Nevi and tumors involving the appendageal structures are also discussed in Chapter 8.

ACNE NEONATORUM

Lesions typical of acne vulgaris are occasionally seen in young infants (Plate XV-D, page 95). The eruption may have its onset any time during the first two years of life, but affected infants seem to separate naturally into two groups: those with onset under three months of age (usually within the first two weeks after birth); and patients with lesions that first occur between three months and two years of life. The first group seems to consist almost entirely of males, whereas in the second group, males are only slightly predominant (Hellier, 1954).

In most cases the papules, pustules and comedones are confined to the cheeks, but the forehead and chin may also be involved. Unlike acne in the adolescent, the back and chest remain clear. A few infants also show deepseated nodules, cold abscesses and cystic lesions which, on resolution, result in pitted scars. The course may be variable with activity decreasing after a few months or persisting one year or longer (Giknis, 1952; Hellier, 1954). The duration and severity of the process seem independent of the age of onset.

The etiology and pathogenesis of infantile acne is not understood. It has been postulated that the pilosebaceous structure in the infant shows a heightened response to elevated levels of maternal hormones, but this hypothesis has never been proved. However, a strong family history of acne is often obtained

and long-term observation of affected infants has suggested that these patients are prone to severe adolescent acne as well (Hellier, 1954).

Although infants with acne generally show no evidence of endocrine disease and have a normal urinary excretion of 17-ketosteroids (Tromovitch, 1963), a careful physical examination of the infant should not be neglected since acne may be a manifestation of a virilizing syndrome. In addition, it is important to inquire about unusual possible exposure to petrolatum, medicated oils or halogenated compounds. These substances may cause a chemically induced acneiform eruption characterized by a profusion of comedones and inflammatory or granulomatous follicular lesions. Eruptions occur at sites of contact and are not necessarily confined to the face (Rook, 1968). Patients with the Apert type of acrocephalosyndactyly, (Fig. 17–2) a syndrome diagnosable at birth, may be expected to develop abnormally widespread acne at puberty, even on arms and legs (Solomon, 1970).

Acne neonatorum will usually respond to the combined use of a kertolytic wash containing sulfur and salicylic acid (Fostex cream), and a mild antiacne lotion (Komed mild; Lotio alba). Frequency of application should be determined by the response to treatment, the presence or absence of peeling and irritation and the complexion of the infant. Fair-complexioned individuals are more likely to suffer from the irritant effects of keratolytic agents.

NAIL DEFECTS

Although abnormalities of the nails are congenital or acquired, virtually all such de-

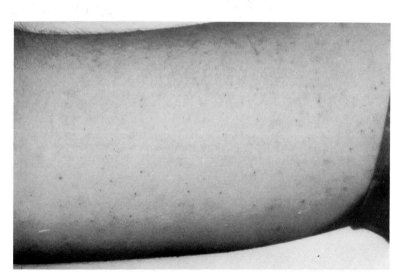

Figure 17–2. Comedones of the arm in the Apert syndrome.

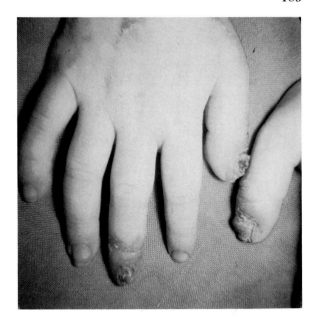

Figure 17–3. Nail involvement in epidermal nevus: ichthyosis hystrix.

fects in the newborn infant fall into the congenital group. Many of these anomalies are also familial and may be a manifestation of a more generalized disorder or syndrome (Figs. 17–1 and 17–3).

A number of descriptive terms have been coined in an attempt to classify nail defects. Very little is known, however, about their etiology and pathogenesis and, in most cases, treatment is not effective. Nevertheless, identifcation of the anomaly in specific morphologic terms is often useful since it can provide a clue to a more widespread disorder. A number of syndromes which include nail defects are listed in Table 17–1.

Congenital Absence of the Nails (Anonychia). This rare defect occurs as an isolated abnormality or in association with digital anomalies (Fig. 17–4). Some cases have been familial, but data is too scant to assess the genetic pattern. Anonychia has also been described with ectrodactyly and is, in this combination, inherited as an autosomal dominant trait. Nails are usually absent on the index and middle fingers and are partially absent on the thumb. Toes are also affected and, in some patients, bizarre defects of the digits occur. In addition, absent nails can be a feature of the nail-patella syndrome (see Chap. 16) or anhidrotic ectodermal dysplasia (see following section).

Atrophic Nails (Onychoatrophia). Atrophic nails result from partial destruction of the nail matrix by trauma, infection or acquired skin diseases but, in the newborn, they are most often a manifestation of a more

Table 17–1. Syndromes Associated with Nail Defects*

I. Total or Partial Absence of Nails; Nail Hypoplasia and Dysplasia

  Acrodermatitis enteropathica
  Anhidrotic (hypohidrotic) ectodermal dysplasia
  Anonychia and ectrodactyly
  Apert's syndrome (acrocephalosyndactyly)
  Cartilage-hair hypoplasia
  Deafness and nail dystrophy (Feinmesser; Robinson)
  Dyskeratosis congenita
  Ellis-van Creveld syndrome
  Enamel hypoplasia and curly hair
  Epidermolysis bullosa
  Focal dermal hypoplasia (Goltz's syndrome)
  Glossopalatine ankylosis, microglossia, hypodontia and anomalies of the extremities (Gorlin-Pindborg)
  Incontinentia pigmenti
  Larsen's syndrome
  Long arm 21 deletion syndrome
  Nail-patella syndrome
  Oto-palato-digital syndrome
  Popliteal web syndrome
  Progeria
  Pyknodysostosis (Lamy-Maroteaux)
  Rothmund-Thomson syndrome
  Skin hypoplasia, nail dystrophy (Basan)
  Trisomy 13
  Trisomy 18
  Turner's syndrome

II. Hypertrophic or Abnormally Large Nails
  Congenital hemihypertrophy
  Familial hyperpigmentation with dystrophy of the nails (Touraine and Soulignac)
  Pachyonychia congenita
  Rubinstein-Taybi syndrome

*Pardo-Costello, 1960; Gorlin, 1964; Sammon, 1968; Smith, 1970; Zaias, 1971.

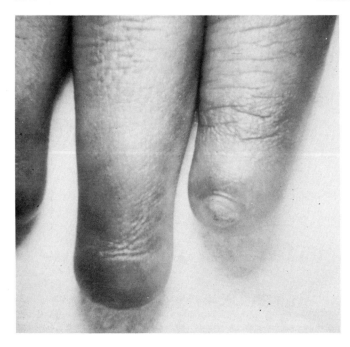

Figure 17–4. Anonychia. (Courtesy of Dr. David Fretzin.)

generalized congenital disorder. Affected nails are diminutive, thin, deformed and often grow extremely slowly. A number of syndromes associated with rudimentary or absent nails are listed in Table 17–1.

Hypertrophy of the Nail. This anomaly is known as onychauxis; where increased curvature is also present the term onychogryposis is used. Affected nails are thickened, elongated and discolored. Often, the nails are twisted like a spiral or hook and resemble the horn or claw of an animal. Subungual accumulations of keratotic debris are usually present. Both types of malformation may be congenital and hereditary, although they more commonly are acquired. Familial onychogryposis has been reported in association with hyperhidrosis, defective dentition, diffuse hyperpigmentation and hypertrichosis (Pardo-Costello, 1960).

Spoon-Shaped Nails (Koilonychia). Usually associated with a hypochromic anemia, spoon-shaped nails also occur as a congenital and hereditary anomaly. Several fingers, or all, show concavity of the nail plate. The toes are less commonly affected. This type of dystrophy has also been reported in combination with anomalies of the hair (Pardo-Costello, 1960).

Racquet Nail. Resulting from an abnormality of the distal phalanx that causes a short, wide nail with loss of its normal curvature, racquet nail usually involves one or both thumbs. The condition may be inherited in an autosomal dominant fashion (Ronchese,

1951). A similar deformity may be seen in inveterate thumbsuckers, but thumbsucking also causes nail ridges, cross-hatching and edema of the paronchial tissues. Another minor defect, *pitting of the nails*, is often attributed to trauma or occurs in childhood as a feature of psoriasis or alopecia areata. A familial form of nail pitting has also been described in which the pits may be noticeable in infancy or fail to appear until later in childhood. The anomaly has been attributed to an unknown but intermittent defect in the nail matrix (Samman, 1968). *Pterygium* is an overgrowth of cuticle onto the nail with partial or total destruction of the nail plate. In the adult this is most commonly due to a degenerative disease or to lichen planus, but it also occurs as a congenital defect.

White Nails (Leukonychia). There are four different forms of this defect: total; partial; striate; and punctate. All but the punctate type may be congenital and hereditary; transmission is by an autosomal dominant gene. All four forms of leukonychia may also be acquired; in these instances, they are usually the result of trauma or an expression of systemic illness. Nonhereditary striate leukonychia may also be seen during the neonatal period. The lines move distally with the growing nail and their distance from the cuticle corresponds to the age of the infant. The striations are shed as the nail grows.

In total leukonychia (Plate XVI-A, page 96) the entire nail plate is white and all the fingernails and toenails are affected. In partial leukonychia the proximal portion of the nail is white, thus obliterating the lunula (the normal white crescent distal to the cuticle), and a distal transverse band of normally pink nail is present up to the free edge of the nail plate. Striate leukonychia is more variable in appearance and may be present as a single white band, as multiple narrow bands involving only a portion of the nail or as bands spanning the entire nail plate. The nail texture is usually normal. Associated appendageal anomalies have been reported but are exceedingly uncommon (Albright, 1964).

Leukonychia is thought to be due to incomplete keratinization of the nail plate, probably occurring secondarily to a maturation defect in its matrix. Periodic disturbances in the nail matrix may account for the striated form of the defect, but in none of these disorders has the mechanism been clearly established.

Separation of the Nail Plate From the Nail Bed (Onycholysis). In this disorder separation begins at the free edge of the nail and slowly progresses proximally so that part, or almost all of the nail plate becomes detached from the nail bed and the nail appears opaque and white. Onycholysis has also been reported as a familial disorder (Samman 1968). In a similar phenomenon, *onychomadesis*, the separation begins proximally and progresses toward the free edge until the nail plate is shed. This type of separation occurs in epidermolysis bullosa and in an unexplained form of periodic nail shedding (Pardo-Costello, 1960).

Beau's Lines. These are single transverse depressions occurring in one or more nails. The lines appear at the lunula and progress with the growth of the nail until they disappear at the free edge. This phenomenon is frequently seen after infectious diseases or other systemic disorders. The defect is thought to be due to an abrupt and temporary depression in the proliferation of nail matrix cells. Numerous insults to the matrix can result in multiple transverse ridges.

Longitudinal Pigmented Bands. Bands of pigmented nail plate are exceedingly common in black individuals and considerably less so in white patients. In some instances they are due to a junction nevus originating in the nail matrix or bed. The pigment carried into the nail plate is seen at any age but, once present, tends to persist. A low potential exists for degeneration into malignant melanoma.

PACHYONYCHIA CONGENITA

The complete syndrome of pachyonychia congenita (Fig. 17–5) consists of thickened, dystrophic nails (Fig. 17–6), keratoderma of the palms and soles, hyperhidrosis, oral leukokeratosis and follicular keratosis (keratosis pilaris). Often, not all the features are present in affected individuals. The disorder is inherited in an autosomal dominant fashion (Joseph, 1964).

The nail dystrophy involving both finger and toenails is usually present at birth or it may develop gradually during the first few years of life. The nails are thickened, tubular and hard, projecting upward at the free edge, while the nail bed is filled with yellow-brown keratotic material. Paronychial inflammation is common and recurrent shedding of the nails can occur. Keratoderma of the palms

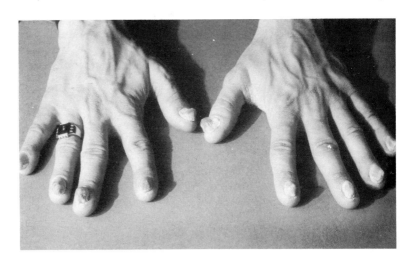

Figure 17–5. Pachyonychia congenita.

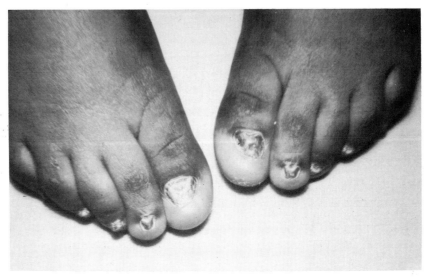

Figure 17–6. Pachyonychia congenita. (Courtesy of Dr. David Fretzin.)

and soles becomes evident during the pre-school years, either focally confined to sites of pressure or more diffusely distributed, with marked maceration and fissuring. Hyperhidrosis of the palms and soles is common, and large painful bullae containing clear, watery fluid can appear on the toes, heels and borders of the feet. Follicular hyperkeratotic papules are frequently present on the extensor surfaces of the extremities, the buttocks, lumbar region, elbows, knees and, less commonly, on the face and scalp (Laing, 1966). If the follicular papules are numerous, hair loss may be an associated finding. White plaques (leukokeratosis) occur on the tongue, oral mucous membrane and larynx. The abnormal epidermis may undergo malignant change during or after the second decade. Less frequent findings include epidermal cysts, corneal dystrophy, natal teeth, scrotal tongue, thickening of the nasal mucosa and tympanic membrane, as well as verrucous skin lesions (Gorlin, 1964).

Examination of a biopsy from the palms or soles typically shows extreme hyperkeratosis with parakeratosis, plugging of the pilosebaceous openings and eccrine pores, and acanthosis with extensive vacuolization of the epidermal cells. The oral mucosa shows a similar hyperplastic epithelium, spongiosis and marked parakeratosis. The ventral portion of the nail is hypertrophied and the nail matrix may show dyskeratosis.

Treatment is relatively ineffective, although keratolytic agents may ameliorate the skin lesions. Avulsion of the nails results only in palliation, amputation of the distal phalanges, although drastic, may be required to restore function.

PARONYCHIA

In the infant, paronychia, or inflammation of the nail fold, is most often secondary to local injury and the wet environment produced by vigorous thumbsucking. Initially, the base of the nail fold becomes swollen and tender. In acute lesions the abscess may point close to the nail plate, requiring incision and drainage. In chronic infections pus may exude intermittently from the nail fold and the nail plate frequently becomes dystrophic. Discoloration of the lateral margins of the nail plate is often seen in infections with *Pseudomonas aeruginosa.* Other causative organisms include *Staphylococcus aureus*, a wide spectrum of bacteria and *Candida albicans.*

Material should be obtained from the nail fold in paronychia for both bacterial and fungal cultures. Bacterial lesions should be treated with soaks and systemic antibiotics, depending on the results of cultures and sensitivity studies. Incision and drainage should be performed when necessary. Candidal paronychia usually responds to topical treatment with a cream or ointment containing nystatin or amphotericin B. The cream should be gently and carefully applied three times a day with a cotton applicator or toothpick in order to fill the gap between the nail plate and posterior nail fold. It is desirable to keep the affected finger as dry as possible since Candida thrives in a moist environment. Detection of the carrier state in the mouth and gastrointestinal tract by cultures of saliva and stools may be important in the occasional infant with refractory paronychia. Such infants may require a course of nystatin suspension to prevent reinfection of the damaged nail. Persistent and repeated candidal paronychia in infancy suggest a more serious underlying disorder, and such infants should be investigated for endocrinopathies and immunologic deficiency syndromes (see Candidiasis; Chap. 13).

THE ECTODERMAL DYSPLASIAS

Ectodermal dysplasia (ED) is often used as a descriptive term for patients with a constellation of defects affecting the skin and its appendageal structures. Since the phrase "ectodermal dysplasia" has been used traditionally to connote one of two specific disease entities (anhidrotic and hidrotic ED), we do not feel that it should be indiscriminately and inaccurately applied to any symptom-complex including ectodermal defects. On the other hand, a number of congenital and hereditary diseases involve abnormal development of one, or several appendages, and may superficially resemble the phenotype of anhidrotic ectodermal dysplasia. As more of these rare syndromes are being studied, it becomes apparent that dysplastic changes can be localized to specific appendages. The pilosebaceous glands, for example, are affected in the OFD I syndrome, and the hair in Marie

Unna hypotrichosis, but the eccrine glands are normal in both conditions. For these reasons it may be preferable to refer to dysplastic changes in a more specific manner, such as pilosebaceous dysplasia, trichodysplasia, epidermal dysplasia, eccrine dysplasia and so forth.

ANHIDROTIC (HYPOHIDROTIC) ECTODERMAL DYSPLASIA

Absence of sweating, hypotrichosis and defective dentition are the most striking features of this inherited disorder, but several other abnormalities are characteristic of patients with full expression of the syndrome (Plate XVI-B, page 96). The facies is distinctive because of frontal bossing and depression of the central face which, as a result of hypoplasia of the maxillary alveolar processes, results in a "dish-face" profile. The nasal bridge is flattened and the columnella is recessed. Eyebrows are absent or sparse and the eyelashes are either absent or fine, delicate, and set in double rows. The skin around the eyes is wrinkled and frequently hyperpigmented (Fig. 17–8). The ears are prominent and may be low set. The lips are thick, everted, and may show pseudorhagades. The chin is also prominent.

The skin over the remainder of the body is thin, dry and hypopigmented; the cutaneous vasculature is often easily visualized due to the translucent quality of the epidermis. The palms and soles are normal rather than thickened as in hidrotic ectodermal dysplasia. A variable degree of alopecia is present in all

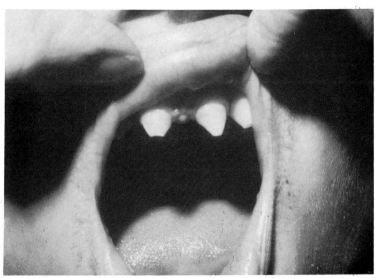

Figure 17–7. Anhidrotic ectodermal dysplasia. Hypodontia and conical tooth formation.

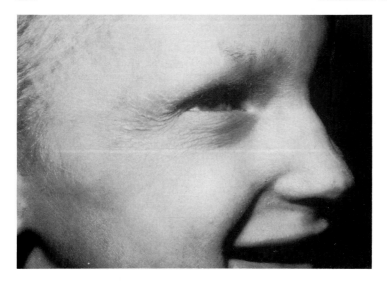

Figure 17–8. Anhidrotic ectodermal dysplasia. Fine wrinkling
around eyes.

patients; the scalp hair is sparse, blond, and fine, often with an unruly appearance. Body hair may also be scanty. Dental anomalies range from total anodontia to hypodontia with defective teeth. The teeth, when present, are widely separated, discolored, peg-shaped or conical (Fig. 17–7). The propensity for caries is great.

The most striking physiologic abnormality is the absence of sweating, which can be demonstrated by a number of techniques: by pilocarpine iontophoresis; with the starch-iodine method; or, by application of an O-phthalaldehyde solution to the skin (see Chap. 4). Severe hypoplasia or absence of the eccrine sweat glands can be confirmed by skin biopsy obtained from the palm, an area normally replete with these structures.

Other glandular structures may also be absent or hypoplastic. Diminished lacrimation has been reported, and atrophic rhinitis due to the lack of nasal mucous glands is a consistent and characteristic finding. A deficiency of glands has been noted in the pharynx, trachea, bronchi, esophagus and duodenum. The paucity of mucous secretion may, in part, account for the tendency of these patients to have recurrent bouts of pneumonia and bronchitis. Dysphagia, hoarseness and intermittent aphonia can also occur. Hypoplasia of the nipples and breast tissue is an occasional finding.

Less constant ancillary findings include conductive hearing loss, gonadal abnormalities, stenotic lacrimal puncta, corneal dysplasia and cataracts. Mental development is usually normal but some degree of retardation has been seen in selected patients.

In most kindreds the disease is inherited in an X-linked recessive fashion. Affected males show full phenotypic expression of the syndrome, whereas carrier females have minor stigmata such as a patchy decrease in sweating, sparse scalp hair or a few missing or dysplastic teeth. The phenotypic variability in carrier females has been attributed to a Lyon hypothesis effect, that is, random inactivation of one X chromosome in each somatic cell of the female early in embryogenesis (Kerr, 1966). Females with the complete syndrome, however, have been carefully documented and, in these families, an autosomal recessive gene appears to be operating (Gorlin, 1970).

Certain clinically applicable techniques aid in delineation of the genetics of this disorder. Frias and Smith (1968) demonstrated diminished numbers of sweat pores, determined by fingertip pore counts, in carrier females. In later evaluations of this technique (Verbov, 1970; Crump, 1971), pore counts did not prove to be as reliable for identification of female carriers as previous studies had indicated. Affected males have markedly reduced or absent sweat pores. In addition, abnormal dermatoglyphics have been noted in this disorder (Priest, 1967). Patients with the complete syndrome show striking ridge disruption on the palms and soles, vestigial palmar patterns, and absent, vestigial or displaced c and d digital triradii; carrier mothers may also display some of these patterns. Unilateral or bilateral high maximal atd angles have been reported in both affected males and carrier mothers (Verbov, 1970).

The most serious effect of anhidrotic ectodermal dysplasia for the patient is marked heat intolerance due to inability to adequately regulate the body temperature by sweating. Undiagnosed infants often undergo extensive investigation for unexplained bouts of fever. Prudent observation of such infants, however, will rapidly disclose correlation of the febrile episodes with upward fluctuations in environmental temperature. Every effort should be made to moderate environmental temperatures by air conditioning. Older children may douse their clothing with water in warm weather and thus cool themselves by evaporation.

Deficient lacrimation can be palliated by the regular use of artifical tears. The nasal mucosa must also be protected by intermittent saline irrigations and application of petrolatum. It is imperative that these children have a thorough dental evaluation during the first years of life, and protheses should be provided even for toddlers so that adequate nutrition can be maintained. Reconstructive procedures can be performed later in life to improve the facial configuration. Affected children are often very conscious of their peculiar appearance and a wig may be required for those with extremely scant scalp hair.

It is now recognized that the incidence of atopic disease, asthma, allergic rhinitis and atopic dermatitis is increased significantly in anhidrotic ectodermal dysplasia (Reed, 1970; Verbov, 1970). Atopic manifestations should be managed as they would be in otherwise normal infants and children (see Chap. 12). Because of the anhidrosis, steroid ointments may not be as effective as creams (Solomon, 1969).

Familial and congenital simple anhidrosis, a recessively inherited disorder, mimics anhidrotic ectodermal dysplasia. These patients also have severe heat intolerance due to absence of the eccrine sweat glands. They are distinguishable by an unremarkable facies and normal teeth and hair (Mahloudji, 1967).

Segmental hypohidrosis may occur in association with pupillotonia and hyporeflexia (*Holmes-Adie syndrome*). Children with this condition may exhibit an inability to regulate body temperature according to changes in ambient temperature and thus can be confused with patients having anhidrotic ectodermal dysplasia (Esterly, 1968).

Ectodermal dysplasia must also be differentiated from *congenital familial sensory neuropathy* (Pinsky, 1966). These patients have recurrent febrile episodes, anhidrosis (despite histologically normal sweat glands),

deep tendon hyporeflexia, insensitivity to pain, self-mutilation impulses, emotional lability, defective intelligence, absence of the axon flare response to intradermal injection of histamine, irregular flushing of the face and an abnormal homovanyllic acid: vanill-mandelic acid ratio. Occasional disturbances in pupillary response and lacrimation have also been noted. An autosomal recessive type of inheritance is probable in this disorder.

HIDROTIC ECTODERMAL DYSPLASIA

This form of ectodermal dysplasia, in which sweating is normal, is characterized by deformity, hypoplasia or absence of the nails, sparse hair and hyperkeratosis of the palms and soles. In contrast to anhidrotic ectodermal dysplasia, the teeth are usually normal, but small teeth and rampant caries are occasionally noted. The disorder is inherited as an autosomal dominant trait (Williams, 1967).

The nails may be thickened and discolored with longitudinal ridging, or alternatively, they may be hypoplastic, thin and brittle. The free edge may be raised from the nail bed and the skin thickened beneath the free edge of the nail, as well as over the knuckles, knees and elbows. The hair on the scalp and body is fine and slow-growing; the eyebrows and lashes are often absent. Histologic examination of sections of a scalp biopsy shows a reduction in the number and size of pilosebaceous follicles. An occasional patient may have cataracts, strabismus, mental retardation or short stature. The facies is normal.

The combination of sensorineural deafness, polydactyly, syndactyly, partial anodontia, conical teeth, dystrophic nails and elevated sweat electrolytes has been described in three generations of a single family (Robinson, 1962). The disorder appeared to be inherited in an autosomal dominant fashion and may be a variant of hidrotic ectodermal dysplasia.

EEC SYNDROME

The associated defects of ectrodactyly, atypical ectodermal dysplasia and cleft lip and palate comprise the EEC syndrome (Rüdiger, 1970). Since the number of reported cases is small, it is difficult to determine whether or not it is a hereditary disorder. The cutaneous features consist of thin, dry, translucent and poorly pigmented integument, mild hyperkeratosis of the palms

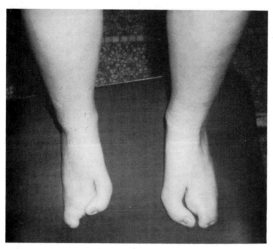

Figure 17–9. Lobster claw deformity of the feet in EEC syndrome. (Courtesy of Dr. Samuel Pruzansky.)

and soles, sparse scalp hair and eyebrows and absent lashes. Other findings include absent lacrimal puncta, strabismus, bilateral cleft lip, median cleft of the palate, granulomatous perleche, a normal complement of teeth, normal nails, and lobster claw deformity of the feet and hands resulting in one definable digit, the thumb or the great toe (Fig. 17–9). Mental and growth retardation occur occasionally. Secretion of eccrine sweat was not detected by sweat tests in Rüdiger's patient; although a skin biopsy was not performed, the child did not appear to suffer hyperpyrexia when exposed to elevated environmental temperatures. Several biopsies from the scalp and hand of three of our patients with EEC syndrome demonstrated a normal complement of sweat glands but sparsity of hair follicles and a greatly diminished number of sebaceous glands. A frequent complication is candidiasis of the lips and tongue (Fig. 14–3).

ELLIS-VAN CREVELD SYNDROME
(Chondroectodermal dysplasia)

This rare syndrome has been found with relative frequency among the Amish population of Lancaster County (McKusick, 1964). Affected individuals are disproportionately dwarfed, with more pronounced shortening of the distal extremities and thickening of the involved bones. Polydactyly, dysplasia of the nails and congenital cardiac malformations complete the syndrome. Cardiac defects occur in approximately 50 per cent of affected individuals, with the most common defect being the presence of a single atrium.

Fusion of the hamate and capitate bones, an almost invariable finding, and erosive changes in the tibia resulting in knock-knees, are also typical. Although the skin, hair and teeth are usually normal, partial anodontia, natal teeth, small teeth and defects in the alveolar ridge with accessory frenula and sparse, fine hair have all been reported. Eccrine sweating is not impaired. Patients without cardiac malformations have a good prognosis for a normal life span.

CONGENITAL ECTODERMAL DYSPLASIA OF THE FACE

In 1963 Setleis and his colleagues described five Puerto Rican children from three different families with a distinctive constellation of defects, all limited to the face. The following features characterize this syndrome: (1) a leonine appearance; (2) absent lashes on either eyelid or multiple rows of lashes on the upper lids and absent lashes on the lower lids; (3) eyebrows which slant sharply upward and laterally; (4) scarring defects in the temporal areas; (5) puckered skin about the eyes; (6) a scarring median ridge on the chin; and (7) a rubbery, hypertrophied nose and chin. The occurrence of identical defects in siblings suggested the possibility of an autosomal recessive disorder.

Jensen (1971) describes two kindreds with the syndrome, one with 20 affected members, and a distribution in the families suggestive of autosomal dominant inheritance. These patients have multiple temporal area defects present at birth that are round or oval, vary in size up to 1 cm, and are sharply demarcated and depressed in relation to the surrounding skin. The skin surface is smooth and transparent, permitting clear visibility of the dermal blood vessels. Vertical linear grooves are conspicuous on the lower forehead, and the eyebrows are sparse over the lateral third. Eyelashes are present and normal, as is the general facial structure. Absence of sweating is demonstrated in areas of temporal lesions. On biopsy the dermis is thin with decreased elastic tissue; the sebaceous glands and hair follicles are absent and the sweat glands are sparse. Similar histologic findings were noted on a skin biopsy from one of Setleis's patients.

It is difficult to decide whether these patients have unrelated disorders or represent clinical variants of a condition which perhaps has genetic heterogeneity. Until further patients have been documented, it would seem most appropriate to consider all such children as having the same syndrome.

DISORDERS OF THE HAIR

A variety of congenital and hereditary disorders is associated with abnormalities of the hair (Porter, 1970). Only rarely does an anomaly of the hair occur as an isolated defect. The hair may be totally absent (alopecia), unusually sparse (hypotrichosis) or overabundant in its growth (hypertrichosis or hirsutism). Changes in color, caliber and fragility can also be detected in many diseases, but these findings may be relatively nonspecific and are only exceptionally diagnostically contributory (e.g., cartilage-hair hypoplasia). Nevertheless, it is useful to perform dissecting microscopic examination of peculiar looking hair and make a histologic examination of the scalp, since the presence of a hair shaft

abnormality may be suggestive of a particular disorder. Structural abnormalities of the hair shaft can often be identified by these procedures. Other studies of hair that are occasionally useful include: amino acid analysis; electron microscopy; polarizing microscopy; scanning electron microscopy; stress-strain curves; and X-ray diffraction curves. The disorders associated with abnormalites of the hair are listed in Tables 17–2 to 17–4.

Table 17–2. Disorders of Hair with Abnormal Morphology

Structural Defects

Arginosuccinicaciduria — monilothrix, trichorrhexis nodosa
Hereditary trichodysplasia (Marie Unna hypotrichosis) — twisted hair
Menkes' syndrome — multiple defects
Monilothrix
Netherton's syndrome — multiple defects (Chap. 11)
Pili annulati
Pili torti
Pili torti and nerve deafness
Trichorrhexis nodosa

Abnormal Color, Caliber and Fragility

Cartilage-hair hypoplasia — small caliber
Citrullinemia — fragile, atrophic bulbs
Congenital trichomegaly with dwarfism, mental retardation and retinal pigmentation. Long brows and lashes
Dyskeratosis congenita — sparse and fine
Hartnup disease — fine, fragile hair (Chap. 16)
Hereditary enamel hypoplasia and kinky hair — abnormal curliness
Homocystinuria — fine, fragile hair
Marinesco-Sjögren syndrome — fragile, brittle, rough hair
Phenylketonuria — fine, light-colored hair (Chap. 16)
Pierre-Robin syndrome — fine, light-colored hair
Tricho-rhino-phalangeal syndrome — sparse hair
Trisomy 21 — fine, light-colored, atrophic bulbs (Chap. 7)
Tyrosinemia — fine, light-colored hair
Woolly hair — abnormal curliness

Table 17–3. Disorders with Hypertrichosis

I. *Generalized*

Congenital lipodystrophy
Cornelia de Lange syndrome
Craniofacial dysostosis with dental, eye, and cardiac anomalies
Hypertrichosis lanuginosa universalis
Hypertrichosis with gingival fibromatosis
Leprechaunism (Chap. 18)
Mucopolysaccharidoses (Chap. 15)

II. *Localized*

Congenital hemihypertrophy with hypertrichosis
Hairy ears
Hairy elbows syndrome
Hairy nevi (Chap. 10)
Ring chromosome E (low hairline)
Trisomy 18 (back and forehead) (Chap. 7)
Turner's syndrome (low occipital hairline)

Table 17–4. Disorders with Hypotrichosis

Anhidrotic (hypohidrotic) ectodermal dysplasia
Atrichia with papular lesions
Combined immunodeficiency syndrome with short-limbed dwarfism
Congenital alopecia
EEC syndrome (ectrodactyly, ectodermal dysplasia, cleft lip-palate)
Goltz's syndrome (Chap. 16)
Hallerman-Streiff syndrome (oculomandibulodyscephaly)
Hidrotic ectodermal dysplasia
Hypotrichosis, syndactyly and retinitis pigmentosa
Incontinentia pigmenti (Chap. 13)
Keratosis follicular spinulosa decalvans
Oculo-dento-digital dysplasia
Oral-facial-digital syndrome
Progeria
Rothmund-Thomson syndrome
Seckel's syndrome
Trisomy A

STRUCTURAL DEFECTS

Pili Torti (Twisted hairs). These hairs are grooved and flattened at irregular intervals because of twisting of the shaft on its own axis. The hairs tend to fracture and break off at the twisted segment, resulting in an apparent absence of growth. The hair may have a spangled appearance in reflected light. Clinically abnormal hair may not be evident until the second or third year of life, alopecia may be present from birth. On microscopic examination, rotation of the hair shaft at irregular intervals is characteristic. Occasionally the hair presents a nodular appearance and, because of an apparent narrowing of the shaft, can be confused with monilethrix hairs. Although many cases are sporadic, the defect does occur in families and can probably be inherited in either an autosomal dominant or recessive fashion. The disorder may remit at puberty.

Concurrent *pili torti and nerve deafness* have been described in a number of children and may constitute a specific syndrome (Robinson, 1967).

Pili Annulati (Ringed hairs). This is a condition in which the hair has 1 to 3 mm bonds of alternating light and dark color in reflected light. The banding is thought to be due to reflection of light from the air-containing cavities in the cortex and medulla of the hair shaft. A few or many hairs may be affected, and a single hair may be banded along the entire shaft or only over a small segment. A familial incidence has occasionally been noted.

Monilethrix (Beaded hairs). This is a herditary defect of autosomal dominant transmission but with variable expressivity. The scalp lanugo hair is normal, but after shedding it may not be replaced by terminal hair (Baker, 1962), or it may be superceded by sparse growth. The new hairs are regularly beaded along the shaft at intervals of about 1 mm; the constricted internodes lack a medulla. Because the hair is excessively brittle it breaks at the internodes, and rarely grows longer than 1 or 2 cm. Although the nape and occipital region are most severely affected, the remainder of the scalp hair, eyelashes, eyebrows and body hair may also be abnormal. Follicular hyperkeratosis is usual, giving the scalp a rough, dry appearance. The diagnosis can be readily made by microscopic examination of the hair shafts. The prognosis is unpredictable since some children experience a remission at puberty.

Arginosuccinic aciduria has been noted in some patients with monilethrix (Grosfeld, 1961), but the specificity of this finding is questionable.

Trichorrhexis Nodosa. In most instances, trichorrhexis nodosa is probably the result of traumatic changes in the hair shafts, although it has been reported in association with arginosuccinic aciduria. The hairs have node-like swellings at irregular intervals along the shaft where the hair readily fractures. On microscopic examination the nodes have the appearance of two interlocking brushes stuck end to end by their bristles. This type of defect can also be seen in patients with other structural abnormalities of the hair and is extremely common in mentally retarded children, who constantly abuse their scalps.

Trichoschisis. A congenital defect characterized by alternating birefringence and a low sulfur content of the hair, trichoschisis has been reported in a single child (Brown, 1970). The hair, peculiar from birth, was sparse, short, and coarse in texture. Fractures of the hair occurred in the nonbirefringent zones. Scanning electron microscopy showed a marked defect of the cuticular layer. Total sulfur content of the defective hair shafts was considerably decreased, as was its cystine-cysteine content.

Marinesco-Sjögren Syndrome

This autosomal recessive syndrome is comprised of moderate growth deficiency, moderate to severe mental deficiency, cerebellar ataxia, weakness, congenital cataracts, nystagmus and dysarthria. The hair is sparse and dystrophic, and narrow bands of incomplete keratinization may be found along the shafts of about 30 per cent of the hairs (Domonkos, 1971).

Menkes Syndrome

Rapidly progressive degenerative disease of the central nervous system manifested by failure to thrive, generalized clonic seizures, absence of motor and mental development, hypertonia, hyperreflexia, irritability, increasing opisthotonus and leg scissoring in association with abnormal hair, are the major clinical features of this syndrome. The hair, scalp and eyebrows are sparse, short, kinky and often poorly pigmented. The microscopic abnormalities are those of pili torti, monilethrix and trichorrhexis nodosa (Menkes, 1962).

The radiologic findings demonstrable in early infancy are bilateral symmetrical metaphyseal spurring of the long bones with normal bone density, diffuse flaring of the ribs anteriorly and excessive wormian bone formation in the parietal region of the skull. Malformation of the cerebral arterial system has also been noted on cerebral arteriography (Wesenberg, 1969). The infant usually dies before the end of the second year; post mortem examinations have disclosed widespread degenerative changes in the cerebrum and cerebellum. The disorder is heritable and transmitted as an X-linked recessive trait. The metabolic defect is as yet unknown.

Hereditary Trichodysplasia
(Marie Unna hypotrichosis)

This isolated structural defect of hair results in a specific type of pattern alopecia (Fig. 17–10). Affected individuals are born with widespread facial milia, sparse scalp hair, eyebrows and lashes, and decreased body hair. The hair is coarse to the touch, like a horse's tail, and is often unruly or frizzy in early childhood. The hypotrichosis resembles male pattern alopecia on the crown and frontal areas; however, the perimeter is also bald so that the scalp resembles that of a monk. Teeth, mucous membranes and nails are normal. Multiple, scattered, horny, follicular plugs and patulous pilosebaceous orifices may be present over the body.

Laboratory studies, including those for urinary amino acids and plasma testosterone, are normal. Histologic examination of the scalp shows an abnormal proliferation of the internal root sheath in many of the follicles. When examined under the dissecting microscope, abnormal hairs are seen to be flat, ribbon-like and twisted at irregular intervals (Fig. 17–11); extensive peeling of the cuticle has been demonstrated by scanning electron microscopy (Fig. 17–12). Intracellular fractures of the cuticular cells, cortical cell fibrils and medullary cells, as well as an increased interfibrillar cortical matrix, are the electron microscopic findings (Solomon, 1972). The disorder is inherited as an autosomal dominant trait.

Cartilage-Hair Hypoplasia

Cartilage-hair hypoplasia was first described in the Amish population (McKusick, 1965), but has now been documented in individuals of other ethnic groups. Affected patients have short-limbed dwarfism and fine, sparse, light-colored hair. Characteristic skeletal findings include a normal head, short, pudgy hands and feet with loose-jointed digits, restricted extension of the elbow, beading of the costochondral junctions, mild to moderate bowing and disproportionate shortening of the legs. Irregularities of the metaphyseal ends of the bony shafts with normal ossification centers (metaphyseal dysostosis) can be demonstrated on roentgenograms. The term "metaphyseal dysostosis" is a misnomer, since biopsies of the costochondral junctions show hypoplasia of cartilage rather than a bony defect.

The scalp hair is sparse, fine and silky and remains relatively short due to its extreme fragility. Eyebrows and lashes may also be sparse and body hair is similarly affected. The hair may be lighter in color than that of other members of the family; the caliber of the hair is reduced and the pigmented core or medulla is absent. The hair has decreased tensile strength but no abnormalities have been detected on amino acid analysis (Coupe, 1970).

Additional variable findings include an absorptive defect of the bowel, congenital megacolon and an increased susceptibility to viral infections, particularly chicken pox, which, in some children, results in death. Chronic neutropenia and defective cellular immunity have been demonstrated in some patients (Lux, 1970). The disorder is inherited as an autosomal recessive trait with reduced penetrance.

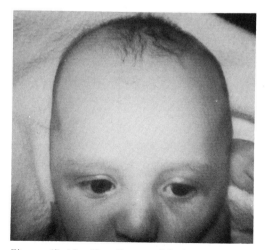

Figure 17–10. Hereditory trichodysplasia (Marie Unna hypotrichosis).

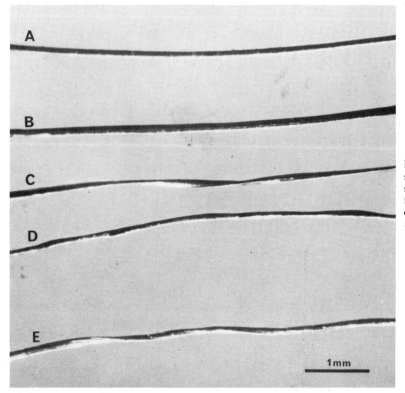

Figure 17–11. Abnormal hair in Marie Unna hypotrichosis, as seen by dissecting microscope. (a) Normal hair; (b) mild flattening of the hair; (c, d and e) twisted hair of increasing severity. (From L. Solomon: J. Invest. Derm. *57*:389, 1971.)

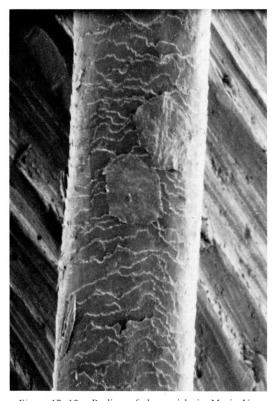

Figure 17–12. Peeling of the cuticle in Marie Unna hypotrichosis as seen with the scanning electron microscope. (From L. Solomon: J. Invest. Derm. *57*:389, 1971.)

Hereditary Enamel Hypoplasia and Kinky Hair

This anomaly has been described as an autosomal dominant disorder. The hair is dark brown, excessively curly and coarse in texture. The nails may be striated and brittle, with a tendency to break and peel, and deciduous teeth have a thin enamel cap. The permanent teeth either lack an enamel cap or have one so thin that it escapes radiologic detection (Robinson, 1966).

Woolly Hair

Localized patches of woolly hair may represent a nevoid change. The hair may be woolly from birth or become abnormal during the first year or two of life. At times the anomaly has a familial distribution.

Trichomegaly

A syndrome of *trichomegaly, pigmentary degeneration of the retina and growth retardation* has been described in a few children. The features of the disorder include intrauterine growth retardation, short stature, poor weight gain, delay in development and osseous maturation and diffuse retinal pigmentary degeneration. The eyelashes and eyebrows are abnormally long and curly. Mental retardation is a variable finding (Corby, 1971).

HYPERTRICHOSIS

Generalized hypertrichosis can be either a temporary normal condition in the newborn (see Chap. 1) or a familial trait. Abnormal hypertrichosis may be generalized or localized.

GENERALIZED DISORDERS

Cornelia de Lange Syndrome

Infants with the *Cornelia de Lange syndrome* can be recognized readily because of their striking constellation of defects and the remarkable similarity in their appearance (Fig. 17–13). Virtually all these children have mental retardation and primordial growth failure, and most have delayed osseous development as well. The head is microbrachycephalic with a high and narrow forehead; the facies is characteristic with anteverted nostrils, a long philtrum, a thin and downcurved mouth and a receding chin. The eyes may have an antimongoloid slant, the eyebrows meet in the mid-forehead, and the ears, although well formed, may be low set. The palate may be high-arched or cleft, the teeth small and

widely spaced. The cry is low-pitched and growling. A variety of ocular anomalies have also been described (Ptacek, 1963).

The cutaneous findings consist of generalized hirsutism that is most pronounced on the back, forearms and forehead, synorphris, a low anterior and posterior hairline and long curly eyelashes which can occur in multiple rows on the upper lids. The skin is dry, or of poor turgor. Persistent, widespread cutis marmorata, coupled with a "cyanotic hue" about the central face is indicative of the cutaneous vascular lability typical of these patients. Defective epidermal ridge patterns have been noted on the finger pads and on the hypothenar eminences. The nipples and genitalia of both sexes are hypoplastic (Schuster, 1966).

Skeletal abnormalities may be pronounced and include syndactyly of the second and third toes, micromelia, phocomelia, clinodactyly, oligodactyly, proximally placed thumbs and flexion contractures of the elbows. Roentgenographic studies may show hypoplasia of the bones of the extremities, low pelvic acetabular angles, a short sternum, a barrel-shaped rib cage and hypoplasia and subluxation of the radial heads (Lee, 1967).

Although the majority of reported cases have been sporadic, several instances of affected siblings have been recorded, suggesting the possibility of an autosomal recessive type of inheritance (Opitz, 1965). Karyotypes are usually normal. There are no consistently abnormal biochemical or hematologic findings.

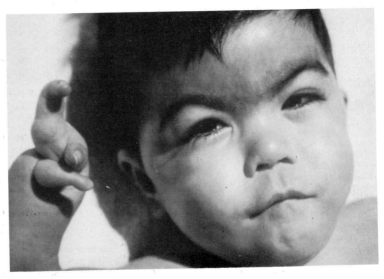

Figure 17–13. Cornelia de Lange syndrome. (Courtesy of Dr. Hermine Pashayan.)

Congenital Hypertrichosis Universalis
(Congenital hypertrichosis lanuginosa)

An exceedingly rare condition, this disorder is heritable and transmitted as an autosomal dominant trait. During the nineteenth century these patients excited great curiosity and many were exhibited in circuses and traveling shows as "dog-faced boys," "human Skye Terriers" and "monkey men." Affected infants may be unusually hairy at birth or may develop hirsutism in early childhood. Virtually the entire skin surface is covered with silky, light colored lanugo hair which may grow to several inches in length; only the palms, soles, dorsal terminal phalanges, labia minora, prepuce and glans penis are spared. Defective dentition is the only associated abnormality and may vary from complete anodontia to absence of only a few teeth. The pathogenesis of hypertrichosis universalis is unknown and no endocrine or metabolic defects have been detected in affected individuals (Suskind, 1971).

Hypertrichosis with Gingival Fibromatosis. This somewhat similar disorder has at times been confused with hypertrichosis universalis. Although these individuals also have generalized hirsutism, the hair is of the terminal, rather than lanugo type. The gingival overgrowth may be so pronounced as to protrude from between the lips. The hirsutism is variable in severity and may be apparent at birth or develop later during childhood (Gorlin, 1964).

The association of *craniofacial dyostosis, patent ductus arteriosus, hypoplasia of the labia majores, dental and eye defects and hypertrichosis* has been reported in two sisters (Gorlin, 1960). The hirsutism was pronounced, especially on the arms, legs and back. The character of the facial anomalies suggested that this entity might be grouped with the "first arch syndromes."

Generalized hypertrichosis is also a feature of *leprechaunism* (Chap. 18) *congenital lipodystrophy* (Chap. 18) and the *mucopolysaccharidoses* (Chap. 15).

LOCALIZED DISORDERS

Circumscribed areas of hairiness may occur within a melanocytic nevus or over spina bifida. Familial varieties have also been described, such as Amish patients with extreme *hypertrichosis of the elbows* noted soon after birth (Beighton, 1970). Hypertrichosis of the back and forehead is seen in *Trisomy 18*

(Chap. 7). A low hairline is characteristic of *Turner's syndrome* and also reported in *ring chromosome E* (Porter, 1970). Infants with *congenital hemihypertrophy* (Chap. 7) may exhibit a marked increase in growth of terminal hair over the enlarged side (Hurwitz, 1971). A tuft of hair in the lumbosacral region may be associated with diastomatomyelia. Abnormal hair growth at other sites may also occur as isolated phenomena.

HYPOTRICHOSIS

Hallerman-Streiff's Syndrome
(Dyscephalia oculo-mandibulo-facialis)

The salient features of the Hallerman-Streiff syndrome are: (1) malformations of the skull and face; (2) dental abnormalities; (3) hypotrichosis; (4) anomalies of the eye; (5) dwarfism; and (6) motor, and occasionally mental, retardation. The head is brachycephalic with prominent frontal and parietal eminences. The anterior and posterior fontanelles are large and frequently remain patent for long periods, as do the cranial sutures. The facial skeleton is small, the nose pinched and bent, resembling a bird's beak, and the jaw underdeveloped (Fig. 17–14). The skin over the scalp, face, and particularly the nose, exhibits striking atrophic changes, allowing the dermal vessels to become clearly visible. The hair is thin and sparse with either frontal balding or patchy alopecia along the coronal and lambdoid sutures. Absence of eyebrows and lashes is also characteristic. The ears may be low set, the lips are thin and small and the palate is highly arched. Natal teeth are common; hypodontia and malformed teeth also occur. The mandible is hypoplastic and the temporomandibular joint has limited mobility.

Frequently occurring anomalous changes in the eye are cataracts, microphthalmia, nystagmus and strabismus. Degenerative retinal disease has also been reported (Hoefnagel, 1965). Proportionate dwarfism with retarded bone development and underdeveloped genitalia are usually present. Chromosomal karyotypes have not shown any consistent abnormalities (Forsius, 1964).

Rothmund-Thomsen Syndrome
(Congenital poikiloderma)

Although the onset of cutaneous signs in this disorder is usually between three and six months of age, lesions have been documented at birth in some patients (Rook, 1959). The initial skin lesions are bright red or pink, shiny tense swellings and reticulated patches of erythema or diffuse areas of erythema resembling sunburn. Rarely, there are a few vesicular lesions. The cheeks are the earliest sites of involvement but later the remainder of the face, ears, buttocks, knees, legs, arms and dorsum of the hands become affected. The erythematous phase is superceded by a poikilodermatous phase. Atrophy is pronounced, giving the affected skin a "cigarette paper" appearance. Circumscribed white macules, dull red telangiectases and irregular or linear areas of atrophy and scaling may be admixed with macular or reticulated pigmentation which usually develops somewhat later. Atrophy and telangiectasia are most prominent on the face and hands, whereas pigmentation is more conspicuous on the limbs. Light sensitivity, at times resulting in a bullous eruption, may be present during childhood.

The scalp hair is sparse and fine and the eyebrows and lashes are frequently absent. Some patients have normal hair at birth, but after it is shed, it is never replaced. Body hair is usually absent from the atrophic areas. The nails may be normal, atrophic or dystrophic. Small or malformed teeth are frequently noted. Ocular lesions include cataracts (usually occurring between the fourth and seventh years) and degenerative lesions of the cornea. Hypogonadism, proportionate dwarfism, small hands and feet with stubby fingers

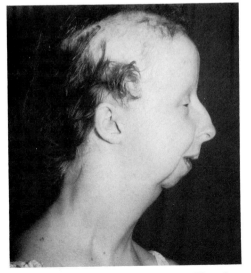

Figure 17–14. Alopecia. Hallerman-Streiff syndrome. (Courtesy of Dr. Samuel Pruzansky.)

and toes, abnormalities of the skull, shortening of the long bones, and changes in bone density are variable features.

No consistent laboratory abnormalities have been recorded. Chromosomal studies have been normal. The disorder is thought to be inherited as an autosomal recessive trait since many affected siblings have been documented and the incidence of consanguinous marriages in affected kindreds is high (Silver, 1966).

Rothmund-Thomsen syndrome must be distinguished from Werner's syndrome (onset in early adulthood), Hallerman-Streiff syndrome, the ectodermal dysplasias, Cockayne's syndrome (onset after six months of life), dyskeratosis congenita (onset after 5 years of age) and progeria. A number of other conditions have also been described in which poikiloderma is associated with an assortment of anomalies. Most of these disorders are excessively rare and may, in fact, be variants of more commonly seen entities.

Oral-Facial-Digital Syndromes
(OFD I and II)

There are two distinct OFD syndromes, genetically heterogenous, but with many malformations common to both. OFD I, (Fig. 17–15), the more common disorder, consists of a lobulated cleft tongue, often containing nodular hamartomas, hypertrophied frenulum, multiple alveolar fibrous bands and clefts, midline cleft of the lip, high arched or cleft palate (Fig. 17–16), a broad nasal root with dystopia canthorum, missing central or lateral incisors, micrognathia, hypoplasia of the nasal alar cartilages and frontal bossing. The digital features include brachydactyly, clinodactyly, syndactyly, polydactyly and radiologically detectable defects in the tubular bones of the hands. Additional and more variable findings include mental retardation, hydrocephalus, trembling, pes equinovarus, kyphoscoliosis and conductive hearing loss. Abnormalities of the cutaneous appendages are frequently present and consist of diffuse alopecia of the scalp (Fig. 17–17) with coarse, brittle, lusterless hair, and fine scaling of the scalp and face. Sebaceous glands are decreased or absent and numerous keratinous cysts localized to the face, scalp, ear pinnae and dorsum of the hands also occur (Solomon, 1970). The cystic lesions may rupture spontaneously, resulting in deep pitted scars. OFD I occurs only in females and is thought

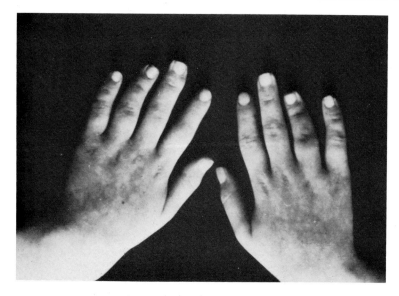

Figure 17–15. Clinodactyly and brachydactyly. OFD I syndrome. (From L. Solomon: Arch. Derm. *102*:598, 1970. © American Medical Assoc. 1970.)

to be inherited as an X-linked dominant trait. The gene is probably lethal in males. The occurrence of the syndrome in females of successive generations, the absence of male-to-male transmission, the increased incidence of abortions and the lack of live-born males in affected sibships all support this postulate.

OFD II syndrome differs from OFD I in that affected patients have a broad bifid nasal tip, bilateral polysyndactyly of the halluces and a normal or flaring alveolar ridge. There are no recorded cutaneous or appendageal changes. In contrast to OFD I, both sexes are affected and pedigree analysis suggests an autosomal recessive type of inheritance (Rimoin, 1967).

Hutchinson-Gilford Syndrome
(Progeria)

This syndrome, probably inherited as an autosomal recessive trait, is characterized by dwarfism and accelerated aging. Affected children may be of low birth weight, have sclerodermatous or cyanotic changes of the mid-face and sculpturing of the nose, but are usually normal during the first year of life (DeBusk, 1972). During their second and subsequent years there is progressive loss of scalp hair, brows and lashes, severe growth retardation and gradual alteration of the facial structure, resulting in a disproportionately small face with a prominent vault, a thin,

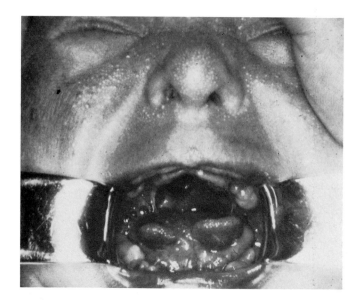

Figure 17–16. Multilobed tongue, bound-down frenulum and uvula in OFD I syndrome. (From L. Solomon: Arch. Derm. *102*:598, 1970. © American Medical Assoc., 1970.)

beaked nose and receding chin. The skin becomes wrinkled and atrophic, often with poikilodermatous changes. The nails are thin, atrophic and brittle. The most striking feature is severe, progressive atherosclerosis involving all the major vessels. Substantial deposits of lipofucsin, a pigment seen in aging cells, is also found in many organs. Death is usual by the middle of the second decade. Fibroblasts obtained from the patients with progeria have been shown to have a limited replicative life span *in vitro*, suggesting that perhaps a foreshortened mitotic potential (Goldstein, 1969) accounts in part for the premature aging (Martin, 1970). This finding has been of major interest in the development of a theory of aging which suggests that cells have a predetermined and definitive number of divisions ("programmed death").

Seckel's Bird-Headed Dwarfism

The features of this syndrome are low birth weight, dwarfism, microcephaly, a bird-like facies with a prominent beaked nose, and multiple malformations, including hypoplastic thumbs, clinodactyly, simian crease, dislocation of the hips, clubfeet, hypoplastic patella, scoliosis, strabismus and genitourinary anomalies. Mental retardation is severe. Sparse scalp and body hair is the only characteristic cutaneous finding. The disorder is inherited as an autosomal recessive trait (McKusick, 1967).

Combined Immunodeficiency Syndrome with Dwarfism and Alopecia

A few infants have been described with lymphopenic agammaglobulinemia, short-limbed dwarfism and various cutaneous abnormalities. Two of these patients were siblings, suggesting a heritable disorder (Gatt, 1969). Both sexes have been affected.

All of the cutaneous abnormalities have not been found in every patient. Four infants had alopecia; in one it was present at birth (Feigin, 1971) and in three it was progressive from birth (Gatti, 1969; Gotoff, 1972). Hypoplastic nails were noted in two infants and defective teeth in one (Gatti, 1969; Feigin, 1971). Two of the infants had thickened, redundant skin which hung in loose folds, particularly over the extremities (Gatti, 1969, Gotoff, 1972 (Fig. 17–18). Generalized chronic scaling, at times associated with erythema, was another prominent feature.

Short-limbed dwarfism differs from achondroplasia on overt clinical and radiologic grounds. Anemia, eosinophilia, depletion of small lymphocytes in the blood and bone marrow and absent plasma cells in the bone marrow are consistent findings. The immunologic deficiency has been characterized by low levels or absence of immunoglobulin, deficient cellular immunity manifested by absent skin reactivity to common antigens and dinitrofluorobenzene (DNFB) sensitization, and depressed lymphocyte transformation in response to mitogens and antigens.

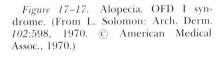

Figure 17–17. Alopecia. OFD I syndrome. (From L. Solomon: Arch. Derm. *102*:598, 1970. © American Medical Assoc., 1970.)

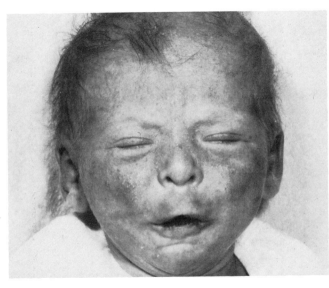

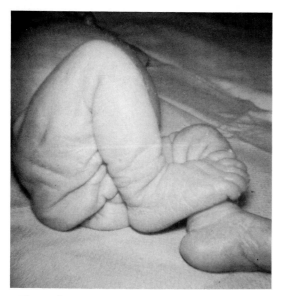

Figure 17–18. Dermatomegaly: folded skin in combined immuno-deficiency disease with short-limbed dwarfism.

All of these infants succumbed to infection during the first few months of life. At autopsy the pathologic changes in the reticuloendothelial system were compatible with observed abnormal immunological findings. A comparison of histologic changes in skin biopsies and post-mortem skin sections shows somewhat variable differences. Most of the specimens showed thickening of the stratum corneum, an atrophic epidermis and a dermal mononuclear infiltrate with involvement of appendageal structures, particularly the hair follicles. Although a slight decrease in elastic tissue was noted in biopsies from infants with redundant skin, this change appeared to be secondary to the inflammatory infiltrate, rather than to a congenital absence of elastic tissue (cutis laxa). A diminution in the number of skin appendages was noted in the autopsy specimen from one patient (Feigin, 1972). Another infant had a peculiar granulomatous reaction with huge foreign body giant cells in both skin and lymph nodes. The disappearance of the granuloma prior to death coincided with shrinkage of the enlarged and palpable lymph nodes and progression of the alopecia (Gotoff, 1972). In two of the infants (Gatti, 1969; Gotoff, 1972), alopecia appeared to be secondary to a chronic inflammatory process involving the pilosebaceous follicles and was not a true ectodermal dysplasia.

Other Causes

Other rare syndromes associated with sparse hair include *hypotrichosis, syndactyly and retinitis pigmentosa* (Albrectsen, 1956) and *keratosis follicularis spinulosa decalvans* (Kuokkanen, 1971). The latter disease becomes apparent during the first few weeks of life and is characterized by hyperkeratotic follicular papules that are most prominent on the face, neck and extensor surfaces of the extremities. There is a progressive loss of scalp hair, eyebrows, lashes and facial lanugo hair. Ocular manifestations include photophobia, blepharitis, ectropion, conjunctival lesions, corneal erosions, myopia and astigmatism. Lenticular cataracts, congenital glaucoma, mental retardation, abnormal hands and mild, generalized aminoaciduria have also been described (Adler, 1969). Full expressivity of the gene is seen only in the male since the disorder is transmitted in an X-linked fashion.

Congenital alopecia can occur as an isolated defect. It is usually inherited as an autosomal recessive trait. The scalp hair is either absent at birth or is shed during the early months of infancy. Teeth and nails are normal. *Atrichia with papular lesions* is a disorder seen only in females. Permanent alopecia follows loss of natal scalp hair and the papular lesions, histologically identifiable as keratin cysts, develop during childhood. One child has also been recorded with *generalized hyperkeratosis, universal alopecia and sensorineural deafness* (Morris, 1969). Accentuation of keratosis in the follicular openings that resulted in prominent spiny projections was an unusual feature.

REFERENCES

Adler, R. C. and Nyhan, W. L.: An oculocerebral syndrome with aminoaciduria and keratosis follicularis. J. Pediat. 75:436, 1969.

Albrectsen, B. and Svendesen, I. B.: Hypotrichosis, syndactyly and retinal degeneration in two siblings. Acta Dermatovener. 36:96, 1956.

Albright, S. D., III and Wheeler, C. E., Jr.: Leukoncyhia. Total and partial leukonychia in a single family with a review of the literature. Arch. Derm. 90:392, 1964.

Baker, H.: An investigation of monilethrix. Brit. J. Derm. 74:24, 1962.

Beighton, P.: Familial hypertrichosis cubiti: The hairy elbows syndrome. J. Med. Genet. 7:158, 1970.

Brown, A. C., Belser, R. B., Crounse, R. G. and Wehr, R. F.: A congenital hair defect. Trichoschisis with alternating birefringence and low sulfur content. J. Invest. Derm. 54:496, 1970.

Corby, D. G., Lowe, R. S., Jr., Haskins, R. C. and Herbertson, L. M.: Trichomegaly, pigmentary degeneration of the retina, and growth retardation. Amer. J. Dis. Child. *121*:344, 1971.

Coupe, R. L. and Lowry, R. B.: Abnormality of the hair in cartilage-hair hypoplasia. Dermatologica *141*:329, 1970.

Crump, J. A. and Danks, D. M.: Hypohidrotic ectodermal dysplasia. J. Pediat. *78*:466, 1971.

DeBusk, F. L.: The Hutchinson-Gifford progeria syndrome. J. Pediat. *80*:697, 1972.

Domonkos, A. N.: Andrews' Diseases of the Skin. 6th ed. Philadelphia, W. B. Saunders Co., 1971, p. 850.

Esterly, N. B., Cantolino, S. J., Alter, B. P. and Brusilow, S. W.: Pupillotonia, hyporeflexia and hypohidrosis: Autonomic dysfunction in a child. J. Pediat. *73*:852, 1968.

Feigin, R. D., Middelkamp, J. N., Kissane, J. M. and Warren, R. J.: Agammaglobulinemia and thymic dysplasia associated with ectodermal dysplasia. Pediatrics *47*:143, 1971.

Forsius, H. and de la Chapelle, A.: Dyscephalia oculomandibulo-facialis. Ann. Paed. Fenn. *10*:Fasc. *4*:1, 1964.

Frias, J. L. and Smith, D. W.: Diminished sweat pores in hypohidrotic ectodermal dysplasia. A new method of assessment. J. Pediat. *72*:606, 1968.

Gatti, R. A., Platt, N., Pomerance, H. H., Hong, R., Langer, L. O., Kay, H. E. M. and Good, R. A.: Hereditary lymphopenic agammaglobulinemia associated with a distinctive form of short-limbed dwarfism and ectodermal dysplasia. J. Pediat. *75*:675, 1969.

Giknis, F. L., Hall, W. K. and Tolman, M. M.: Acne neonatorum. AMA Arch. Derm. *66*:717, 1952.

Goldstein, S.: Lifespan of cultured cells in progeria. Lancet *1*:424, 1969.

Gorlin, R. J. and Pindborg, J. J.: Syndromes of the Head and Neck. New York, McGraw-Hill, 1964.

Gorlin, R. J., Chaudhry, A. P. and Moss, M. L.: Graniofacial dysostosis, patent ductus arteriosus, hypertrichosis, hypoplasia of labia majora, dental and eye anomalies—a new syndrome? J. Pediat. *56*:778, 1960.

Gorlin, R. J., Old, T. and Anderson, V. E.: Hypohidrotic ectodermal dysplasia in females. A critical analysis and argument for genetic heterogeneity. Z. Kinderheilk. *108*:1, 1970.

Gotoff, S. P., Esterly, N. B., Gottbrath, E., Liebner, E. J. and Lajvardi, S. R.: Granulomatosis reaction in an infant with combined immunodeficiency disease and short-limbed dwarfism. J. Pediat. *80*:1010, 1972.

Grosfeld, J. C. M., Mighorst, J. A. and Moolhuysen, T. M.: Arginosuccinic aciduria in monilethrix. Lancet *2*:789, 1964.

Hellier, F. F.: Acneiform eruptions in infancy. Brit. J. Derm. *66*:25, 1954.

Hoefnagel, D. and Benirschke, K.: Dyscephalia mandibulo-oculo-facialis. Arch. Dis. Child. *40*:57, 1965.

Hurwitz, S. and Klaus, S. N.: Congenital hemihypertrophy with hypertrichosis. Arch. Derm. *103*:98, 1971.

Jensen, N. E.: Congenital ectodermal dysplasia of the face. Brit. J. Derm. *84*:410, 1971.

Joseph, H. L.: Pachyonychia congenita. Arch. Derm. *90*:594, 1964.

Kerr, C. B., Wells, R. S. and Cooper, K. E.: Gene effect in carriers of anhidrotic ectodermal dysplasia. J. Med. Genet. *3*:169, 1966.

Kuokkanen, K.: Keratosis follicularis spinulosa decalvans in a family from Northern Finland. Acta Dermatovener. *51*:146, 1971.

Laing, C. R., Hayes, J. R. and Scharf, G.: Pachyonychia congenita. Am. J. Dis. Child. *111*:649, 1966.

Lee, F. A. and Kenny, F. M.: Skeletal changes in the Cornelia de Lange syndrome. Amer. J. Roentg. *100*:27, 1967.

Lux, S. E.: Chronic neutropenia and abnormal cellular immunity in cartilage-hair hypoplasia. New Eng. J. Med. *282*:231, 1970.

Mahloudji, M. and Livingston, K. E.: Familial and congenital simple anhidrosis. Amer. J. Dis. Child. *113*:477, 1967.

Martin, G. M., Sprague, C. A. and Epstein, C. J.: Replicative life-span of cultivated human cells. Lab. Invest. *23*:86, 1970.

McKusick, V. A.: Dwarfism in the Amish. Trans. Ass. Amer. Physicians 77:151, 1964.

MuKusick, V. A., Eldridge, R., Hostetler, J. A., Ruangwit, U. and Egeland, J. A.: Dwarfism in the Amish, II. Cartilage-hair hypoplasia. Bull. Johns Hopkins Hosp. *116*:285, 1965.

McKusick, V. A., Mahloudji, M., Abbott, M. H., Lindenberg, R. and Kepas, D.: Seckel's bird-headed dwarfism. New Eng. J. Med. *277*:279, 1967.

Menkes, J. M., Alter, M., Steigleder, G. K., Weakley, D. R. and Sung, J. H.: A sex-linked recessive disorder with retardation of growth, peculiar hair and focal cerebral and cerebellar degeneration. Pediatrics *29*:764, 1962.

Morris, J., Ackerman, A. B., and Koblenzer, P. J.: Generalized spiny hyperkeratosis, universal alopecia, and deafness. Arch. Derm. *100*:692, 1969.

Opitz, J. M., Segal, A. T., Lehrke, R. L. and Nadler, H. L.: The etiology of the Brachmann-de Lange syndrome. Birth Defects Reprint Series, National Foundation. PE-RS *16*:22, 1965.

Pardo-Costello, V. and Pardo, O. A.: Diseases of the Nails. 3rd ed. Springfield, Charles C Thomas, 1960.

Pinsky, L. and DiGeorge, A. M.: Congenital familial sensory neuropathy with anhidrosis. J. Pediat. *68*:1, 1966.

Porter, P. S. and Lobitz, W. C., Jr. Human hair: A genetic marker. Brit. J. Derm. *83*:225, 1970.

Priest, J.: Dermatoglyphics in ectodermal dysplasia. Lancet *2*:1093, 1967.

Ptacek, L. J., Opitz, J. M., Smith, D. W., Gerritsen, T. and Waisman, H. A.: The Cornelia de Lange syndrome. J. Pediat. *63*:1000, 1963.

Reed, W. B., Lopez, D. A., and Landing, B.: Clinical spectrum of anhidrotic ectodermal dysplasia. Arch. Derm. *102*:134, 1970.

Rimoin, D. L. and Edgerton, M. T.: Genetic and clinical heterogeneity in the oral-facial-digital syndromes. J. Pediat. *71*:94, 1967.

Robinson, G. C. and Johnson, M. M.: Pili torti and sensory neural hearing loss. J. Pediat. *70*:621, 1967.

Robinson, G. C., and Miller, J. R.: Hereditary enamel hypoplasia: Its association with characteristic hair structure. Pediatrics *37*:498, 1966.

Robinson, G. C., Miller, J. R. and Bensimon, J. R.: Familial ectodermal dysplasia with sensori-neural deafness and other anomalies. Pediatrics *30*:797, 1962.

Ronchese, F.: Peculiar nail anomalies. Arch. Derm. Syph. *63*:565, 1951.

Rook, A., Royden, D. and Stevanovic, D.: Poikiloderma congenitali. Rothmund-Thomson syndrome. Acta Dermatovenereol. *39*:392, 1959.

Rüdiger, R. A., Haase, W. and Passarge, E.: Association

of ectrodactyly, ectodermal dysplasia and cleft lip-palate. Amer. J. Dis. Child. *120*:160, 1970.

Samman, P. D.: The nails. *In* Rook, A., Wilkinson, D. S., and Ebling, F. J. G. (eds.): Textbook of Dermatology. Philadelphia, F. A. Davis Co., 1968, p. 1426.

Schuster, D. S., and Johnson, S. A. M.: Cutaneous manifestations of the Cornelia de Lange syndrome. Arch. Derm. *93*:702, 1966.

Setleis, H., Kramer, B., Valcarcel, M. and Einhorn, A. H.: Congenital ectodermal dysplasia of the face. Pediatrics *32*:540, 1963.

Silver, H. K.: Rothmund-Thomson syndrome: An oculocutaneous disorder. Amer. J. Dis. Child. *111*:182, 1966.

Smith, D. W.: Recognizable Patterns of Human Malformation. Philadelphia, W. B. Saunders Co., 1970.

Solomon, L. M. and Altman, A.: Percutaneous steroid absorption in anhidrosis. J. Invest. Derm. *53*:454, 1969.

Solomon, L. M., Esterly, N. B. and Medenica, M.: Hereditary trichodysplasia: Marie Unna's hypotrichosis. J. Invest. Derm. *57*:389, 1972.

Solomon, L. M., Fretzin, D. and Pruzansky, S.: Pilosebaceous abnormalities in Apert's syndrome. Arch. Derm. *102*:381, 1970.

Solomon, L. M., Fretzin, D. and Pruzansky, S.: Pilosebaceous dysplasia in the oral-facial-digital syndrome. Arch. Derm. *102*:596, 1970.

Suskind, R. and Esterly, N.: Congenital hypertrichosis universalis. *In* Bergsman, D. (ed.): The Clinical Delineation of Birth Defects. Vol. 12: Skin. Baltimore, Williams and Wilkins Co., 1972, p. 103.

Tromovitch, T. A., Abrams, A. A. and Jacobs, P. H.: Acne in infancy. Amer. J. Dis. Child. *106*:230, 1963.

Verbov, J.: Hypohidrotic (or anhidrotic) ectodermal dysplasia — an appraisal of diagnostic methods. Brit. J. Derm. *83*:341, 1970.

Wesenberg, R. L., Gwinn, J. L. and Barnes, G. R., Jr.: Radiological findings in kinky hair syndrome. Radiology *92*:500, 1969.

Williams, M. and Fraser, F. C.: Hydrotic ectodermal dysplasia-Clouston's family revisited. Canad. Med. Ass. J. *96*:36, 1967.

Chapter Eighteen

DISEASES OF THE SUBCUTANEOUS TISSUES

Only a few disorders of subcutaneous tissue are evident during the neonatal period and these occur with relative infrequency. Absence of adipose tissue is a striking feature of two rare syndromes, congenital lipodystrophy and leprechaunism. Although a widespread decrease in subcutaneous fat may also be seen in dysmature infants, or occasionally in infants with multiple congenital anomalies, this deficiency does not occur to as great a degree as does congenital lipodystrophy or leprechaunism. Sclerema neonatorum and subcutaneous fat necrosis are more common disorders of adipose tissue and they are usually identifiable by their characteristic clinical and histologic features. Cold panniculitis is most often seen in late infancy or early childhood but should be considered in the differential diagnosis of any neonate with a confirmed history of prolonged cold exposure. Weber-Christian panniculitis has been reported in only one newborn infant; however, this disorder will be discussed briefly because the skin lesions may resemble those of subcutaneous fat necrosis.

SCLEREMA NEONATORUM AND SUBCUTANEOUS FAT NECROSIS

There is considerable confusion in the literature regarding the relationship of these two entities. Many authors have combined both disorders under one heading, whereas others have believed them to be separable on the basis of morphology, histology and etiology (Marks, 1962). Textbooks of pathology, including several that focus on the fetus and newborn (Potter, 1952; Macgregor, 1960), as well as those pertaining only to the skin (Lever, 1967), reflect conflicting opinion. Also, reports of patients with mixed clinical and pathological pictures have further complicated the issue. However, more recent evidence, although still too insufficient to allow formulation of firm conclusions, indicates that the biochemical abnormality in the subcutaneous tissue may be identical in the two disorders. Both are noted within the first three months of life with the average onset occurring at a few days of age.

Sclerema Neonatorum

Sclerema neonatorum most frequently affects the preterm or debilitated newborn. Diffuse hardening of the subcutaneous tissue results in a tight, smooth covering that feels bound to the underlying structures. The skin is cold, stony hard and nonpitting. The joints often become immobile and the face acquires a mask-like expression. The duration of the disorder is variable, but persistence of sclerematous changes beyond a two-week period is uncommon in surviving infants. Affected patients may be seriously ill with sepsis, pneumonia, gastroenteritis or multiple congenital anomalies. Instability of body temperature, weakness, poor feeding, apneic spells, respiratory distress, cyanosis, convulsions and other neurological signs frequently complicate the course of the disease. Some observers believe that sclerematous change is a nonspecific sign of grave prognostic significance rather than a primary disease, and that recovery depends solely on the outcome of treatment for an underlying disorder (Warwick, 1963). The mortality rate is high (Levin, 1961), since many infants die shortly after the onset of sclerema.

An increase in serum urea nitrogen and potassium and a decrease in carbon dioxide content has been noted in infants seriously ill with sclerema (Levin, 1965). The specificity of these data may be questioned, however, since electrolyte imbalance is common in severely stressed infants. Histologic examination of the subcutaneous tissue is not diagnostic since edema and thickening of the connective tissue septa are usually the only findings.

The differential diagnosis includes generalized edema, Milroy's disease and Turner's syndrome. Edema neonatorum (see Chap. 2) can be distinguished by its predilection for dependent parts and by easy pitting on pressure. Milroy's disease is confined to the legs, and it is apparent at birth in an otherwise healthy infant. The edema of gonadal dysgenesis is localized to the hands and feet and may be associated with other stigmata, such as webbed neck, shield-shaped chest, congenital heart disease and a negative chromatin pattern in cells obtained by buccal smear. Scleroderma and scleredema adultorum probably do not occur in the newborn period.

Subcutaneous Fat Necrosis

The lesions of subcutaneous fat necrosis are more localized and sharply circumscribed (Fig. 18–1). They vary in size from small nodules to large plaques. The sites of predilection are the cheeks, buttocks, back, arms and thighs, although lesions have been described in other locations. The involved tissue has a nonpitting, stony consistency and may have an uneven lobulated surface with an elevated margin separating it from the surrounding normal tissue. The overlying skin may have a reddish or violaceous hue. Subcutaneous fat necrosis is a self-limited disease; resolution occurs over a period of weeks to months, and residual atrophy or scarring are unusual in uncomplicated cases (Plate XVI-C).

On occasion the skin lesions become the sites of extensive calcium deposition, and in some patients hypercalcemia has been observed as an associated finding. Soft tissue dystrophic calcification can be demonstrated

by roentgenography. When the skin lesions are heavily calcified, the contents often liquify and drain spontaneously. The drainage material is usually sterile, but scarring may take place. Refusal to feed, vomiting, hypotonia, irritability, fever and failure to thrive may complicate the clinical course. Rarely, calcification of the viscera may occur (Sharlin, 1970). Hyperlipemia has also been reported in one instance (Weary, 1966).

On gross examination the subcutaneous tissue is hard, and white, with a consistency like tallow. Histologic findings most often conform to a single description. The subcutaneous fat contains a granulomatous reaction with an infiltrate composed of foreign body giant cells, fibroblasts, lymphocytes and histiocytes. The fibrous septae are thickened by edema and increased vascularity. The necrotic fat cells contain sheaves of acicular crystals which are dissolved with routine fixation and embedding, leaving characteristic clefts. The results of lipid-stained frozen sections have been inconsistent. Rarely, a similar histologic involvement of visceral fat has been noted at autopsy (Flory, 1948).

Cold exposure and hypothermia are frequently invoked as causative factors in sclerema and subcutaneous fat necrosis, although there is little documentation of this occurrence. Since maintenance of normal body temperature is a common problem in the healthy preterm infant, it seems unlikely

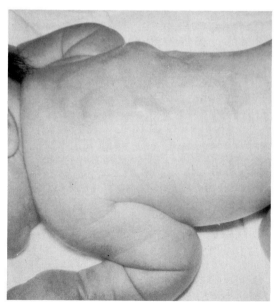

Figure 18–1. Subcutaneous fat necrosis. (Courtesy of Dr. David Fretzin.)

that moderate hypothermia alone is responsible for these disorders. In a series of 70 infants with "cold injury" (Bower, 1960), not only was the presence of sclerema poorly correlated with lowered body temperature, but a few infants were found to have the condition during the summer months when they could not have been exposed to severe cold. Both sclerema and subcutaneous fat necrosis have also been attributed to obstetrical trauma, asphyxia and peripheral circulatory collapse. Although these may be predisposing or contributory factors, it is unlikely that the etiology of these diseases can be explained entirely on this basis.

Early chemical studies of fat in sclerema (Harrison, 1926) demonstrated a higher melting point and a slightly lower iodine value when compared to normal newborn fat. The anisotropic crystals seen in the sections were shown to consist of neutral triglycerides, probably palmitin or stearin (Plate XVI-D). On the basis of these findings it was postulated that the ratio of saturated to unsaturated fatty acids was raised in sclerematous fat, resulting in decreased amounts of olein and greater quantities of palmitin and stearin. The data of Horsefield and Yardley (1965) also support this thesis. These authors studied the fat from an affected infant by thin layer, column and gas chromatography and demonstrated an increased ratio of saturated to unsaturated fat attributable to a specific increase in palmitin and stearin, with a decrease in oleic acid. X-ray diffraction patterns of fatty acid crystals were also suggestive of the triglyceride structure with a high palmitic acid content. Another such analysis of sclerematous fat (Kellum, 1968) confirmed the altered ratio of saturated to unsaturated fatty acids, but no deviation from normal was found in the content of oleic acid.

Normal prenatal adipose tissue contains small numbers of needle-like crystals dispersed throughout the fat cells. These occur in two forms: very small crystals deposited without definite patterns (A crystals); and larger crystals (B crystals), which are arranged in rosette formations (Prokš, 1966). In a study of four infants with sclerema neonatorum, crystal morphology and histopathology of the subcutaneous fat were correlated (Prokš, 1966). X-ray diffraction patterns indicated that both the A and B crystals were composed of triglycerides of palmitic and stearic acid. It was then postulated that excessive formation of the smaller A crystal could cause the less common clinical picture of sclerema; histologic examination of

the fat would show only edema of the fibrous septae since these crystals apparently do not incite an inflammatory response. Recrystallization of A crystals, provoked by unknown etiologic factors, might result in the formation of larger B crystals, a granulomatous reaction in the subcutis and clinical lesions of subcutaneous fat necrosis.

The management of infants should include correcting fluid and electrolyte imbalance and constant monitoring of body temperature. Sepsis and other associated disorders should be treated promptly and intensively. Systemically administered corticosteroids have been advocated for some cases of sclerema, but indications for their use are unclear. Furthermore, in a controlled study, treatment with corticosteroids did not significantly alter the mortality rate (Levin, 1961).

Careful needle aspiration of fluctuant areas of fat necrosis prior to rupture may diminish subsequent scarring. Infants with hypercalcemia and subcutaneous or visceral calcium deposits may require restriction of oral calcium intake, omission of vitamin D from the diet and systemic corticosteroid therapy.

CONGENITAL LIPODYSTROPHY SYNDROME

The congenital lipodystrophy syndrome, a constellation of defects involving several organ systems, is often detectable at birth because of its striking cutaneous findings. Early signs consist of generalized hyperpigmentation and hypertrichosis, as well as complete absence of adipose tissue. A number of patients have also had a velvety thickening and intense hyperpigmentation of the skin of the neck, axillae, groin, umbilicus, popliteal and antecubital fossae (Brubaker, 1965). Histologic sections taken from these areas show hyperkeratosis, papillomatosis and increased melanin throughout the epidermis—features consistent with the diagnosis of acanthosis nigricans. There are few detailed descriptions of affected infants, but some dermatologic features appear to be consistent in older children, including thick, curly scalp hair, low hairline, accentuated hyperpigmentation of the knuckle skin, palmar and plantar creases, and deeply pigmented macules, papules (presumably nevi) and skin tags scattered over the body (Brubaker, 1965). Mucous membranes are not involved.

As the affected infants grow, their appearance and habitus become even more distinctive. The face is gaunt, with coarse features and a large tongue, and the overall appearance of the body is one of excessive muscularity due to absence of subcutaneous tissue. The superficial veins are prominent and thickened. Hirsutism becomes more pronounced, with thick, curly scalp hair growing almost to the eyebrows and increased amounts of hair on the face, trunk and extremities. Pubic and axillary hair do not appear before puberty. The skin is coarse, dry and hyperpigmented. Linear growth is markedly accelerated, but premature bony maturation curtails height. Clitoral and penile enlargement have been noted at birth (Seip, 1959, 1963), but neither increased gonadotropin levels nor excessive adrenal androgen secretion have been found (Senior, 1966). An elevated level of plasma human growth hormone, which responded abnormally to induced hyper- and hypoglycemia, has been reported in one patient (Gordon, 1971).

A protuberant abdomen secondary to hepatomegaly is a constant feature. Splenomegaly and esophageal varices are occasionally present. Portal cirrhosis and fatty metamorphosis of the liver are progressive, and some infants have died of hepatic failure within the first year of life (Seip, 1959). Hyperglycemia is a characteristic consequence but may not be evident until later in childhood; it is nonketotic in type and refractory to insulin therapy (Senior, 1964). Hyperlipemia also occurs frequently with the increase in lipids that is almost always confined to the neutral triglyceride fraction. Central nervous system manifestations include dilitation of the cerebral ventricles, mental retardation and epilepsy (Reed, 1965). Renal and cardiac enlargement have also been noted, but, in most patients, the cause has been obscure. Corneal opacities, hyperproteinemia and hyperinsulinemia are occasionally associated features.

Children of both sexes and several sets of siblings with this syndrome have been described. The incidence of consanguinity is high in families with affected children. Pedigree information therefore supports a claim for an autosomal recessive type of inheritance. The metabolic defect responsible for congenital lipodystrophy has not yet been determined.

LEPRECHAUNISM

Less than 10 infants with this rare syndrome have been described. All have had intrauterine growth retardation, absence of adipose tissue and a characteristic elfin facies. The head appears disproportionately large, the chin is pointed, the lips are thick, the ears are low set and protruding, the nose is broad and upturned and the eyes are widely spaced and prominent. A thick coat of downy lanugo hair covers the body but is most striking over the face. The skin hangs in loose folds and the body has a wasted appearance due to both the decrease in muscle mass and the lack of adipose tissue. Diffuse bronzing of the skin and cutis gyrata of the hands and feet were noted in one infant (Patterson, 1962), and hyperpigmentation of the palmar and plantar creases was seen in another (Evans, 1955). Hypertrophy of the nipples, labia minora and clitoris has been present in all the females and enlargement of the phallus occurs in most males.

The bone age has been found to be markedly retarded in all patients. A low fasting blood sugar and a prolonged response to exogenously administered insulin have been found in some affected infants. Generalized aminoaciduria is a variable feature (Patterson, 1962; Salmon, 1963), and urinary 17-ketosteroids may be elevated (Kálló, 1965).

These infants usually suffer from severe infections and die in infancy. The most consistent post mortem findings include hyperplasia of the islets of Langerhans, abundant deposition of glycogen and iron in the liver, large cystic ovaries and atrophy of lymphoid tissue. The occurrence of the disorder in siblings and the frequency of consanguinous marriages in families with affected infants suggest an autosomal recessive type of inheritance (Donahue, 1954; Salmon, 1963; Kálló, 1965). It has been postulated that an overproduction of estrogen may account for some of the clinical and laboratory findings (Kálló, 1965).

COLD PANNICULITIS

In contrast to other types of cold-induced lesions, this particular cutaneous response to cold exposure is seen most frequently in young infants and children (Haxthausen, 1941; Rotman, 1966), and rarely in adults (Solomon, 1963). Although the cheeks are the most common site of involvement, identical lesions have been produced in other areas by application of ice. Warm, erythematous, indurated plaques appear in a few hours to a few days following the episode of cold exposure. On histologic examination of the lesions, the pathology is found to be confined to the dermal-subdermal junction and subcutaneous fat. The changes observed include slight thickening of the vessel walls, a perivascular infiltrate of lymphocytes, histiocytes, and polymorphonuclear leukocytes and aggregations of lipid from rupture of fat cells (Duncan, 1966). The inflammatory response subsides gradually over a period of two to three weeks. Temporary postinflammatory hyperpigmentation at the site of involvement may be apparent for an additional few weeks.

Lesions may be reproduced in susceptible infants by application of ice to the forearm (see Chap. 4) for a two-minute period (Solomon, 1963). The response at the test site may be delayed for several days. Cold agglutinins, cold hemolysins, cryoglobulin, and cryofibrinogen have been absent in all infants so evaluated. The peculiar susceptibility of some young infants to cold-induced lesions of this type may be related to a biochemical difference in composition of their adipose tissue.

Weber-Christian Panniculitis

Nodular nonsuppurative panniculitis, usually a disease of the adult female, has been reported in a few children and one newborn infant (Vestermark, 1966). Typical lesions are dull red, well-defined and tender nodules which may be mobile or adherent. They vary in size from 1 to 6 cm. The most common sites of involvement are the thighs and legs; however, the arms, trunk, and face may also be affected. The lesions erupt in crops and resolve gradually over a period of weeks, leaving atrophic scars. Occasionally, the visceral fat may also be involved. Hepatomegaly, relapsing fever, alterations in the white blood count and an elevated erythrocyte sedimentation rate are inconstant associated findings.

The nature of the primary process is unknown, but it is thought by some to be a type of vasculitis. Biopsy of an early lesion shows an inflammatory infiltrate with many polymorphonuclear leukocytes. During the intermediate stage foamy macrophages, giant cells and lymphocytes are prominent.

Supportive treatment will usually suffice, although corticosteroid therapy has been advocated for severe and widespread disease. Healing is by fibrosis.

REFERENCES

Brubaker, M. M., Levan, N. E., and Collipp, P. J.: Acanthosis nigricans and congenital total lipodystrophy. Arch. Derm. 91:320, 1965.

Donohue, W. L. and Uchida, I.: Leprechaunism. A euphemism for a rare familial disorder. J. Pediat. 45:505, 1954.

Duncan, W. C., Freeman, R. G., and Heaton, C. L.: Cold panniculitis. Arch. Derm. 94:722, 1966.

Evans, P. R.: Leprechaunism. Arch. Dis. Child. 30:479, 1955.

Flory, C. M.: Fat necrosis of the newborn. Arch. Path. 45:278, 1948.

Gordon, H., Pinstone, B. L., Leary, P. M. and Gordon, W.: Congenital generalized lipodystrophy with abnormal growth hormone homeostasis. Arch. Derm. 104:551, 1971.

Harrison, G. A.: An investigation of sclerema neonatorum with special reference to the chemistry of the subcutaneous tissues (Part II). Arch. Dis. Child. 1:123, 1926.

Harrison, G. A. and McNee, J. W.: An investigation of sclerema neonatorum with special reference to the chemistry of the subcutaneous tissues (Part I). Arch. Dis. Child. 1:63, 1926.

Haxthausen, H.: Adiponecrosis e frigore. Brit. J. Derm. 53:83, 1941.

Horsfield, G. J. and Yardley, H. J.: Sclerema neonatorum. J. Invest. Derm. 44:326, 1965.

Kálló, A., Lakatos, J. and Szijártó, L.: Leprechaunism (Donohue's syndrome). J. Pediat. 66:372, 1965.

Kellum, R. E., Ray, T. L. and Brown, G. R.: Sclerema neonatorum. Arch. Derm. 97:372, 1968.

Lever, W. F.: Histopathology of the Skin. Philadelphia, J. B. Lippincott Co., 1967.

Levin, S. E. and Milunsky, A.: Urea and electrolyte levels in the serum in sclerema neonatorum. J. Pediat. 67:812, 1965.

Levin, S. E., Bakst, C. M. and Isserow, L.: Sclerema neonatorum treated with corticosteroids. Brit. Med. J. 2:1533, 1961.

Macgregor, A. R.: Pathology of Infancy and Childhood. London, E. and S. Livingstone, Ltd., 1954.

Marks, M. B.: Subcutaneous adipose derangements of the newborn. Amer. J. Dis. Child. 104:122, 1962.

Patterson, J. H. and Watkins, W. L.: Leprechaunism in a male infant. J. Pediat. 60:730, 1962.

Potter, E. L.: Pathology of the Fetus and the Newborn. Chicago, Year Book Medical Publishers, Inc., 1952.

Prokš, C. and Valvoda, V.: Fatty crystals in sclerema neonatorum. J. Clin. Path. 19:193, 1966.

Reed, W. B., Dexter, R., Corley, C. and Fish, C.: Congenital lipodystropic diabetes with acanthosis nigricans. Arch. Derm. 91:326, 1965.

Rotman, H.: Cold panniculitis in children. Arch. Derm. 94:720, 1966.

Salmon, M. A. and Webb, J. N.: Dystrophic changes associated with leprechaunism in a male infant. Arch. Dis. Child. 38:530, 1963.

Seip, M.: Lipodystrophy and gigantism with associated endocrine manifestations. A new diencephalic syndrome? Acta Paediat. 48:555, 1959.

Seip, M. and Trygstad, O.: Generalized lipodystrophy. Arch. Dis. Child. 38:447, 1963.

Senior, B. and Gellis, S. S.: Syndromes of total lipodystrophy and of partial lipodystrophy. Pediatrics 33:593, 1964.

Sharlin, D. N. and Koblenzer, P.: Necrosis of subcutaneous fat with hypercalcemia. A puzzling and multifaceted disease. Clin. Pediat. 9:290, 1970.

Solomon, L. M. and Beerman, H.: Cold panniculitis. Arch. Derm. 88:897, 1963.

Vestermark, S.: Weber-Christian syndrome in a newborn. Acta Paed. Scand. 55:432, 1966.

Warwick, W. J., Ruttenberg, M. D. and Quie, P. G.: Sclerema neonatorum—A sign, not a disease. J. Amer. Med. Ass. 184:680, 1963.

Weary, P. E., Graham, G. F. and Selden, R. F., Jr.: Subcutaneous fat necrosis of the newborn. South. Med. J. 59:960, 1966.

Index

Note: Page numbers in *italics* indicate illustrations; **boldface** indicates illustrations in color plates; (t) indicates table.